THE RISE OF
THE MEDICAL PROFESSION

A STUDY OF COLLECTIVE SOCIAL MOBILITY

NOEL PARRY and JOSÉ PARRY

CROOM HELM LONDON

Croom Helm Ltd, 2-10 St. John's Road, London SW11

ISBN: 0-85664-224-X

This book is dedicated to our parents, Muriel Parry and the late Charles Parry, and Sybil and Nesbit Robinson. Also to Louise and Daniel Parry.

Printed in Great Britain by Biddles Ltd, Guildford, Surrey

CONTENTS

R
487
P37

59015

ACKNOWLEDGEMENTS

This study has been a long time in the making. We wish to thank
Professor Stephen Cotgrove who provided the initial impetus for a
study of the medical profession when the senior author was a student at
the Regent Street Polytechnic in 1960, and for his acknowledgement
of the concept of occupational strategy which he used in his book *The
Science of Society* (1967).

Thanks are due to the London School of Economics where the
senior author was a research student from 1961-3, and to the
Leverhulme Foundation and the Ministry of Education which awarded
a Leverhulme Scholarship and a State Scholarship respectively for part
of the preliminary research. The late Professor R.M. Titmuss tried
valiantly in his role of supervisor to reduce the research to manageable
proportions but these efforts were obstinately resisted, which is why
the completion of this project has taken so long.

During the years in which the study has been more or less in progress
numerous colleagues and students have contributed to its development.
In particular Alan Dawe and Professor Anthony Coxon, who were
colleagues at the University of Leeds and former students such as
Robert Witkin and Norman and Valerie Ellis, deserve special thanks.
The project in its present form has been undertaken at the Hatfield
Polytechnic where the contribution of Jolyon Flowers and Daphne
Johnson, who worked closely with the senior author on other projects,
was especially valuable. The encouragement of Gabriel Newfield, Dean
of Social Sciences, and the Sociology Academic Group have been much
appreciated, as well as the Polytechnic's contribution of resources
especially the funding of a research assistantship for Jose Parry.

Our book could not have been produced without the dedicated and
skilled assistance of the library staff at the Hatfield Polytechnic, most
particularly Eve Buckle and Joan Gray. Equally the competence and
forbearance of the secretaries who were engaged on the production
of the typescript, with all the attendant problems that entails are
beyond praise. We gratefully acknowledge the contribution of Peggy
Cohn, Molly Thorn and Pat Hawkins in this regard.

Our contacts with sociologists working in other institutions have
been a fruitful source of inspiration. Frank Parkin and Derek Allcorn
at the University of Kent; Sydney Holloway, Ivan Waddington,
Terence Johnson, and Professor Ilya Neustadt at the University of
Leicester; and Michael Rustin, Barrie Newman and Jean Donnison at
the North East London Polytechnic. The selection of the names of
particular individuals and the exclusion of others must always be
invidious and we wish to acknowledge the contribution of those who
contributed to seminars at the above institutions and at British

Sociological Association Conferences and Study Groups where we have given papers. Needless to say, the views expressed in this book are essentially our own, and errors are not to be attributed to any of the persons mentioned above.

INTRODUCTION

There is one sense in which it is possible to say that all intellectual work is work in progress and that the act of laying down the pen in the case of writing a book is an arbitrary one. The development of ideas, the introduction of new evidence, the integration of the whole work on more rigorous principles yielding more coherence and consistency, is always a possibility. The fact is that any book takes some time to write, and in our case, the development of concepts and ideas through the reading of other people's work has to an extent altered and shaped the enterprise as we have gone along. We believe that the signs of development in our book give evidence of the living struggle we went through in its production. The approach in this book has been developed over a long period. It addresses the starting problem – how to relate the study of professionalism to class theory – and places it within a wider context of a general thesis about collective social mobility. It contains also the fruits of our researches into the history of the English medical profession. We feel that class theory can only benefit by such an approach which examines the neglected subject of the middle class. It is curious that theorisation about the middle class has been inadequate. It may be that the very fact that most sociologists are themselves middle class means that this issue is taken for granted in a way that does not apply to studies of either the working class or the upper class. In any case, the dominance of Marxist perspectives in which the thesis of polarisation tends to preclude interest in the middle class may be one reason why there has been little careful study of its role or significance. In addition the debate about class has tended to operate on the terrain of Marxian analysis even where particular writers are not Marxist, but are concerned with the refutation or modification of Marxist theory, for example along Weberian lines. Our detailed study of that archetypal middle-class occupation, medicine, forced us – grounded as we were in the historical evidence – to cope more directly in sociological terms with the issues arising from the existence and role of the middle class in modern society.

It is perhaps fitting that our book should be published at a time when disquiet among the middle classes is high in an era of inflation and militant unionism, and when perhaps, for the first time in a quarter of a century, that class in British society feels itself acutely threatened. Among the middle-class occupations there is perhaps none which has experienced the trauma of a challenge to its legitimacy in recent years more acutely than the medical profession. Currently it feels itself to be a profession in crisis, a crisis which it takes to represent that of the middle class as a whole. It is our hope that this book will serve to illuminate the nature of the current crisis and to explain in some measure the character of it.

John Rex has been a leading exponent of the view that sociology must combine a theoretical with a historically-grounded approach. It is a requirement for the sociologist, Rex affirms, for him to be steeped in the social reality which he is studying, particularly history, in order to avoid sterile theorisation as an end in itself. It has been our aim to contribute to theoretical sociology through a sociologically informed history. We wish also, by this approach, to contribute to the sociological understanding of social policy. The inspiration of the work of David Lockwood, unbeknown to him, has been an example for many years, and likewise also, more recently, the writing of Anthony Giddens. Both of these scholars have achieved, in their particular studies, the application of the criterion of an historically-grounded sociology which we would hope to emulate.

PART I

1. SOCIAL MOBILITY AND CLASS STRUCTURE – THE ORTHODOX APPROACHES

Collective social mobility, a term used by Everett Hughes, (Hughes 1971:368) has been a neglected aspect of social stratification in Western countries, though sociologists have often noted its significance in the traditional caste system of India (Srinivas 1967:552). Collective social mobility it will be argued is an important feature of Western societies. The study of this phenomenon will assist in deepening our understanding of our own society and throw light on debates in sociology – such as the one about *embourgeoisement*. This debate, together with the study and measurement of individual mobility, has been one of the larger areas of research interest in sociology in the last twenty-five years. It has been of the greatest moment in defining the scope of the subject in terms of an established tradition of research not least in Britain.

In 1954 a book was published, edited by David Glass, reporting on a major set of related research projects. In his introduction (Glass 1954:3) Glass says:

> 'the programme as a whole is concerned with the processes of social selection and differentiation which are at work in Britain, with the formation of social strata and with the nature, composition and functions of those strata. Such problems are central to the study of social structure; they are of direct concern both for the development of sociological theory and for the formulation of social policy.'

The object of the study was to be the 'middle classes' because as he said 'save in respect of their early history "the middle classes" of Britain have not been much exposed to investigation'. He went on to say that 'the core of the general investigation is the study of social mobility in Britain – of the extent of movement in social status or social position by individuals of diverse social origins' (1954:5).

The method was modelled on demography and used statistical techniques, in particular the index of association, to measure intra-generational social mobility. Valuable information was provided about the extent of self-recruitment in the various social classes and in certain occupations i.e. medicine. The social class index used was the Hall-Jones scale. It may be observed that among the possible items for research cited in the aims only some have actually been investigated. In such an ambitious programme this is not surprising, but what is interesting is the selection of items which have actually been researched as opposed to those which were left out. These give an indication of the purposes and priorities of the researchers.

Glass himself explicitly states further on in his introduction what his preconceptions and priorities were when he decided to 'step outside the frame of the studies contained in the present volume and put forward personal views which are explicitly "loaded" in that they have a value basis' (1954:22). 'Certainly', he said, 'it is one of the postulates of a democratic and egalitarian society that ability, whatever its social background shall not be denied the chance to fulfil itself' (1954:25). He states that there are two primary reasons for wishing to see a higher degree of social mobility in the community. These are to increase economic and social efficiency and to improve the lot of the individual by making sure that there are fewer square pegs in round holes and thus greater personal fulfilment. Rather than stepping outside the frame of the study, as Glass puts it, these remarks point up the reasons why it took a particular form. Reflected there are the assumptions of liberalism and social democracy which was the established radicalism of the day. The doctrine of equality of opportunity was embodied in the 1944 Education Act and the idea of the 'career open to all the talents' was an accepted objective. The removal of barriers preventing access to education would, it was hoped, assist in the achievement of this aim.

The focus of attention was on the individual and on his talents and his fulfilment. The measurement of the opportunities and achievements of individuals was done by a process of aggregation. The methods employed neatly match the objects of the study. A shrewd observer may notice that the methodological tool, the index of association, is in fact a logical analogue to the classical economic notion of the perfect market. The liberal assumption that talented people may be born in any stratum of society was also basic to the study. It is the reason why statistical randomness is equated with 'perfect mobility'. The index of association is a measure of the extent of self-recruitment in any actual society. or to put it round the other way, it is a measure of the extent to which there is deviation from the standard of perfect mobility. Glass and his co-workers claimed that this is purely a methodological device with heuristic value only. Value-neutrality as a precept guiding the work of the sociologist was then regarded as both more feasible and more desirable than it is today. However, the reader will notice that Glass's methodology is at least not inconsistent with his stated values. It is clearly his belief that a society which approximates most closely to perfect mobility is a better society than one in which the incidence of mobility is small. We contend that Glass's approach is limited by the individualism which arises from his ideological assumptions and it is not surprising therefore that in setting the scene for much future work on social mobility, the movement of groups was left out of account.

American studies have also been influenced by the same starting assumptions and have defined their conception of the problems of social mobility and methods of investigating it in a similar way. Pitirim

4

Sorokin's *magnum opus* on social mobility was published in the United States in 1927, although the author was in fact a distinguished Russian émigré. Introducing the subject in the preface he says 'our society is a mobile society *par excellence*. An intensive shifting of individuals from position to position and a great circulation of social objects in horizontal and in vertical directions are probably the most important characteristics of contemporary Western society. To them is due its dynamic character.' In an earlier book *The Sociology of Revolution* he studied the abnormal forms of social mobility. However, in *Social Mobility* he states his intention 'to give a general theory of vertical mobility of individuals and social objects' (Sorokin 1927:preface).

He defines social mobility as follows:

> 'by social mobility is understood any transition of an individual or social object of value — anything that has been created or modified by human activity — from one social position to another. There are two principal types of social mobility, horizontal and vertical. By horizontal mobility or shifting, is meant the transition of an individual or social object from one social group to another situated on the same level. Transitions of individuals, as from the Baptist to the Methodist religious group, from one citizenship to another, from one family (as a husband or wife) to another by divorce or remarriage, from one factory to another in the same occupational status, are all instances of social mobility. So too are transitions of social objects, the radio, automobile, fashion, Communism . . . within the same social stratum' (1927:133).

Sorokin is aware also of changes in geographical location as an aspect of social mobility. He explains that 'shifting' of these kinds may take place without an individual changing his social position in the vertical direction. He goes on

> 'by vertical social mobility is meant the relations involved in a transition of an individual (or a social object) from one social stratum to another. According to the direction of the transition there are two types of vertical mobility: ascending and descending, or social climbing or social sinking. According to the nature of the stratification, there are ascending and descending currents of economic, political, and occupational mobility, not to mention other less important types. The ascending currents exist in two principal forms; as an infiltration of the individuals of a lower stratum into an existing higher one; and as a creation of a new group by such individuals and the insertion of such a group into a higher stratum instead of, or side by side with, the existing groups of this stratum' (1927:133-34).

There are processes of downward mobility, which correspond with these but in addition there is the possibility of the 'disintegration [of a group] as a social unit'.

Sorokin is well aware of the importance of collective social mobility. He suggests that the question 'of social ascending and descending, the rise and fall of groups, must be considered more carefully' (1927:134). He gives some historical examples – the Indian caste system is one case where the superior caste of Brahmins did not always hold the position of indisputable superiority which it has maintained during the last 2,000 years. He points out that if 'the group as a whole being is elevated, all its members, *in corpore* through this very fact, are elevated also' (1927:134). Other cases he mentions are those of the social ascent of the Christians during and after the reign of Constantine the Great and, in the Middle Ages, the elevation of the communal bourgeoisie and the Gilda Mercatoria. Referring to the question of social descent, he cites both the Romanoffs and their ruling class and the Hapsburgs. He suggests as a contrary example the case of those members of the Communist Party in Russia who, after the revolution, were elevated *en masse* into the place of the former Czarist aristocracy. In Western industrial societies, he mentions the rise of the groups associated with the oil and automobile industries.

Sorokin recognises that there may be a type of immobile stratified society in which vertical social mobility is nil. This means that within such societies there is no ascending or descending, no circulation of its members so that every individual is for ever attached to the social stratum in which he was born.

> 'Such a type of stratification may be styled as absolutely closed, rigid, impenetrable or immobile. The opposite theoretical type is that in which vertical mobility is very intensive and general . . . Such a type of stratification may be styled open, plastic, penetrable or mobile. Between these two extreme types there may be many middle or intermediary types of stratification'

(1927:137-138). Sorokin argues that although democratic societies are believed to be characterised by more intensive vertical mobility compared with that of non-democratic ones, they are in fact not necessarily more open in this sense than autocratic societies; the channels of mobility may simply be different. Extensive social mobility is not guaranteed simply by the existence of democratic elections or the widespread belief that the social position of the individual ought not to be ascribed at birth. Neither of these, nor the idea of equality of opportunity or freedom from prejudice occasioned by judicial or religious obstacles necessarily produce high rates of individual mobility. No society in fact is absolutely closed, or conversely, free from transition from one social stratum to another.

Sorokin discusses channels of vertical circulation such as the army, the church, the school, governments and political groups, professional organisations, wealth-making organisations and the family. Questions which have been much researched and debated since his day concern the mechanisms of social testing. One of these – the school – he chooses to discuss in some detail from the point of view that it is a selective and distributing agency (1927:188). He argues that the school is an agency which 'leads not so much to an obliteration of mental and social differences as to their increase . . . [it] is a machinery [for] the stratification of society, not of "levelling" or "democratisation" ' (1927:189-190).

Returning to the subject of vertical mobility in Western societies, Sorokin sets an example for later studies, such as that associated with David Glass, by focussing on the extent of inter-occupational and intra-occupational mobility and in particular he asks the question, to what extent does the occupational status of the father determine that of his children. In caste society, Sorokin says, there is an established set of privileges adhering in caste groups which confers the right to the performance of a definite occupation on an hereditary basis. In modern Western society, by contrast, the occupational status of parents plays a more modest part in determining that of their children. Sorokin states that the transmission of occupational status seems to be much less in Western societies than a hundred per cent. In his view contemporary occupational groups are far from rigid. He notes the probability that the transmission of occupational status is not equal in all occupational groups. He also seeks to show with such evidence as is at his command, that there is a considerable fluctuation of inheritance of occupations in different social groups. He further suggests (1927:419), quoting F. Chessa,[1] that 'hereditary transmission of occupation is stronger in those occupations which demand a greater technical experience and specialisation or a more or less large amount of money for their performance than in the occupations which do not demand either of these conditions'.

On the subject of the liberal professions, (again following Dr Chessa) Sorokin proposes that hereditary transmission of occupations tends to be higher in those professions which are connected with social honour and privilege and which are also characterised by stability and durability, or again those which require intensive intellectual work. He makes the point that these conclusions are tentative and need to be tested by further studies. Following up the evidence he has presented, Sorokin suggests some 'tentative inferences' (1927:426-7). He says

'other conditions being equal, first, within the same occupation the more qualified and better paid strata shift less intensively than the less qualified and more poorly paid groups; second, members of occupations which disappear shift more intensively than members of occupations which develop and prosper; third, unskilled labour is more mobile than skilled labour; business and professional groups (their higher strata) are likely to be still more stable even than the group of skilled labour' (1927:427).

Another interesting proposition put by Sorokin is that 'the closer the affinity between occupations, the more intensive among them is mutual interchange of their members; and *vice versa* . . .' (1927:439).

From our point of view, it is important to notice that all of these statements which anticipate much of the later research on social mobility do not deal adequately with the question of group mobility, but always focus on the transposition of individuals from occupation to occupation. It is very relevant to our argument to notice that in his section on professional organisations as channels of vertical circulation, there is no conception of the possibility of collective mobility via professionalism. On the contrary, he argues that

> 'as the entrance to these organisations (professional organisations) has been relatively free to all who displayed a corresponding ability, regardless of the status of families, and as an ascent within these institutions has been followed by . . . elevation in the social position of a corresponding individual, therefore, many scientists and scholars, lawyers and literary men, artists and musicians, painters and architects, sculptors, physicians, and players, dancers, and singers, born in humble families, have climbed up through this channel' (1927:174).

This quotation underlines the fact that Sorokin holds the long accepted view that the professions are vehicles through which individuals obtain upward social mobility. There is no conception in his work of the idea we are advancing, namely, that professionalism is itself an important type of collective action which may be used as a strategic mechanism to elevate the social position of a whole occupational group.

Speaking of what he regards as 'the Golden Rule of distribution of individuals', he says,

> 'in the ideal mobile society individuals must be distributed according to their capacity and ability, regardless of the position of their fathers. Such a social distribution where everybody is placed at his proper place, seems to be the best. At least since ancient India and China, through Plato and Aristotle, up to the present democracies, this type of social distribution of individuals has been recognised as the most desirable. And, it seems, only an ideal mobile society can realise it. In an immobile society, only extremely fortunate racial purity may to some extent approach such a type. But such purity cannot prevent the appearance of children dissimilar to their parents, [therefore] even an exclusively fortunate immobile society has to deviate from the ideal rule. In an ideal society, such children are at once shifted to the positions corresponding to their ability' (1927:530).

Sorokin takes the view that within mobile societies, since there is a system of open positions and greater competition for the higher places among candidates . . . 'the relatively weaker individuals are eliminated or ousted by the relatively stronger ones'. This process by which the weak posterity of prominent parents is forced downward and stronger men of humbler origin climb up, ensures that 'the whole social structure is permanently cleansed from the inappropriate dwellers of its different storeys' (1927:532).

He distinguishes between this form of 'normal vertical mobility', which facilitates a more appropriate social distribution of individuals and an alternative form, which occurs in anarchical or revolutionary times and which, in his view, is quite blind and unselective.

Sorokin is well aware of the arguments for and against an open society which maximises opportunities and chances for social mobility. Indeed, he rehearses the arguments in his book. His position is, however, different in some respects from many of the liberal or social democratic writers on social mobility. These hold the view that the maximisation of social mobility is desirable as a means of achieving a more egalitarian and less class-ridden society. For Sorokin, social mobility is important precisely because it is a defence of social order. Thus potential revolutionaries who are given the opportunity to rise and are incorporated in the ruling group are transformed from leaders of revolution into protectors of social order. In this way 'mobility permanently robs the revolutionary factions of their possible and capable leaders' (1927:533-4). This, then, appears to be the principle reason why Sorokin supports the 'open society'.

Sorokin suggests two important conditions for the creation of such a society. They are 'an equality in the starting point of children and an equality of chance'. He goes on to argue that

'as we cannot know *a priori* who are talented and the nature of those talents, we must test them. In order that the testing be fair it is necessary that children start from the same point, equipped more or less equally, and given equal chances in "their life race". Only under such conditions of equality may be determined those among them who are "good runners" ' (1927:530).

Another condition he lays down is that the testing institutions and methods be adequate. Sorokin's difficulty in attempting to marry his conservatism with American liberalism is apparent in the following quotation:

'it is somewhat difficult to decide whether mobile or immobile societies have been nearer to their ideal rule of social distribution of individuals. We know some mobile socities, and the United States of America may serve as an example, in which the social distribution of individuals has been very satisfactory. But we know also some immobile societies, like India, where social distribution has been not altogether bad. The objective fact of an unquestionable supremacy of the Brahmins during 2,000 years is a very convincing test of their adequacy for their social position regardless of whether we like the caste-system or not. Surely, stupid men, without money and organisation, cannot keep such exclusive domination for so long a time' (1927:531).

Sorokin's work on social mobility contains a rich variety of propositions rather loosely put together and not all of which are logically compatible with one another. The central theme is a contrast between egalitarian and elitist perspectives on the organisation of society. The egalitarian model is developed in some detail both in terms of methodological suggestions for future research and concepts which have been influential in later studies of social mobility. It is possible to discern a treatment of issues such as race and intelligence in a manner which is by now traditional in one strand of psychological theory. In certain parts of the book, readers of Eysenck and Jensen will find themselves in a familiar intellectual environment. In other chapters one may see the basis upon which sociologists like Glass were to build their research. Glass's operationalisation of concepts and his development of methods by which social mobility can be more accurately measured are both premised upon a commitment to the open society. Sorokin, in spite of the enthusiasm of the émigré confronting a hospitable American democracy, is nevertheless profoundly ambivalent about the benefits of the 'open society'.

Lipset and Bendix (1959) in an influential book took a more pessimistic view about the extent of social mobility in American society than Sorokin had been inclined to do. Perhaps the overriding effect of their study was to undermine the myth that America, among industrial societies, was the most egalitarian compared with the old highly stratified and class conscious countries of Western Europe. The tenor of the argument is, however, familiar: it is that America is failing to live up to the ideals of an open society in which each and every individual may realise his talents through his own achievement. They discerned powerful constraints over opportunities arising particularly from the existence of a self-perpetuating class structure. As with Glass, the methods they employed and the sources they quoted were almost exclusively based on the measurement of individual mobility and the result was a discussion of statistical aggregates. There is little reference to the phenomenon of collective mobility. Indeed, the only major passage devoted to the matter occurs at the end of the book where the situation in caste societies is discussed. The authors define their enterprise in the following way:

> 'when we study social mobility we analyse the movement of individuals from positions possessing a certain rank to positions either higher or lower in the social system. It is possible to conceive of the result of this process as a distribution of talent and training such that privileges and perquisites accrue to each position in proportion to its difficulty and responsibility. An ideal ratio between the distribution of talents and the distribution of rewards can obviously never occur in society, but the approximation to this ideal or the failure to approximate to it, lends fascination to the study of social mobility' (1959:2).

It is evident that this position is highly similar to that of David Glass.

In another considerable study of social mobility produced in the United States but the subject of which is Italian society (Lopreato and Hazelrigg 1972:115), the authors assert that in the analysis of class theory and class dynamics, there are two cardinal variables — class consciousness and social mobility. They remark that 'it is no exaggeration to say that the history of any class structure is to a large extent the history of the interplay of these two great social forces'. Arguing along Marxian lines, they propose that

> 'class consciousness refers to the social-psychological process underlying the transformation of the *Klasse an sich* into the *Klasse für sich* [Marx 1955:150]. Thus, the working class is viewed as going through a series of steps which lead to its organization into a political party powerfully situated to engage in concerted action against the enemy class. Class consciousness, in short, is an associative variable.
>
> 'By contrast, social mobility is largely a *dissociative* variable. To be sure, Marx had viewed the decline of the "middle strata" into "the working masses" as an important factor in the political development of the proletariat. However, in the literature that has developed in part as a reaction to Marx's extreme thesis of proletarianization, mobility is properly seen as the crucial variable interfering with the formation of classes. Mobility bears an interesting conceptual relationship to migration: it abstracts some people from a population (a class) and adds them to another. This process of abstraction and addition, which is everywhere continuous, keeps the social classes in a state of uninterrupted resocialization and reorganization' (1972:115).

The bulk of Lopreato's very substantial work is devoted to the study of these two processes of class dynamics in Italian society.

We take a view different from Lopreato, namely that social mobility is not by any means always a *dissociative* variable, but rather that it is frequently linked with class consciousness through the mechanism of collective social mobility. In this sense it is often an *associative* variable. Lopreato's work is for us another example of the manner in which the prescriptions of liberal individualism have become incorporated in sociology and have dominated studies of social mobility.

Returning now to a consideration of some of the developments arising from the research programme whose aims, as we mentioned earlier, were specified by Glass in his book *Social Mobility in Britain* we note its crucial influence on certain studies published in Britain during the 1950s and 60s. Research on the measurement of educational opportunity and the detailed study of several occupational groups were among the enterprises thus generated.[2] Connected with this programme there were sociologists with a prime concern to inform their empirical investigations with a theoretical basis drawn from the founding fathers,

11

especially from Marx and Weber. David Lockwood, for example, looked at social mobility by way of taking issue with the Marxian thesis about the proletarianisation of the blackcoated worker (Lockwood 1958). Already in the 1930s a study had been done of the clerical worker in London. This was at the time of the world economic slump. The author adopted a Marxist position and concluded that 'the economic assimilation of clerks to the proletarian level can no longer be a matter of doubt' (Klingender 1935:200-01). Lockwood, on the contrary, suggested that the class consciousness of the clerk — specifically his identification with the middle class — could survive even an equalisation of money income with the skilled manual worker (1958:211).

The debate centered on a key proposition of Marx's theory. This states that under capitalism an increasing polarisation and homogenisation of classes was to be expected. Marx drew attention particularly to the divisive nature of the relations between men in the labour market due to the unequal distribution of property. He realised that the existence of property owning and propertyless groups would warp the nature of the bargain struck between those owners who bought labour and those ordinary workpeople who had nothing to sell but their labour power. Marx stressed the fact that considerations of economic power could not be eliminated from the market place by the implementation of policies founded upon the economic theory of the Manchester School. He saw that market relations were based on unequal power relations which enabled some men to exploit the services of others. Specifically the weakness of the position in which the proletarian found himself lay in the fact that he would not be able to withhold his labour from the market — he had to labour to live. It was one of Marx's predictions that the group of propertyless workers would find themselves in a situation, which, due to the de-skilling of craftwork, would eventuate in their downward social mobility and consequent assimilation into the class of unskilled workers. This would produce an increasing homogeneity of all propertyless workers. Differences between such seemingly diverse groups as craftsmen and labourers, peasants and factory workers, clerks, teachers, and other propertyless groups, would be expected to disappear (Marx, Engels 1968:C.M.). They would move from a situation of objective propertylessness through to a common consciousness of their situation, and finally to collective action directed to changing the existing state of affairs in their own collective interest. For Marx, as Lockwood says 'the increasing impoverishment, insecurity, and caste-like character of the propertyless class would, according to this theory, override the internal differences and provide the principal dynamic of the class system of late capitalism' (Lockwood 1958:203). Stemming from Marx's political commitment to the abolition of capitalism was his belief that interests held in common by those without property would be focussed upon the overthrow of capitalism and its institutions.

During the middle decades of the twentieth century a different view has been widely held. A number of influential writers have suggested that, contrary to the Marxian prediction, the propertyless proletarian class was becoming increasingly diversified. They provide evidence that there has been a growth of skills rather than diminution of them. In addition, the role of the state in the management of the economy and in welfare provision has according to this view blunted the fluctuations and crises which Marx anticipated and which he believed would be important in the emergence of class consciousness and hence in the downfall of capitalism. Lockwood for his part stressed

'the important truism that all those who fall into the category of propertyless contractual labour do not necessarily share an identical market situation . . . As a consequence, any empirical study of class consciousness must begin by taking into account actual differences in the market situations of propertyless groups. To define such differences out of existence at the very beginning as being irrelevant to the long-run development of class alignments and class consciousness is nothing less than an abdication from sociological understanding. Variations in class identification have to be related to actual variations in class situations and not attributed to some kind of ideological aberration or self-deception' (1958:203).

Lockwood analysed the variation of class situations by utilising the concepts of class as market, work, and status situation respectively. These concepts were taken from the work of Max Weber (Gerth and Mills 1948:181-91). Lockwood contrasted the position of the black-coated worker with that of the manual worker. In particular he focussed on the problem of class consciousness and he dealt especially with the difficulty presented to the Marxian theory by the reluctance, historically speaking, of white collar workers to identify with their proletarian brothers. He demonstrated that the concept of 'false class consciousness' utilised by Marxists to explain the behaviour of clerical workers is really a political and ethical gambit rather than a sociological one. As Lockwood put it 'although he shares the propertyless status of the manual worker, the clerk has never been strictly "proletarian" in terms of income, job security and occupational mobility' (1958:204). Lockwood demonstrated in particular the ways in which the variety of actual market situations can be the basis of differences of interest *within* the propertyless class.

The point which we wish to make is this. Lockwood's clerks undoubtedly had a commitment to individualism expressed in their reluctance to engage in collective action. Lockwood, following an established sociological tradition, assumes that commitment to individualism is perhaps the principal defining characteristic of the middle class. The clerks, who identify with the middle class, are said to be simply reflecting the established and institutionalised middle class values. If Lockwood were to be true to his own theoretical and methodological principles he would, we believe, not make such an assumption. Instead he would look at the variation in the class positions, specifically the market situations, of the various occupations usually regarded as middle class. This was precluded by the scope of his study. Lockwood's analysis of the special characteristics of the market, work, and status situations of the clerical worker allow him to explain the unusual degree of individualism which characterises them (as opposed to the ideal-typical collectivism of the working class). What he appears not to realise is that the individualism of the clerk may be untypical of other sections of the middle class who also are themselves committed to collective action albeit of a type different from working class unionism. It is for this reason that Lockwood is able to assume that the ideology of individualism is characteristic of middle class belief and practice, and that social mobility is consequently so much a phenomenon of the individual that collective mobility may be safely ignored as an object of study.

Subsequently, in a collaborative project (Goldthorpe *et al* 1968 a:2) Lockwood turned his attention to another variant of the problem. After World War II, a long period of economic boom and of full employment dispelled for most observers the plausibility of the belief that clerical workers were becoming proletarianised. The alternative thesis which became widely accepted was that the affluent worker, whether skilled or semi-skilled was being assimilated into the middle class. The Affluent Worker Studies attempted a refutation of the idea that the sheer economic equivalence of the affluent manual worker with the lower echelons of the middle class (such as the clerical worker) would cause manual workers to become fully assimilated members of the middle class. The proposition that such a process of assimilation was taking place became known as the *embourgeoisement* thesis.

In their study of the affluent worker Goldthorpe and Lockwood distinguished between the economic, normative, and relational aspects of class and they suggested that all three elements, taken together, were essential to the understanding of the process of assimilation. Their observation of affluent manual workers and of white collar workers in Luton showed that such assimilation was not happening. Indeed the authors predicted that there was little likelihood that assimilation would occur in the forseeable future. Moreover, they argued that the working class was not experiencing a simple breakdown of traditional community as some writers had suggested, but rather that the new worker was moving in the direction of "instrumental collectivism" — collectivism, that is to say, which is directed to the achievement of individuals' private goals outside the workplace' (Goldthorpe 1968 a:106). By this they meant that manual workers were coming to behave more like 'economic man' in terms of their instrumental relationship to work. The same instrumental orientation was to be found in relation to trade unions and to the class party of working people — the Labour party. Outside work the decline of working class community was manifested in an increasing privatisation of life characterised by home-centredness.

Among white-collar workers a parallel, but even stronger movement, was taking place towards 'instrumental collectivism'. Increasingly, unionism was becoming a feature of the lives of lower middle class people. At the same time, they continued to be distinguished from affluent manual workers by their commitment to a different set of social norms and by the particular form of their 'relational' patterns of interaction with friends and colleagues. It was especially characteristic that non-manual workers manifested much higher rates of participation in voluntary associations. Goldthorpe and Lockwood argued that there was a process of class convergence taking place, characterised by 'instrumental collectivism', but they stressed that this was in no way to be confused with the process of assimilation of working people into middle class life. The distinction between manual and non-manual work continued on their evidence to remain a predominant feature of the British class structure.

A reading of both the *Blackcoated Worker* and the *Affluent Worker Studies* (Lockwood 1958, Goldthorpe 1968/69) underlines the central importance in contemporary sociology of conceptions of social class which connect individualism particularly to the middle class and collectivism to the working class. The method employed is that of ideal-type analysis commended to sociologists by Max Weber (Gerth and Mills 1948:59-60). In order to be able to judge the characteristic differences between the 'middle class' and the 'working class', Goldthorpe and Lockwood decided as they put it: 'to make our own ideas in this respect as clear and explicit as possible.' This was a sensible preliminary in a study which set out to judge whether assimilation of one class to another had or had not taken place. They go on, 'we attempted, in the light of available empirical material, to represent these two perspectives in ideal-type form as a preliminary to the analysis of our research findings' (Goldthorpe 1969:118). For them the traditional working class perspective involves a dichotomous conception of the social order in which society is divided into 'them' and 'us'. This division is rooted in power and authority and was seen by those who experienced it as permanent and virtually unbridgeable. Also, social circumstances were regarded as immutable and expectations relatively fixed. The chief economic conception is of the maintenance of a certain standard of living and lifestyle, not of continuous improvement. The idea of putting up with one's lot and making the best of it, is very much to the fore because the world is regarded as very little under the control of the individual. Fatalism is the major orientation 'insofar as it is felt that purposive action can be effective, the emphasis is placed on action of a *collective* kind aimed at the protection of collective

15

interests – trade unionism being, of course, the most developed form' (1969:119). Mutual aid and group solidarity are highly valued in the face of the problems created by living in a market economy. Individual action is constrained by social controls which operate to sanction those who would make themselves 'a cut above the rest'. Aspirations are confined to achievements within the context of working class values and life styles.

Turning to the middle class perspective Goldthorpe and Lockwood admit that 'we have far less research material to guide us. However, that which is available suggests, with some consistency, a configuration of beliefs and values that is in almost point by point contrast with the working class pattern' (1969:119-20). The middle class conception of social order is a hierarchical one. Society is seen as divided into strata differentiated in terms of the lifestyles and the associated prestige of their members. The system is seen as 'relatively open' and those with ability and relevant moral qualities such as perseverance and determination can, and do, move upwards. A man is judged very much on the basis of what he makes of himself. The individual is regarded as having 'an obligation to assume responsibility for his own life and welfare and to *try* to "get on in the world" as far as he can' (1969:120). Typically the expectation in the middle class is of continuous improvement in economic terms as well as status and style of life. Allied with this is an orientation toward the future, to planning ahead, and to making sacrifices in the present while deferring gratification to the future. This is a matter not merely of expediency but is a moral injunction.

'The middle-class social ethic is thus an essentially individualistic one: the prime value is that set on individual achievement. Achievement is taken as the crucial indicator of the individual's moral worth. However, achievement is also regarded as a family concern: parents feel an obligation to try to give their children a "better start in life" than they themselves enjoyed, and then anticipate that their offspring will in turn attain to a still higher level in the social scale' (1969:120-21).

Goldthorpe and Lockwood are aware that the ideal-type approach may 'overstate the degree of divergence that may often in fact be found as between specific working-class and middle-class groups. For example, within the traditional working-class one could point to the "respectable artisan" who sets great store on a well regulated existence and on looking ahead, and who has white-collar ambitions for his children; or on the other hand, to the lower middle-class "ritualist" – to use Merton's term – who has drawn in his horizons and has in effect rejected the obligation to continue to strive for material success [Merton 1957:149-53]. Nevertheless, the empirical evidence that is reflected in the ideal-types makes it clear enough that quite basic class differences in aspirations and in their conceptual contexts do exist' (1969:121).

16

In the *Blackcoated Worker*, the manual working class had been used as the comparative group against which the relative position of the lower-middle-class clerical employee was assessed. The debate about affluence involved a shift of focus from the middle class to the working class side of the manual non-manual boundary. The new worker was contrasted with the traditional worker and with the middle class clerk. In the *Affluent Worker Studies*, a contribution was made to the debate between Marxists and anti-Marxists which had been going on for a hundred years. Goldthorpe and Lockwood brought a greater degree of theoretical sophistication and empirical rigour to the study which was their contribution to the debate. The issue was about the significance of the working class and of working class consciousness in the development of capitalist society. Whereas in the *Blackcoated Worker* Lockwood had shown why the proletarianisation of clerical grades was not occurring, in the *Affluent Worker,* the thesis that affluent working men were being assimilated into the middle class was challenged and itself shown to be far from the straightforward matter which influential writers had maintained in the 1950s. Both the proletarianisation thesis and its counterpart, the *embourgeoisement* thesis, are in fact species of a general argument about predominant trends of mass social mobility in advanced industrial societies. Goldthorpe and Lockwood have demonstrated that the process of social mobility can usefully be placed in a wider context where questions about social mobility are afforded greater significance precisely because they are posed in relation to competing theories about the nature of social stratification in industrial society itself.

Each theory has made certain assumptions about the nature of social mobility. Marx's conception of the development of class society contained within it a theory of social mobility which focussed on the downward mobility and downward assimilation of those in the middle stratum into the proletariat. The decline of skills, and the increasing homogeneity of labour (whether by hand or brain) brought about by the mechanisation and routinisation of work were assumed to be basic to the process. Where this was combined with the cutting back of wages to subsistence level and the consequent polarisation of classes, Marx suggested that eventually the middle stratum would be assimilated into the proletariat, and would by reason of this provide part of the impetus to revolution (Marx, Engels 1968: C.M.). Klingender's thesis, as we have seen, exemplifies precisely this Marxist argument. The counter-Marxist view has stressed the alternative possibility of mass upward social mobility in capitalist society. Democratic socialism, which appears to involve a compromise between liberalism and socialism, contains the notion that by gradual reform especially of the educational system it will be possible to increase the rate of social mobility of individuals between classes. By this means the hold of class divisions in society would be gradually weakened. The Marxist argument concerning the polarisation of classes has led to very considerable

17

interest in the study of both the ruling class and the working class.[3] The position of the middle class is of less concern and interest to Marxist writers precisely because of the theoretical position which suggests that the future lies with the proletariat. It is, after all, the working class not the middle class which according to Marx is destined to fulfil an historic role in the overthrow of capitalism. In Marxian theory dissociative forces will polarise society and thus tear the middle class apart. Some will remain as the 'lackeys' of the capitalists but the majority will be forced eventually into an assimilation with the workers.

In the light of this theory it is little wonder that Marxist writers have turned to the concept of false class consciousness to explain why certain groups such as clerical workers have not as yet been fully assimilated into the working class movement. As we have seen this is exactly the problem which Lockwood set out to explore. He inherited the long established belief that the most salient characteristic of the middle class has been their commitment to individualism; a view which, we believe, masks the importance of the phenomenon of collective social mobility. The clerical workers, whom Lockwood studied, came closest to exemplifying individualism in action. We suggest that certain core elements of the established middle class, such as the professions themselves, often follow modes of collective action.

Lockwood and Goldthorpe concentrated their attention upon the margin between classes – they were concerned with the boundaries between the lower middle class (white-collar workers) and the upper end of the working class (skilled manual workers). We contend that an analysis confined to the margins around this particular class boundary is likely to divert attention away from an understanding of the nature of middle class life, particularly in its central business and professional groups. One aim of our book is to demonstrate that the characterisation of the middle class as thoroughly and archetypically individualist is mistaken. On the contrary, we use historical evidence to support our thesis that the development of the middle class in English society has been very much dependent on collective action and collective social mobility. In order to demonstrate that collective social mobility has been an important and viable process we shall look not simply at groups of people at the margin between classes, such as clerical workers or manual workers, but at core elements of the middle class. We think that Goldthorpe and his colleagues have perhaps been influenced too much by the assumptions of earlier students of social mobility, including David Glass. Studies of social stratification linked with social mobility have, in our view, been dominated by the essential individualism of liberal social theories which tend to shut out the considerations of the importance of collective action, not least in regard to the middle class.[4]

Notes

1. Sorokin has taken this quotation from F. Chessa, *Trasmissione. Ereditaria dei Professioni.*
2. Examples of work in this tradition are Asher Tropp, *The School Teachers,* and J. Banks, *Prosperity and Parenthood,* Olive Banks, *Parity and Prestige in English Secondary Education,* Jean Floud, *The Schoolteachers,* Halsey, *The British Academics,* Kelsall, *Recruitment to Several Professions.*
3. See for example, W.L. Guttsman, *The British Political Elite,* MacGibbon 1963. S. Aaronovitch, *The Ruling Class: a Study of British Finance Capital,* Lawrence and Wishart 1961.
4. At the time of writing the substantive findings of the Oxford Occupational Mobility Inquiry have not yet been published. This major study based at Nuffield College and supported by the Social Science Research Council is unlikely to provide *direct* evidence about collective social mobility because, as far as we understand, it is a development of the studies of individual social mobility undertaken by Glass. Two preliminary publications concerning methods and approaches on the one hand, and a reconsideration of mobility in Britain on the other, are already available. (Hope 1972, Ridge 1974).

2. PROFESSIONALISM AND SOCIAL CLASS – I

This chapter and the next are closely linked by the single theme of professionalism and social class. We are first concerned to explore in some detail the development of a body of writing about the professions sub-divided by several rather different approaches. Then to draw attention to the marked lack of interest in the relationship between the study of the professions and class theory. Even in the case of writers who have explicitly claimed that they intend to examine the professions and class we find paradoxically that they typically fail to do so. We suggest that the reasons for this are bound up with the inadequacy of the approach through the individualistic perspective of the traditional studies of social mobility, an approach which has been conceived of as the appropriate link between professions and class. Continuing this theme in the following chapter we contend that an alternative way of exploring the problem is via the concept of collective social mobility. We examine the contribution of several writers whose work provides a foundation for the development of such a new approach while recognising that none have as yet clearly perceived the problem or posed it in a manner which would admit of an adequate theoretical link between the professions and the theory of class structure.

One of the most important quantitative changes in the occupational structure has been the rapid increase in the twentieth century of white collar, service and professional occupations. Difficult as it is to decide on a satisfactory definition of the term 'professional', quantitatively the evidence of rapid growth is such as to brook no argument although 'the overall increase obscures the quite marked variations within the professional group' (Marsh 1965:138). Qualitatively, professionalisation has been regarded as a very significant development. It has been said that 'an industrialising society *is* a professionalising society' and the reader may find it somewhat surprising then, that the widespread assertion of the importance of professional occupations has not been matched to a similar extent in theoretical analysis at least at the macro-sociological level (Johnson 1972:9). It is true that one strand of social thought has strongly supported the idea that ours is a technocratic society in which the professional with his expertise, the organisation man, and the manager are more and more involved in the centres of power (Galbraith 1968:378-87). Nevertheless, Johnson makes it clear that 'the numerous attempts to identify emerging elites have, in general, been quite separate from the problems associated with the sociology of the professions' (Johnson 1972:9). Although a substantial and increasing sociological literature has emerged concerning the professional occupations, a review of these studies shows that they have been mainly concerned, as Ben David recognised, with the micro-sociological or social-psychological aspects of professionalisation (Ben David 1963-4:251). A number of excellent studies have been undertaken concerning the socialisation of novices into professional occupations, for example Becker (1961). There are, however, rather fewer which attempt to deal with the relationship between the professions and social class. Ben David's own work is only apparently an exception. Prandy's study of professional employees (Prandy 1965) is one of the few which directly confronts the problem of class and the professions.

In origin, it has been argued, the sociology of the professions was engaged with two fundamental questions. These are: to what extent are professional occupations a unique product of the division of labour in society; and is it correct to say that the professions perform a special role in society whether economic, political or social? Marx, in his analysis of the division of labour, argued that the professions were occupations of a secondary and derivative character because of their negative contribution to surplus value. Recently sociologists have turned away from the direct analysis of the division of labour itself, and concentrated instead upon issues of individual social mobility. Thus, Johnson suggests, the notion that the professions might be a 'special' product of the division of labour has been lost (Johnson 1972:10). The main effort of sociologists has been directed instead to the definition of the key attributes of a profession as such. In evaluating the definitional exercises which 'litter the field', Johnson finds himself bound to make the harsh judgement that these have been 'largely sterile'. He points out that the basic assumption that the professional occupations are unique is never opened to debate, but rather is safely hidden from scrutiny. It is this assumption which is used to justify the existence of 'the sociology of the professions' as a specialist field and which therefore is held to be the basis of a distinct body of theory and research. The other and larger question as to whether or not the professions perform a special role in industrial society has, in Johnson's view, been split up into such small and 'manageable' parcels for research that it is impossible to reconstruct an adequate answer. The outcome has been a failure to bridge the gap which has opened between research findings and the original theoretical problems posed by the rapid growth of the professions in industrial society. In particular, the relationships of the professions to the changing distribution of power has been neglected (Johnson 1972:18).

There have been two conflicting themes underlying the debate about the role of the professions in industrial society. The supporters of economic liberalism, economists in particular, have tended to see in the professions a monopolistic conspiracy against the public. On the other hand, the critics of unrestrained economic liberalism have often discerned in the professions a type of 'moral community' which will provide just that element of collective interest which can transcend the unbridled self-seeking which they regard as an essential feature of capitalist society.

Emile Durkheim was an early sociological contributor to the view that professional associations were an important precondition for stability and a source of consensus in industrial societies. He argued that the organisation of occupations as professions would act as a desirable alternative to the excesses of *laissez faire* individualism which he regarded as the basic cause of anomie in industrial society. Professional occupational communities, he averred, were moral communities and they, rather than the individual, should directly elect representatives to government (Durkheim 1957:29-41). On the other hand the exponents of economic theory have argued that the professions have a tendency to dangerous monopoly and hold unwarranted power in the community in the service of their own selfish interests (Lees 1966).

In the period between the two world wars, there was a considerable vogue for the ideology of professionalism in a variety of forms. R.H. Tawney (1972:106-11) argued, like Durkheim, that economic individualism was destructive both of community and of the community interest. In his view professionalism, with its stress on the ethics of 'moral community', could be used to counter the ubiquitous individualism of a capitalist society. Carr-Saunders and Wilson strongly urged this viewpoint saying that the professions are a major force for stability in society and are a defence against 'crude forces which threaten steady and peaceful evolution' (Carr-Saunders 1933:497). Some fascist governments between the two world wars adopted the principle of the corporative state. This involved direct representation of occupations and professions in government. In the Italian case such forms of representation were built into the Constitution (Lyttelton 1973:306-12; Cassels 1959:55-62).

According to some writers the professions have been increasingly threatened by the growth of large scale bureaucratic organisation in both government and private industry. A continuing theme has been that they are among the few remaining bulwarks against bureaucratic encroachment on the freedoms already gained for the individual citizen in an earlier liberal era (Lewis and Maude 1952). R.A.B. Butler made the point in this way

> 'society in the future may become progressively intolerant of voluntary professional institutions especially if they are the bulwark of private practice, and yet be oblivious to the truth that in these institutions resides a most precious liberty essential to the health of a civilised society' (Bennion 1969:*ii*).

These ideas have also been projected onto the international stage. Professional institutions are an 'important stabilising factor in our whole society and through their international associations they provide

22

an important channel of communication with the intellectual leaders of other countries, thereby helping to maintain world order' (Lynn 1963:653).

The growth of bureaucracy and the rationalisation of the modern world have long been an important issue in sociology. Johnson points out following Parsons, that

'Weber did not distinguish radically between the consequences of professionalisation and bureaucratisation and specifically linked the process of bureaucratisation with the development of specialised professional education. He saw both processes as expressions of the increasing rationalisation of Western civilisation' (Johnson 1972:15).

The difference between the political and social contexts in which the professions grew up in continental Europe, especially in France and Germany, (compared with Britain and the USA) is crucial. The particular social and political structure of Imperial Germany, in which Weber lived and worked, helps us to account for the fact that he did not conceive of a conflict between professionalism and bureaucracy (MacRae 1974:37). The 'free professions' were, rather, a characteristic development of Britain and the United States. Paradoxically, they were a typical product of the age of *laissez faire*. Both Weber and Carr-Saunders saw the professions as bringing 'knowledge to the service of power'. Weber saw the professional specifically as a technical 'expert' subordinated to the bureaucratic machine, not as belonging to an 'independent' professional association which might itself act as a constraint upon the exercise of bureaucratic power (Giddens 1972:22).

Since the late nineteenth century an increasing proportion of professionals are no longer independent consulting practitioners but rather employees of large scale public and private bureaucracies. C. Wright Mills is one among those who have regarded the professions as succumbing to a 'managerial demiurge' (Wright Mills 1956:112). R.K. Merton has expressed the view that professional technocrats are men whose vision is excessively narrowed by over-specialisation within the context of a complex division of labour, they have a 'trained incapacity' for dealing with issues, especially social issues, which lie outside the purview of their discipline (Merton 1964:569). Thorstein Veblen, touching on the same theme in another way, had argued that the engineer would emerge as leader in contemporary society because as a professional technocrat he alone would have the necessary knowledge and capacity to run a modern complex industrial system. In this sense the engineer would be the natural decision-maker in industrial society (Veblen 1921:33). Paul Halmos has distinguished a group of professional occupations characterised by 'a service ethic'. He claims that such an ethic was originally characteristic of only certain professions, such as social work and medicine, which were concerned to bring about a transformation in 'the psycho-social personality of the client'. This ethic of personal service has spread, so be believes, to many other occupations and has become the basis for a new moral uniformity which may be found at work in the industrial societies irrespective of their manifest political ideology or governmental structure (Halmos 1966:5).

Whatever the political and moral perspectives of sociologists who have studied the professions there has been one predominant sociological theme within the field; namely, professionalisation. While it is conceded that there are many variations to be found in the nature of professional practice, organisation and attitude among the occupations loosely known as the professions, the main thing they share in common, according to this view, is a process, the process of professionalisation. Some occupations such as social work or teaching are considered not yet to have travelled far along the road to full professionalisation. Others, such as medicine or law, have arrived, or at least are close to arrival, at the destination of 'full professionalisation'. Johnson makes the point that this approach assumes too much about the selected 'professionalising' occupations and fails to place the problem in the wider context of class structure and the distribution of power. There is no attempt at the classification of modes of occupational control.

There is no doubt that Johnson is also right when he points to the lack of agreement among the contributing scholars about the determinants of professional status. In the confusion thus generated, he does however discern two broad approaches to the professions: these he calls the 'trait' model and the 'functionalist' model respectively. In practice, there is a strong tendency on the part of particular authors to blend elements of the two approaches, but for the sake of clarity Johnson keeps them distinct. In the case of the 'trait model', a list of core attributes representing the common characteristics of professional occupations is put forward. The alternative approach is functionalist in character. Generally, rather than attempting to provide an exhaustive list of traits, only those elements are considered which are thought to have a functional contribution for the maintenance of society as a whole or to the relationship between professional and client. Millerson's work is most closely identified with the trait model (Millerson 1964:3-5) and Johnson's chief criticism is that there is a failure in this approach' 'to articulate theoretically the relationships between the elements' (Johnson 1972:24). For example, is there a direct causal relationship between the expansion of systematic theory in the body of knowledge belonging to a profession on the one hand and the level of authority exercised by it on the other? Johnson also points out that there is some lack of clarity over the question of the levels of analysis used by the trait theorists themselves. Altruism, for example, is said to be characteristic of the professional role but it is not always obvious whether altruistic motivation is also being imputed to the professional man. Again, while the service ethic may be part of professional ideology there is no necessary relationship between this and the actual behaviour of practitioners. In short, it appears that traits may be added or subtracted at will from the model, in an arbitrary manner, because of the lack of logical and theoretical coherence among the traits. The lack of a firm theoretical basis also encourages the mistake of accepting the professionals' own definitions and evaluations of themselves at face value. There is too little questioning of the extent to which professional rhetoric about community service and altruism may be but a legitimation for professional privilege. Johnson contrasts this view with that of the liberal economic standpoint of the Monopolies Commission's Repo on Professional Services (1970) which drew the conclusion that a number of the restrictive practices carried on by professional groups, justified on the basis of community welfare, looked in fact 'rather [like] arrangements for making life easier for practitioners at the expense, one way or another, of their clients' (Johnson 1972:26).

Another criticism which Johnson levels against the trait model, is that the method is fundamentally ahistorical. The model of professionalisation characterised by a list of 'traits' suggests a rigid unilinear process of change. It is imposed on the diversity of historical variations in occupational development and anything which does not fit it is either discarded or at best regarded as deviant. Finally, Johnson identifies what he regards as the gravest weakness of both the 'trait' and 'functionalist' approaches. He tells us that

'these models are not definitions of occupations at all but specify the characteristics of a particular institutionalised form of occupational control. This confusion between the essential characteristics of an occupation and the characteristics of a historically specific institutionalised form of its control is the most fundamental inadequacy of both "trait" and "functionalist" approaches to the study of the professions' (Johnson 1972:27).

Clearly if these criticisms are accepted, and we find them cogent, then the further extension of the trait approach is unlikely to be useful. The process of professionalisation is understood by some writers as a determinate sequence of historical events through which any professionalising occupation must pass in identical stages. This approach which has been called 'the natural history of professionalism' is presented by scholars such as Caplow and Wilensky. Johnson points out that the sequence offered by Wilensky is historically specific and bound to the culture of its authors, namely, the United States. A comparison with England which has a much closer cultural and historical affinity with the United States than many other societies, belies Wilensky's assertion. Similarly, the countries of the British Commonwealth, which also have close historical affinities with Britain, have been shown by Johnson's own research to differ in this respect (Johnson 1973:281-306).

A Canadian sociologist, Everett Hughes, who worked for many

years in Chicago, is justly recognised as perhaps the major contributor to the foundation of modern occupational sociology (Hughes 1971:364-407; Daedalus 1963:655-68). At one time he asked the question 'is this occupation a profession?' but later commented that he realised the falsity of the question and went on instead to ask 'what are the circumstances in which people in an occupation attempt to turn it into a profession, and themselves into professional people' (Vollmer and Mills 1966:V). Johnson's view is that this approach avoids some of the pitfalls of trait theory but is still wedded to the concept of professionalisation. He says:

> 'we avoid the sterility of definition-mongering and instead focus on two of the major empirical phenomena of our times; group mobility through occupational upgrading and the expansion of professionalism as a result of the growth of occupational group consciousness. However, when either of these processes is identified with professionalisation it remains incumbent on the analyst to state unequivocally what the nature of the process is and to have some idea of its end-state. In short, the claims for this approach are vacuous unless we are clear what a "claim" for professional status entails. What is being claimed? What are the claimants aiming for? What are the consequences of such claims and under what conditions are they likely to be successful? All too often this form of analysis is taken as a short-cut to an explanation of professionalisation. That is to say, it is assumed that the claims for professional status are themselves *the* major conditions for professionalisation. What sources of power are available to an occupational group making such claims is a question of crucial significance which again is often ignored' (Johnson 1972:31-2).

We are entirely in agreement with the approach suggested by these questions, which, within the limits of our work we explore in subsequent chapters.

The second major theoretical approach to the sociology of the professions is that of functionalism. It is characterised by a higher degree of abstraction and greater parsimony; Barber, who is an exponent of this perspective argues that the sociologist should concentrate on the *differentia specifica* of professional behaviour. In his view there are 'four essential attributes' of professionalism: viz. a high degree of generalised and systematic knowledge; a primary orientation to the community interest rather than to individual self-interest; a high degree of self-control of behaviour through codes of ethics internalised in the process of work socialisation and through voluntary associations organised and operated by the work specialists themselves; and a system of rewards (monetary and honorary) that is primarily a set of symbols of work achievement and thus ends in themselves, not means to some end of individual self-interest (Barber 1963:671).

What distinguishes Barber's work from that of the trait theorists is that he argues that knowledge confers power over nature and society and that it is therefore functional to society that knowledge be used in the interest of the community. Barber wrongly assumes that people equipped with knowledge, or institutions furthering knowledge, will naturally serve community rather than individual interests. Society, he suggests, ensures this by rewarding the practitioners of knowledge with above average levels of remuneration and status because the performance of their occupation is highly valued. Johnson is perhaps wise to say that he will not debate the tautologies generated by this form of functional argument but the criticisms which have been launched at functionalist theory in general are pertinent. The central functionalist assumption of societal unity built on an accepted set of shared cultural values must be called into question. It is not clear that every class or interest group in society values knowledge to the same extent and thus that professional occupations are indisputably to be regarded as equally valued throughout society. Neither is it necessarily true that professional groups will promote the community interest or that if they do they will be rewarded for doing so.

Talcott Parsons, who is an important exponent of the functionalist point of view, can also be criticised, but not quite with the ease with which it is possible to deal with less sophisticated versions of function-alist theory. He virtually ignores considerations of interest-group con-flict and power within the professions, but this omission stems from the fact that it is a weak point more generally in his sociological theory (Johnson 1972:35). We are able to offer some evidence in our subse-quent chapters which suggests that in medicine, teaching, and related occupations there has been no simple process of the 'automatic' unfolding of the division of labour, but rather that the latter must be considered in terms of the institutionalised outcome of power conflicts. The influence of the Durkheimian approach to sociology, with its stress on the importance of the division of labour, has been paramount in the sociological study of the professions. It is also a fundamental influence in Parsons' sociology considered as a whole. Durkheim regarded the increasing division of labour as potentially dangerous for the integration or 'solidarity' of society. Literally, it could be divisive and in its abnormal forms produce the breakdown of social order. For Durkheim, and for later writers, including Johnson, the division of labour is a fundamental mechanism of social change. Adam Smith's concept of the division of labour was used by Parsons and conjoined with biological evolutionism to develop his concept of 'functional differentiation' (Parsons 1951). It is clear that this concept is merely the principle of the division of labour writ large which is then applied to the other three sub-systems, which Parsons distinguishes, in addition to the economic sub-system. The evolution of societies, in Parsons' view, develops from a situation in primitive societies where the four major functional

problems are met,[1] if only barely, by an undifferentiated social system.
Subsequently through the differentiation of structures the basic
requirements of society are more adequately and efficiently met because
differentiation involves greater specialisation (Parsons 1961:219-39).
We believe that Parsons' evolutionary theory of social change postulates
an 'automatic' process of differentiation at two levels: the material,
(including the technological) and the cultural, (including the automatic
working out of the logic of particular value systems). This type of
theory has been called 'preformist' by Etzioni because all the potentialities of the fully developed society are said to be contained in its original
state (Etzioni 1964:482-5). Parsons believes that the basic functional
problems of society are far more efficiently served in a highly
differentiated (industrial) society than in a primitive undifferentiated
one. In the work of Parsons and his followers there is a courageous
attempt to address the classic philosophical problem of sociology,
namely the question of the relationship between material conditions
and ideology, and their relative causal priority in the explanation of
sociological phenomena. Parsons evidently believes that he has solved
the problem, or at least gone a long way towards a solution (Parsons
1951:428-79). His critics beg to differ with him. There is a tendency in
Parsons to suggest that at the cultural level a process is at work by
which the logic or rationality of the value system of society is working
out in an 'automatic' way, in parallel to the automatic advancement of
the division of labour, (or more broadly, functional differentiation)
at the level of the social system.

In common with most sociological writers, Parsons and his followers
in fact sometimes seem to attribute causal priority to values and
sometimes to material factors, especially technological ones. It is
unsurprising, therefore, that the same contradictory tendency exists in
sociological writings on the subject of the professions. Carr-Saunders
and Wilson, for example, appear to rely at times upon a version of
technological determinism with regard to the division of labour. This is
especially so when they speak about the proliferation of new techniques
and skills. As they put it

> 'science advances and techniques multiply. In the long run
> technical advance implies an increase in the number of those
> doing more or less specialised intellectual work relative to the
> number of those who are engaged in manual labour or in un-
> specialised intellectual routine . . . Thus, taking the long view,
> the extension of professionalism over the whole field seems in
> the end not impossible' (Carr-Saunders and Wilson 1933: 493-4).

For our part, we do not regard the division of labour as in any sense an
automatic process but one which is deeply influenced by the interests
and activities of individuals and associations. Specialism in medicine, or
any other profession, is developed with an eye to the main chance.

Attempts are made to seize opportunities and achieve control over markets, remuneration and status. Frequently more highly specialised occupations are dominated, in particular institutional contexts, by less specialised managers or professionals, who are themselves more highly remunerated and have higher status. The 'politics' of change are usually ignored by Parsons or sometimes viewed as temporary constraints upon the unfolding process of differentiation. Fundamentally, the argument betrays a commitment to the liberal view that 'change is progress' which is allied with the functionalist dynamic implied in the process of structural differentiation.

We have already had occasion to draw attention to the period between the world wars in which professionalism was put forward as part of an alternative middle-class ideology in substitution for the increasingly discredited doctrines of *laissez faire*. The professions were said to embody the dynamic principle of the advancement of knowledge, not merely its preservation. Knowledge was regarded as an evolutionary force and the professions were thought of as an advanced manifestation of the division of labour, the vanguard of science and technology.

In the European politics of the 1930s one theme was a belief in the moral superiority of professionalism, a belief which was to some extent shared by those of both left- and right-wing persuasions whether in corporatist or democratic states. Nevertheless, as Ben-David points out 'theorizing about the professions arose in different settings and took different forms in the United States and Britain on the one hand, and in continental Europe on the other' (Ben-David 1963-4:248). In the Anglo-Saxon countries some of the older professions such as physicians and lawyers achieved considerable power and influence and consequently became a model for other occupations endeavouring to obtain similar privileges. In this context questions arose about the nature of the professions and the justification and basis for their privileges. In societies such as these, where the doctrines of liberalism had eroded the idea of restrictions upon entry into the occupational world, the special demands of the professions for formal qualifications were an obvious exception to the rule. Such exceptions required explanation. As we have already seen, Carr-Saunders and Wilson felt that the professions represented a new and emerging type of occupational structure transcending the capitalist relationships of production through the use of collective control and regulation rather than the search for individual profit in competition.

Many, not least the professions themselves, especially in England, propagated the belief that professional men were not interested in making money (unlike businessmen) but were altruistically motivated to the service of their fellowmen. In fact the English idea that the professional is disinterested where money is concerned, arises from the aspirations of the professional men in the nineteenth century to adopt the high status image of the gentleman, who because he was (at least notionally) endowed with a private income could afford to disdain gross pecuniary interests.

On the continent the situation was different. In the case of Italy, no ethical rules pertaining to advertising or mores which involve an apparent disdain for money have been adopted.[2] Parsons, writing from the vantage point of the United States of America, clearly finds the English idea of the moral superiority of the professional, based upon the supposed rejection of the profit motive, to be quite incongruous in the American context, where in fact, the making of money still remained socially admirable rather than stigmatising. This helps us to explain the particular position which Parsons took with respect to the professions. His theory was infused with the doctrines of liberalism and while he regarded the individualism of economic theory as posing the fundamental methodological problem of sociology as a discipline (he believed he had transcended it), he did not see it as a 'political problem' as European writers did. There was no need for Parsons to regard the professions as engendering a new social ideology or as in some sense 'superior', as the Europeans were inclined to do. In the United States because the 'profit motive' was, for the most part, socially acceptable among workers as well as businessmen and professionals, he was able to regard motivations of professional people and businessmen alike within a common framework of values which stressed individual achievement and success. For Parsons, professionals do no more than share with people in other occupations, the values and orientations of a market society. The altruism which other writers stressed as an essential feature of the professions was for him no more than a necessary set of additional norms required to make the intimate relationship between professional and client actually function (Parsons 1954:34-49). A good example, he thought, was the case of the doctor-patient relationship which required what he quaintly called privileged access to the body (Parsons 1951:451). Professional ethics and etiquette, he argued, are specific to that kind of context and are not generalised to other relationships in the wider society. 'Accordingly, Parsons did not see in professional roles and associations indications of the rise of a new, more collectivistic type of class' (Ben-David 1963-4:248).

A fundamental difficulty in Parsons' theory is, as we have seen, the characterisation of social evolution in terms of the pattern-variable scheme which turns out to be both over-simplified and paradoxically, therefore, somewhat confusing. For example, his assumption that ascription and achievement are mutually exclusive categories so that the more a society moves towards achievement the less it utilises ascription, is patently a gross over-simplification to say the least. This may be illustrated by noticing that in medicine there is a high level of ascription and achievement at the same time, as indicated by high levels of self-recruitment in the profession.

In fact Parsons' pattern-variable scheme is a thinly-disguised ethical theory which rests on the social, political and economic doctrines of nineteenth-century liberalism. Parsons is in no way being cynical about professional men when he says that they are not different from business men; rather he is arguing that the growth of managerial roles in business will lead to their professionalisation and that the moral imperatives of business and the old professions will converge. This has elsewhere been embraced in the concept of the managerial revolution but could also be called the professional revolution (Burnham 1945:73). Parsons finds plenty to admire in the ethical imperatives which he attributes to these groups, whom he sees at the vanguard of progress. For him they incorporate the values on the right-hand side of his pattern-variable scheme, namely they are directed towards achievement, they are effectively neutral; and their work is functionally specific, moreover their values are regarded as universalistic rather than particularistic. These are quintessentially the professional values and indeed are, in Parsons' terms, the very embodiment of 'rationality'.

In truth the difference between Parsons and other writers of this period on the professions is more apparent than real, because the question of the altruism of the professional seems in the end not to be an issue between them. What is shared between Parsons and these writers, namely the doctrines of liberalism, are of overriding importance, the resultant debate therefore continues in the sphere of ideology. The fact that the men who write about the professions are usually professionals has meant that they have a tendency to project the justificatory ideology of professional men and their organisations. There was little conscious attempt by the professional to distance himself from professional institutions and undertake a cool appraisal as he would of, say, the House of Lords or trade unions. Only in the 1970s is such a development gaining momentum.

Carr-Saunders and Wilson turn out, on close reading, to have anticipated Parsons.

> 'We may therefore suppose that, under a system of large scale commercial and industrial organisation, all those who occupy the important positions will gradually come within professional associations, or at least under professional influences . . . what is relevant to our discussion is that the incompatibility of profit-making with professionalism is ceasing to be an obstacle in the way of the spreading of professionalism throughout the world of business ' (Carr-Saunders and Wilson 1933:493).

In fact the disappearance of the old-style entrepreneur and the coming of the new-style manager who has 'little personal concern with profit' and, who in addition has a specialised technique, anticipates Burnham's thesis of 1941 (Burnham 1945). Again the similarity between Parsons (1954:34-50) and the co-authors just quoted above is quite striking.

'If evolution goes this way, what changes in the structure and functioning of society may be expected to follow? . . . Opportunities for specialised training are being gradually extended to all, and we may therefore look forward to a system of careers open to trained and tested talent. This should be a factor making for social stability since it tends to reduce social injustice . . . [and] should lead to greater efficiency. More important than this would be the effect upon the world of business where the drive to see the professional technique fully and effectively used would provide a non-self-regarding motive' (Carr-Saunders and Wilson 1933:494).

Rather than disagreeing with each other Parsons and Carr-Saunders and Wilson are taking issue with the doctrine of egoism in classical utilitarian theory. Parsons argues that professionals, such as doctors and business men, are both constrained by a set of norms which preclude them from taking

'the immediate financial advantage to be derived from a particular transaction. Orientation is rather to a total comprehensive situation extending over a considerable period of time . . . the difference may lie rather in the "definition of the situation" than in the typical motives of the actors as such' (Parsons 1954:43). Again 'the conflict is not generally a simple one between the actor's self-interest and his altruistic regard for others or for ideals, but between different components of the normally unified goal of "success" each of which contains both interested and disinterested motivation elements [thus] the typical motivation of professional men is not in the usual sense "altruistic", nor is that of businessmen typically "egoistic" ' (1954:45).

Parsons argues that there is little basis for postulating any important difference of motivation between the two, but rather that differences exist, at the level of institutional patterns. Carr-Saunders and Wilson argue similarly that the professions with their character of free-vocational associations 'moulded by the responsibility of preserving, developing, and applying an elaborate technique' are devoted by virtue of their moral qualities to the public good. Clearly they see professional institutions as having the qualities necessary to resolve the conflict in utilitarian thought between self-interest and public interest. This is not the case where trade unions are concerned which Carr-Saunders and Wilson characterise as self-regarding (Carr-Saunders and Wilson 1933:493). It becomes evident that both Parsons and Carr-Saunders and Wilson regard the professions as a means of reducing conflict. For Parsons they have a 'tension management' function and for Carr-Saunders and Wilson they are a fortification against anarchy. Professionalisation of elite positions and as a means of reducing conflict. For Parsons they have a 'tension management' function and for Carr-Saunders and Wilson they are a fortification against anarchy. Professionalisation of elite positions and of middle positions in the hierarchy of industrial society, especially business commerce and government, will, they believe, save our society from destruction.

The work of Parsons and his school focussed attention on the function of the professions for the maintenance of balance or equilibrium in the social system. Although sharing many similarities with the American micro-sociological tradition of occupational sociology, Parsons' analysis still relates professions, as Ben-David points out, to the total social structure even though not by means of a theory of social classes. He reports that there has been 'a growing divorce between sociology and the broad spectrum of problems which arose in connection with the phenomenal growth of professions and professionalism in present day societies' (Ben-David 1963-4:253). Parsons' analysis of the doctor-patient relationship is focussed wholly at the micro-sociological level. It is defined in terms of concepts such as 'functional specificity' and 'affective-neutrality' which are far from 'value-free' as he seems to assume. The professional-client relationship is explored within a framework which leaves it isolated from the wider pressures of class, organisational context and other relevant factors. Generally speaking, Parsons and other functionalist writers are neglectful of the richness of historical evidence and are thus apt to assume too much. We, for our part, have consciously turned to historical material which we feel strengthens our own sociological approach.

T.H. Marshall thought, rather like Carr-Saunders, that the professions were a new class with new interests. He believed that unlike other and earlier social classes the professions were uniquely concerned with 'social efficiency' and in this sense could be said to transcend partisan interest and might therefore be a class to find 'for the sick and suffering democracies a peaceful solution of their problems' (Marshall 1939:170). Karl Mannheim argued similarly that the intelligentsia were a free-floating, disinterested class. (He defined the group roughly in terms of those who had received a university education.) Within this class were the professionals and the whole formed a distinctive stratum in society with a special role (Mannheim 1936:137-43). Mannheim's claim was that, because of their education, they were able to free themselves from specific class ideologies and therefore were in a position to mediate in the peaceful settlement of class conflict. This conception is in many respects similar to that suggested by Carr-Saunders and Wilson and by Marshall although the line of reasoning by which it was reached is different. Geiger (1949) was highly critical of Mannheim's thesis. He offered evidence to suggest that the class of intellectuals or professionals were by no means detached from a committed ideological position in class society and consequently the existence of distinct class interests could be discerned.

Ben-David makes the important point that subsequent to the debate between Mannheim and Geiger 'only occasional reverberations of the question whether professional people did or did not constitute a sociologically distinct class can be found in recent sociological literature' Post-war writers of both the left and right, politically speaking, like C. Wright Mills and Lewis and Maude, tend to be more concerned with another problem, namely that 'professional people and intellectuals are getting absorbed and assimilated into the bureau-cratic context of white-collar work. This they fear might endanger the values of intellectual independence and moral responsibility which professionals and intellectuals have traditionally represented' (Ben-David 1963-4: 249). Ben-David highlighted the change of direction when he observed that 'the class nature of the professions has become a peripheral issue in sociology'. He also stated his convic-tion that the 'analysis of the professions in terms of class theories thus seemed to have led to a dead end' (1963-4:250). Our thesis starts boldly with a rejection of this standpoint and our book, we hope, marks a new departure from an old theoretical perspective.

In the important articles written by Ben-David himself he tells us that it is not his intention to draw up a list of professions or to define the term but rather to explore the 'various points of view from which the so-called professions have been studied, with a view to identifying the phenomena and problems associated with them'. There are in existence many histories and descriptions of particular professions, Ben-David tells us, most especially of the well-established ones such as medicine and law, but until the 1930s there were few studies written by sociologists or from a sociological perspective. It is true that Max Weber's writings 'about types of legal functionaries, his essays on science and politics as professions' as well as some other studies are exceptions to the rule, but they are few. Although the professions as a group of occupations were not the object of systematic sociological study their growth had 'aroused some sociological and quasi-sociological speculations much earlier. The middle classes in general, and the white-collar workers and the professions in particular, did not fit any of the then prevailing conceptions of social class.' According to class theory,

'classes were groups with economic interests clearly defined by the property relations or calculable economic life chances in a capitalist society. Employers and manual workers fitted easily into these categories, and the older middle classes could be explained away as vanishing remnants of the society of estates. But the growing number of white-collar workers and professionals neither fitted the definitions nor could be dismissed as a passing phenomenon. Professional people, writers and artists were, from the point of view of the prevailing class theories, particularly disturbing phenomena, since their relationship to the industrial order was even less clearly defined than that of the other white-collar groups.

In empirical studies of the class structure the problem was partially glossed over by lumping together professionals with other white-collar workers in a residual category of "new" middle classes. This was of little help for the theoretically minded and, indeed, there was little connection between theorizing about the meaning and consequences of the growth of the new white-collar groups and empirical descriptions of the changing class sytem as a whole' (Ben-David 1963-4:247-8).

An important theme in the pre-war sociological literature on the professions deals with the question of 'overcrowding'. It was asserted that in many cases overcrowding was due to political and social causes, such as the striving of the emancipated lower middle classes, women, or of previously subject peoples to catch up with the others. There arose, therefore, disequilibrium due to institutional causes. There were education systems geared to status and equivalent political arrangements representing the values of a society of 'estate trained' intellectuals who were unprepared for the occupational roles of developing modern economies. Ben-David noted that this perspective had not been adopted in more recent work and intended his own study to approach the problem from this point of view. He felt that there was ample justification for taking up once again the question of the place of the professions in the class structure. Surprisingly he addressed himself however, not to the effect of professionalism on class structure as such but rather to a comparative analysis of the growth of the professions in different countries. His endeavour was directed to providing an explanation of the nature and extent of any differences discovered. Professionalism 'is thus treated first as a dependent rather than an independent variable' (Ben-David 1963-4:255). The

'impression is that entry into the professions and elites during the recent past has been shaped by two opposite forces. On the one hand there has been everywhere a deliberate tendency to abolish class privileges which had previously restricted the entry into these positions. But on the other hand, the effect of these has been limited by the equally growing emphasis on the need for higher educational qualification for entry . . . The trend of the professionalization of the elites, in general, at least to the extend that higher education becomes increasingly a necessary qualification for obtaining such positions in practically any field constitutes therefore one of the most important barriers to social mobility today.

'This may sound like a paradox, since the substitution of educational qualification for title and money is usually regarded as the most important means of ensuring equality and social justice. It has indeed ensured equality of opportunity for the middle classes, but not, or not yet, for the lower ones' (1963-4:283-4).

Ben-David concludes his survey of the growth of the professions in different countries by saying that 'the participation of various classes in this growth explains the discontinuity in the sociological study of professions' which he had observed earlier. The macro-sociological approach of the pre-war years had sought to establish the place of the professions in class systems viewed in Marxian or Weberian terms. Defining classes as essentially economic interest groups, the writers of this period

'assumed that there is a political ideology and strategy universally characteristic of each such group. The question as they posed it was, therefore, what was the peculiar interest, and the ideology and strategy following from it, characteristic of the professions, and how, furthermore, would the emergence of this new group affect the class system, until then conceived as composed of capitalists, workers and peasants' (Ben-David 1963-4:296).

Ben-David goes on to say that

'clearly there is nothing in this model which explains or even helps to order the facts here explored. The model which is relevant to these data is one little used by sociologists, that of Schumpeter [Schumpeter 1951:133-221]. According to him the key to an understanding of the state of society is mobility. Or more specifically, 1) the study of emerging new social functions enabling people to occupy important positions in society through exploiting previously unnoticed opportunities, rather than by deposing the incumbents of existing positions; and 2) the recruitment of the people entering into the new positions. The existing classes of society consisting of relatively stable people adhering to established interest cum status groups — whether situated on the top, the bottom, or the middle of the status hierarchy — only serve as a background to the process of mobility. It is not their interests and conflicts which propel social change. They can obstruct mobility and hold up change, but change itself occurs through the discovery of new functions, and the mobility of people to and through the new roles reflecting these functions' (1963-4:296).

Ben-David believes that in the light of Schumpeter's theory

'the place of the professions in the social stratification of modern societies becomes easily discernible. They are a group of newly-created roles, carrying out novel and most rapidly expanding social functions, thus providing new opportunities for social advancement and self-fulfilment in work. As a result they have become the ideal occupational goal for youth, and the most highly valued group of occupations in scales of occupational prestige. They have taken in these respects the place of the self-made entrepreneur, which in its turn has replaced the nobleman-landlord and the knight as the occupational ideal of Western societies' (Ben-David 1963-4:296-7).

Adopting this point of view Ben-David directs his attention, not to the professions as such, unless defined in the loosest possible terms, (in fact he uses the very general definition contained in the Concise Oxford Dictionary), but rather to the whole group who go through some form of university or similar higher education. Having analysed this stratum in a number of countries and made a comparison of the findings, his concluding article is then devoted to a consideration of the evidence about social mobility drawing on available empirical research. In this way he was drawn into the perspective of those concerned with the measurement of individual social mobility, which we examined in Chapter 1, and we find that although he appears to be aware of the likely importance of collective social mobility in general, and professionalism in particular, his perspective and method of approach leads him to neglect an analysis of these important phenomena. He is overwhelmed by the dominant sociological assumptions of the day. This outcome is perhaps made almost inevitable by his rejection of the class theories of an earlier tradition and his reliance on the strictly empiricist concepts of class contained in the social mobility studies. Although his endeavour was directed to the study of the professions in the class systems of present day societies, his lack of an adequate theoretical framework to cope with professionalism in relation to class leaves him in the end with little to say on this the central question which his title poses.

In the 1960s, after Ben-David had published his study of the professions, (apart from the continuing dominance of the micro-sociological approach) there was a tendency to focus on professional ideology. We have already noted the contribution of Halmos on the ideology of the personal service professions 'whose principal function is to bring about changes in the body or personality of the client' (Halmos 1970:22).

The work of Prandy marked a return to class theory and linked it with a study of ideology which he says

> was too much concerned with the overall historical view to pay sufficient attention to what he thought of as the transient peculiarities of the class structure in capitalist society. The major omission was a consideration of the middle class, a weakness upon which most critics have laid great stress. Marx was not unaware of the existence of the middle class; in one work indeed he makes the criticism of Ricardo that "what [he] forgets to mention is the continual increase in numbers of the middle classes", who "rest with all their weight upon the working class and at the same time increase the social security and power of

the upper class" ' (Prandy 1965:32).
On the other hand he often seems to be predicting the decline of the middle class, for example, in his statement that the lower stratum of the middle class sinks gradually into the proletariat. Prandy suggests that perhaps the real reason why Marx was not particularly interested in the middle class is

> 'that it has no place in his theory of social change, to which his theory of social class is so closely bound. For the course of history only two classes are of any importance. Nevertheless, this omission weakens the utility of the theory for explaining the behaviour of middle class groups, such as technologists in modern society.'

Prandy notes that for Marx

> 'class relationships are inherently ones of conflict, for the interests of the two groups (capital and labour) are opposed and incompatible. Such a relationship is therefore qualitatively different from other differences between groups, which arise from the division of labour' (1965:33).

Prandy believes that it is too restrictive to interpret Marx's theory as explaining merely revolutionary types of social change.

> 'It seems much more useful to accept that class conflict may be more or less acute, and may even in some cases become institutionalised. . . . In view of the social changes which have taken place since Marx's time it is necessary to question his emphasis on the ownership of property or rather capital, as the basis for social class under capitalism. Again there is no need to deny the partial truth of Marx's theory, but to accept that it is only partial. The ownership of capital may be one of the bases of social class, but as Dahrendorf has shown, there are many good reasons for treating this as one example of a more general class situation' (1965:33-4).

The other dimension of stratification arises from status and as Lockwood points out the concept of false class consciousness is valueless in explaining why certain groups do not behave in accordance with their apparent class interest. Status situation is determined by the specific, positive or negative social estimation of honour, and may be understood in terms of particular styles of life rooted in patterns of consumption. In fact this is an admitted over-simplification since not merely consumption of goods but things like family background and occupation affect status. But Weber thought it was necessary to use both concepts, that is class and status because, as he put it, 'class distinctions are linked in the most varied ways with status distinctions. Property, as such, is not always recognised as a status qualification, but in the long run it is and with extraordinary regularity' (Gerth and Mills 1948;187). It is paradoxical, Prandy notes, that it is Marx, who seemed to be unaware of the idea of status, who can best provide a solution to this problem. He rejected any theory which gave ideas an independent existence, since, as he believed, the social being of man determined his consciousness. Each class, in fact, creates its own ideology but not all ideologies are equally accepted in society because the power of the ruling class to impose its own ideology is of pivotal importance to the Marxian argument. Whether or not one agrees that economic power is the only source of social power, one must nevertheless accept that it is an important source of power in society.

> 'That stratification by both class and status is found in modern society [Prandy thinks] cannot be doubted. Unfortunately, sociologists have tended to emphasise only one or the other, often trying to prove that only one of them is real and that the other is a sociological imposition on the facts. As Lipset and Bendix have said "discussions of different theories of class are often academic substitutes for a real conflict over political orientations" ' (Prandy 1965:37).

Turning to the question of class consciousness Prandy makes his position clear when he says

> 'class consciousness can be seen as, in fact, a consciousness of the class system, and as leading to behaviour which is associated with [a class] view of society. Lack of class consciousness means not that it is "false", but that it does not exist at all. There is no identification with the wrong class, but a rejection of a class view of society in favour of a status view. It may be objected that the former is more real than the latter, being based in objective fact rather than in mere subjective judgements, but such objections subordinate sociology to philosophy or politics. This is a good example of a situation in which what men define as real is real in its consequences' (1965:38).

Prandy's view is that class and status are in reality two separate ideologies and he proposes that the study of a middle class occupational group, such as professional employees, provides an excellent case for testing the hypothesis.

> 'Since they are not situated at either extreme of the class-status continuum, they are most likely to hold views and exhibit behaviour which are a mixture of the class and status types. Being in the middle they are the most obviously subject to pressures from both directions.'

For this purpose it is most useful to look at the organisational associations representing this middle group and to see to what extent there is a difference between those with a trade union and those with a professional orientation. As he puts it 'we must discuss the ways . . . trade unionism and professionalism are related to the concepts of power, class and status respectively' (Prandy 1965:42). Prandy argues that professionalism is a specific sub-type of status ideology. Status ideology can of course exist independently of professionalism but 'the professional association is important as a concrete expression of this ideology among certain groups'. In general, Prandy's aim was

> 'to show how the differing employment situations in which
> scientists and engineers are placed influences their attitudes and
> behaviour in the direction of a class or a status ideology,
> represented on the one hand by trade unions and on the other by
> professional associations.'

Under modern conditions, he asks how far does there exist 'a confusion of ideologies [of] status elements in trade unions and class elements in professional associations' (1965:47).

Apart from Prandy's work, the study of professionalism and social class continued to be neglected in the 1960s. During the early 1970s a change of orientation in the sociological studies of the professions was evident. Several articles contained in Jackson (1970), especially Turner and Hodge on 'Occupations and Professions', Leggatt on 'Teaching as a Profession' bear witness to this. Turner and Hodge suggest as a future task 'the analysis of occupations rather than upon professions or professionalizing occupations alone'. They also insist that the focus of study should be the

> 'analysis of the changing degree of control exercised over these
> [occupational] activities by various parties and of the relation of
> these parties to one another [which] can provide a significant
> contribution to understanding the way in which occupations
> crystallize, continue to operate, and change. It is necessary to
> relate occupational activities to the wider social structure before
> they can be meaningfully interpreted' (Turner and Hodge
> 1970:49).

They then go on to stress the importance of the division of labour in understanding these processes. They do not, however, explicitly deal with the relationship between professionalism and social class, though they touch upon the 'regulation of working and market conditions' (1970:40). On the other hand they stress the significance of occupational control, particularly citing the case of medical practition practitioners. This becomes an important concept in the debate from about 1970 onwards as we shall see (Freidson 1970).

Johnson's theoretical perspective in common with many other studies of the professions starts from a Durkheimian concern with the social division of labour (Durkheim 1964) and following Turner and Hodge he develops a typology of occupational control. He tells us that

> 'in all differentiated societies, the emergence of specialised
> occupational skills, whether productive of goods or services,
> creates relationships of *social and economic dependence* and,
> paradoxically, relationships of *social distance*. Dependence upon
> the skills of others has the effect of reducing the common area of
> shared experience and knowledge and increases social distance;
> for the inescapable consequence of specialisation in the
> production of goods and services is unspecialisation in
> consumption. This consequence flows from the crystallisation

and development of all specialised occupations. While
specialisation creates systematic relationships of interdependence,
it also introduces potentialities for autonomy. It is social distance
as a product of the division of labour which creates this
potentiality for autonomy, but is not to be identified with it'
(Johnson 1972:41).
Social distance creates uncertainty (indeterminacy) and power relationships resolve this in favour of one or other party.
Johnson thinks that because the level of indeterminacy is variable it has
important consequences for the extent to which occupations can
become autonomous. Occupational autonomy will depend, in particular,
upon the 'resources' available to one occupation compared with
another which will be useful in imposing its own definition of the producer-
consumer relationship. Success will depend on the extent of access by
an occupational group to 'wider bases of social power'. In Johnson's
view an important factor 'producing variations in the degree of
uncertainty and, therefore, the potentialities for autonomy is the
esoteric character of the knowledge applied by the specialist'. He
recognises that social distance 'does not . . . automatically increase . . .
with the increase of specialisation' and specialist knowledge. For
example the professional may deliberately use the process of
'mystification' in order to increase social distance and thus his own
autonomy and control over practice. 'Uncertainty is not, therefore,
entirely cognitive in origin but may be deliberately increased to serve
manipulative or managerial ends' (1972:42). Johnson's assertion

> 'that an occupational group rarely enjoys the resources of power
> which would enable it to impose its own definition of the
> producer-consumer relationship suggests that *professionalism*
> as defined in the literature is a peculiar phenomenon. It is only
> where an occupational group shares, by virtue of its membership
> of a dominant class or caste, wider resources of power that such
> an imposition is likely to be successfully achieved, and then only
> where the actual consumers or clients provide a relatively large,
> heterogeneous, fragmented source of demand. A polar opposite
> of this situation is where there is a single consumer — a patron
> who has the power to define his own needs and the manner in
> which he expects these to be catered for. In order to determine
> the variations which are possible in forms of institutionalised
> control of occupational activities . . . it is necessary to take
> account of the wider resources of power which are available to an
> occupational group and also to focus upon the producer-consumer
> relationship in so far as this is affected by the social composition
> and character of the source of demand' (Johnson 1972:43).

In addition Johnson suggests that another factor is important:

> 'occupational activities vary in the degree to which they give rise
> to a structure of uncertainty and in their potentialities for
> autonomy. It is this factor which provides an explanation of why
> it is that some occupations rather than others achieve self-

regulation and even why they draw recruits from groups who already command alternative resources of power. Certain occupations are associated with particular acute problems of uncertainty, where client or consumer judgement is particularly ineffective and the seeking of skilled help necessarily invites the intrusion of others into intimate and vulnerable areas of the consumer's self- or group-identity. Medical practice, for example, intrudes into areas of social taboo relating to personal privacy and bodily functions, as well as areas of culturally defined ritual significance such as birth and death' (Johnson 1972:43).

Johnson goes on to suggest that 'historically, various social mechanisms have arisen to "manage" these areas of social tension which present problems of social control'. He cites a form of traditional control through blood relationship and contrasts this with the use of 'contract' in the free market of modern times. For Johnson professionalism must therefore be seen as one form of institutional control in the occupational context which is associated with 'changing power relations'.

'Professionalism, then, becomes redefined as a peculiar type of occupational control rather than an expression of the inherent nature of particular occupations. A profession is not, then, an occupation, but a means of controlling an occupation. Likewise, professionalisation is a historically specific process which some occupations have undergone at a particular time, rather than a process which certain occupations may always be expected to undergo because of their "essential" qualities' (1972:45).

With these considerations in mind Johnson then proposes a typology of institutionalised orders of occupational control which 'in a more developed form, apply to all occupations, [but] for the purpose of the present argument the discussion will be restricted to those occupations conventionally regarded as professions'. In drawing up a typology, Johnson says 'it has been found useful to focus on the core of uncertainty – the producer-consumer relationship. There are three broad resolutions of the tension existing in the producer-consumer relationship which are historically identifiable.' Johnson's first type he calls collegiate control which 'is exemplified by the emergence of autonomous occupational associations' based on a situation in which the 'producer defines the needs of the consumer and the manner in which these needs are catered for'. Johnson discerns 'identifiable sub-types of collegiate control namely professionalism and guild control'. Professionalism he sees as a 'product of social conditions present in nineteenth-century Britain and guild control [as] one of the phenomena associated with urbanisation in late mediaeval Europe' (Johnson 1972:45-6).

A second resolution of the uncertainty inherent in the relationship between consumer and producer is the one in which the consumer 'defines his own needs and the manner in which they are to be met'.

This type includes both oligarchy and corporate forms of patronage as well as types of communal control. The third type of relationship, postulated by Johnson, he calls the 'mediative type'. One form of this is capitalism

> 'in which the capitalist entrepreneur intervenes in the direct relationship between the producer and consumer in order to rationalise production and regulate markets. No less significant, however, is *state mediation* in which a powerful centralised state intervenes in the relationship between producer and consumer, initially to define what the needs are, as with the growth in Britain of state welfare policies' (1972:46).

Johnson takes account of the way in which types of institutional control of occupations will be determined by prior historical developments of the occupation in question 'for example, an occupation which emerged in nineteenth-century Britain may bring with it into the twentieth century many of the symbols and organisational characteristics of *professionalism* even though *professionalism* may be in decline and new institutional forms of control emerging' (1972:47).

The main advantage of Johnson's approach is that it brings to the fore the question of power. Although, like other students of the professions, he starts from the division of labour he rejects any conception of an automatically unfolding process of specialisation dividing types of work on wholly 'rational' principles. He urges that power and control are of great importance in the actual structure of professional occupations, most especially in the relationship between producer and consumer. On the other hand, in our opinion, he rather overplays the importance of the producer-consumer relationship as the fundamental dimension of professionalism (Parry 1973:30). The central contribution of his book is the typology of consumer-producer relationships and this leads him rather to neglect what we regard as fundamental to professionalism, namely the relationship between colleagues expressed in 'colleges' and professional associations which, via the use of distinctive methods, enable control over the supply of professional services to the market. Control over clients has, in our view, been historically less important. Some occupations which are *not* strongly organised as professions nevertheless have elaborate forms of collective control over clients (including some measure of legal control). If we take the case of medicine, neither the Royal Colleges, nor the British Medical Association nor even the General Medical Council have been primarily interested in the professional-client relationship (1973:31). They have, however, been very much concerned about the relationship between the medical profession and rival occupations which they have set out to control. It appears that the intention has often been to drive them from the market for medical services or subordinate them to the medical profession in a defined and regulated way. The medical profession in England and America has sought autonomy and dominance in a field which it has itself largely determined. Thus Johnson is, in our view, under a misconception with regard to his notion of 'collegiate control'. The college has always been a group of peers organised to pursue some collective end. It was certainly *not* primarily concerned to control clients.

Equally, Johnson's attempt to define capitalism as mediation by the entrepreneur-capitalist between the producer and consumer has only limited value. It is true that in the case of colonialism, in which he has a special interest, the commercial capitalist buys goods in one market and sells in another, and in that sense can be said to mediate between the producer in one location and the consumer elsewhere. On the other hand, especially in the early days of capitalism, the producer and industrial capitalist-entrepreneur were usually one and the same person. Under these circumstances the capitalist is not a mediator in Johnson's sense. Neither can the large modern company which both produces and markets its own goods be said to play the role of mediator between producer and consumer, though some specialist finance houses do nothing else. In the context of capitalism, we feel, Johnson places too much reliance on his concept of mediation.

Johnson proposes another application of the concept; namely, the state as mediator between producer and consumer. Certainly the state does play this role to a growing extent in the realm of consumer affairs or in price control policies. We are doubtful, however, whether the concept of mediation is so very useful in the case of the welfare state which he explicitly cites. In the context of the National Health Service the state has not been especially concerned with the client's own definition of his needs, but rather has had a marked tendency to accept the definition of the needs of the client articulated by the profession (Parry 1973:32).

We suspect that Johnson's definition of occupational sociology, especially of professionalism, in terms of the producer-consumer relationship is too much influenced by a conception arising in economic theory, and for this reason is too limiting to be an adequate sociological model. Likewise, the notion of the state as 'mediator' arises from the political philosophy of nineteenth-century economic liberalism and is reminiscent of the view of the state as 'ringmaster', balancing competing interests. However, the chief limitation of Johnson's book, from our point of view, is that he fails to relate his conception of occupational control to a theory of social class.

Notes

1. The four functional problems are: goal attainment, adaptation, integration and latency.
2. We are grateful to Dr Maurice North for drawing our attention to this difference.

3. PROFESSIONALISM AND SOCIAL CLASS – II

Johnson's theoretical position which was among those we examined in the last chapter is closer to ours than most others and has some affinities with an earlier article by the senior author in which it was suggested that 'we should broaden the scope of our attention to include all classes of occupational groups' (Parry 1963:15). It was noted that 'if men in different occupational groups have in view the same general end, namely security at work, why is it that the methods they employ seem to differ from one occupation to another?' An answer was sought by looking at the available means of influence which

> 'differ systematically from one occupational group to another and this depends in turn upon whether the group in question owns property and employs others, is itself employed or is an independent and largely self-employed group. Thus trade unions, professional associations or businessmen's associations use different modes of influence to control their work situations and markets' (1963:15-6).

In the same article it was suggested

> 'that with the growth in size and complexity of our market economy, and the consequent development of old occupations and the birth of new ones, we can observe a widespread aim to control the work situation. Businessmen or doctors, as well as skilled manual trade unions have tried to rig the market to make it more secure for themselves. The control of peers in one's occupation, or of the boss in the case of employees . . . have been brought about by different methods of influence.'

In the case of doctors, it was noted that

> 'standards of education and legislation were employed to control entry and that the organisation of the buyers of medical care forced doctors to attempt control of their work situation which they have achieved successfully. The study of the methods of influence employed by different occupational groups, the reasons for their use, and the consequences, offer [the possibility of] an explanation of the success of some groups in attaining control of the work situation and the relative failure of others' (Parry 1963:19).

The piece we have just quoted was short but it was perhaps the first harbinger of the later studies, such as those of Prandy, Johnson and Freidson among others who have sought to redirect the sociological study of the professions away from the micro-sociological approach and back toward the macro-structural level. The article also suggested the possibility that class theory might be useful in the explanation of the significance of the professions in the social structure. In that sense it is at variance with Ben-David's notion that class theory leads to a dead end when used as a framework for the study of the professions. On the contrary, in this respect the article has an affinity with Prandy's work (1965) in which were utilised the concepts of class and status drawn from class theory. Whereas Prandy polarised the concepts of class and status and raised the level of debate to one concerned with contrasting ideologies, the analysis in the article (Parry 1963) was founded on the idea that status could be raised through collective control of the work situation and thus of the market. We believe that the distinction between class and status introduced by Weber was intended to relate the 'status position' of each group to its basic 'class position'. For us a justifying ideology, whether it is in Prandy's terms a 'class' or 'status' one, can only be understood by referring first to the structural situation of an occupational group (or set of such occupations sharing a common class position) to see what the possibilities of that situation are and the strategies and tactics which are used by the groups in any attempt to control their situation. In Prandy's work, it seems to us, there is a gap where the analysis of class structure should be. What we are offered, essentially, is a study only of ideology.

Freidson, like Johnson and other writers, starts his important contribution with a consideration of the concept of the division of labour. Dealing specifically with the 'dominance' of the medical profession among the occupations inhabiting the field of medical care he says 'I shall use the concept of division of labor in a way that is not conventional in sociology'. He suggests that it should be treated 'as a social organization of interrelated occupational groups that divides among them in an orderly way a complex of work activities'. The division of labour is thus conceived 'as an organized social structure'. Freidson proceeds by dramatising 'the structural characteristics of the health-related division of labor (comparing it) with those of formally constituted bureaucratic organizations'. He believes that

> 'in much of modern life the organizing principle of bureaucracy is such an important source of social order that it is thought to lead to client and worker dissatisfaction, the division of labor around health services, organized by the principle of professional dominance, provides an order similar to that of bureaucracy and seems to be as responsible for the pathologies of the system as is bureaucracy' (Freidson 1970:128-9).

Freidson reaffirms that the

> 'principle of bureaucracy — orderly, systematic administrative procedures designed to ensure that work is done efficiently, honestly and fairly, is one of the chief organizing principles of modern society. In contrast to "bureaucracy" we have the word "profession". This word is almost always positive in its connotation, [unlike bureaucracy] and is frequently used to

46

represent a superior alternative [to it]. Unlike "bureaucracy" which is disclaimed by every organization concerned with its public relations, [the title] "profession" is claimed by virtually every occupation seeking to improve its public image. When the two terms are brought together, the discussion is almost always at the expense of bureaucracy and to the advantage of profession' (1970:129-30).

Freidson notes that in the litereature over the years there has been a marked emphasis on the differences between the two. We have already seen that Parsons was aware that Max Weber in his treatment of rational-legal bureaucracy failed to distinguish between the authority of administrative office and that arising from expertise (Parsons 1964:58-60). Gouldner, following Parsons, suggested that bureaucratic rules may be less effective in ordering work in organisational contexts than rules based on expertise (Gouldner 1964). A number of other writers taking up these suggestions have stressed that 'expertise and professions' are taken together and 'equated by virtually all writers, with a flexible, creative, and equalitarian way of organizing work, while bureaucracy is associated with rigidity and mechanical and authoritarian ways' (Freidson 1970:130).

There are two problems which Freidson discerns and which are overlooked by this approach. Firstly, it is wrongly 'assumed that technical expertise unlike "arbitrary" administrative authority is in some way neutrally functional' and therefore provides a basis for authority which automatically produces co-operation and obedience as well as the efficient attainment of goals. Freidson's general argument is

> 'that the authority of expertise is in fact problematic, requiring in its pure functional form the time-consuming and not always successful effort of persuading others that its "orders" are appropriate. As a special kind of occupation, professions have attempted to solve the problem of persuasion by obtaining institutional powers and prerogatives that at the very least set limits on the freedom of their prospective clients and that on occasion even coerce their clients into compliance. The expertise of the professional is institutionalized into something similar to bureaucratic office' (1970:130-1).

Secondly, Freidson suggests

> 'that the division of labor is a social organization distinct from any external or artificial authority imposed on it by administrators. The social organization is constituted by the relations that occupations within a division of labor have to one another. Such relations are not only determined by the functional interdependence of those relations but also by the formal social relationships of the occupations themselves. The social organization of the division of labor is especially distinctive, when

occupations with a special professional status are involved.
Indeed, a division of labor ordered by professionals rather than
by administrative authority contains within it mechanisms and
consequences similar to those described as the pathologies of
bureaucracy' (Freidson 1970:132).

Following this line of argument Freidson notes that in the health field
'many of the rigid, mechanical, and authoritarian attributes, and much
of the inadequate coordination said to characterize the health services,
may stem more from their professional organization than from their
bureaucratic characteristics' (1970:132-3).

Like Johnson, Freidson is aware that much attention has been
focussed upon the question of 'what [is] the best definition of
"profession" '. He believes that as a result little attention has been paid
to 'the most critical of . . . underexamined elements . . . related to the
organization of practice and the division of labor'.

'Such elements are critical because they deal with facets of
professional occupations that are independent of individual
motivation or intention, and that may, as Carlin had suggested for
law, [Carlin 1966] minimize the importance to behaviour of the
personal qualities of intelligence, ethicality, and trained skill
imputed to professionals by most definitions' (1970:133).

The key to such institutional elements of professions, Freidson believes,
lies in the concept 'autonomy'. Autonomy means, 'the quality or state
of being independent, free, and self-directing'. In the case of professions,
autonomy apparently refers most of all to control over the content and
the terms of work. The professional is self-directing in his work.
Freidson's view is that from the notion of self-direction or autonomy
can be derived 'virtually all the other institutional elements that are
included in most definitions of professions' (Freidson 1970:134). An
occupational group which has obtained some legal or political position
of privilege which prevents encroachment by other occupations; which
can control the production and application of knowledge and skill in
the work it performs; and has an extended period of education
controlled by the profession itself in exclusively segregated professional
schools, as well as a code of ethics 'or some other publicly waved
banner of good intentions; (these) are elements of autonomy of the
professions'. As Freidson puts it 'most of the commonly cited attributes
of the professions may be seen either as consequences of their
autonomy or as conditions useful for persuading the public and the
body politic to grant such autonomy' (1970:135).

Turning to the question of autonomy and dominance in the division
of labour, Freidson tells us that in his view autonomy is not a simple
criterion for there are many occupations in which autonomy is derived
either from the esoteric nature of the craft — he cites cases such as
night club magicians or circus acrobats — or from the segregated nature
of the work, such as cab drivers or lighthouse keepers. This latter case

is an example of what he calls autonomy by default. In these cases there are 'no formal institutions in existence that serve to protect the occupation from competition, intervention, evaluation, and direction by others'. 'In short', he avers, 'organized autonomy is most stable and relevant to professions' (1970:136).

Freidson directs our attention to the fact that within the complex division of labour in the field of health care we find that only medicine itself, apart from dentistry, is truly autonomous. Only the members of the medical profession have

> 'the authority to direct and evaluate the work of others without in turn being subject to formal direction and evaluation by them. Paradoxically, its autonomy is sustained by the *dominance* of its expertise in the division of labor. It is true that some of the occupations it dominates – nursing for example – claim to be professions, as do other groups that lack either organized autonomy or dominance, such as schoolteachers or social workers. But surely there is a critically significant difference between dominant professions and those others who claim the name but do not possess the status. While the members of all may be committed to their work, may be dedicated to service, and may be specially educated, the dominant profession stands in an entirely different structural relationship to the division of labor than does the subordinate profession ... In essence, the difference reflects the existence of a *hierarchy of institutionalized expertise*' (Freidson 1970:136-7).

Freidson goes on to point out that the complex organisations such as hospitals which are criticised for de-humanising the experience of the patient or client are usually attributed with the faults of bureaucratic organisation. He argues that equally this may flow from the introduction of professional organisation and professional dominance in the division of labour. As he succinctly puts it 'in medical organizations, the source of a client's alienation is professional rather than bureaucratic authority' (1970:143).

Freidson defines professionalism in terms of 'three major sets of attitudes, values, or orientations: one set addressed to the professional ideals of knowledge and service, one to the professional occupation and the life-career it provides, and one to the character of professional work' (1970:152). He goes on to suggest that 'while members of *most* occupations seek to be free to control the level and direction of their work efforts, it is distinct to professionalism to assert that such freedom is a necessary condition for the proper performance of work'. In essence Freidson's argument is

> 'that the weaknesses to be found in professions are not mere flaws that can be corrected by recruiting better men, improving their training, and organizing their work more effectively. They cannot be eradicated by the profession itself. Those weaknesses

are consequences of the fact that men cannot be led to serve an occupation by becoming committed to its ideals alone. They must also become committed to a concrete career and to concrete, historically located institutions. And in the case of professionals they also develop a sense of pride based on a typical conception of the special nature of their work. All three things compose professionalism, and in their interaction they produce the characteristic weaknesses of the professions' (Freidson 1970:155).

Summing up his position Freidson says that he has chosen to use the term profession 'first . . . to refer to a way of *organizing* work rather than, as is common, to refer to an *orientation* toward work or a body of *knowledge*'. By that criterion we might distinguish

'between what are commonly (and . . . meaninglessly) called professions and those professions that are dominant, directing others in a division of labor and being themselves autonomous, subject to direction by no other. Medicine is one of those dominant professions. Expertise institutionalized into a profession is not, as much writing seems to assume, an automatically self-correcting, purely task-oriented substitute for "arbitrary" bureaucracy. Expertise establishes office and hierarchy analogous to that of bureaucracy. The definition of the work — that is, how the client should behave and what others should do — is a partial expression of the hierarchy created by the office and of the ideology stemming from the perspective of the office as well as of the purely technical character of the work itself' (1970:157-7).

Freidson says

'unlike the bureaucrat, who may on occasion attain autonomy *by default*, the professional has gained *organized autonomy* and is not bound by rules that stand outside his profession. His performance, however, can produce the same barriers to communication and co-operation within a functional division of labor, the same structures of evasion, and the same reduction of the client to an object which has been attributed to bureaucratic organization. In the name of health the client may be stripped of his civil status, a status which is as much if not more an element of his welfare than his health. But unlike bureaucratic practices, which in rational-legal orders are considered arbitrary and subject to appeal and modification, professional practices are imputed to have the unquestioned objectivity of expertise and scientific truth, and so are not routinely subject to higher review or changed by virtue of outside appeal. There is no generally accepted notion of due process for the layman — client or worker — in professional organization.'

The crux of the matter is that

'expertise is not mere knowledge. It is the practice of knowledge, organized socially and serving as the focus for the practitioner's commitment. In this sense, it is not merely mechanical skill which, like the cog of a machine, automatically fits itself into Durkheim's organic order. The worker does not see his work as merely different from another's He develops around it an ideology, with the best of intentions, an imperalism that stresses the technical superiority of his work and his capacity to perform it. This imperialistic ideology is built into the perspective that his training and practice create. It cannot be overcome by ethical dedication to the public interest because it is sincerely believed in as the only proper way to serve the public interest. And it hardens when an occupation develops the autonomy of a profession and a place of dominance in a division of labor and when expertise becomes an institutional status rather that a capacity' (Freidson 1970:159-60).
'The para-professional worker is, then, like the industrial worker, subordinated to the authority of others. He is not, however, subordinated solely to the authority of bureaucratic office, but also to the putatively superior knowledge and judgement of professional experts' (1970:144-5).

Freidson from our point of view offers a conception of the missing link between class theory and professionalism through his examination of the ways in which the division of labour can be influenced and manipulated by a powerfully organised occupation. Certain occupations achieve a dominant position in a particular field, or in society at large. Freidson himself does not make the connection with class theory and this is understandable as it is of little concern to his thesis. For us the formation of occupational associations and organisations concerned with the exercise of control over the market must be understood also to incorporate Freidson's thesis that such an occupation is normally dominant in a particular division of labour and by virtue of that distorts such a division from any conception of an 'ideal type' shaped by technological or economic imperatives alone. The powerful influence of dominant and well-organised occupations is, in our view, of great significance for class theory. We have argued in the last chapter that sociological research on the professions has generally failed to make the important connection between class theory and professionalism and in this sense the relevance of professionalism has not been understood by sociologists.

Anthony Giddens for example was able to write recently in an important book on the theory of class structure, that 'although there certainly are controversial problems of sociological analysis posed by the existence of the professions, professionalisation does not offer major difficulties for class theory' (Giddens 1973:186). He relies upon a reference to Johnson's work to substantiate his point. As we have seen

Johnson himself does not make the connection between professionalism and class theory. Giddens believes that other sources of differentiation within the middle class are much more important. For our part we feel that Giddens is rather dismissive of the significance of the professions and that this is related to his failure to notice that collective social mobility is itself a key phenomenon in the class structure of industrial society. His discussion of social mobility is conventional in the sense that it only treats individual mobility, measured either inter-generationally or intragenerationally. The importance which Giddens apparently places upon the phenomenon of 'closure' in the process of class structuration might well, in our view, have led him to take a greater interest in professionalism because certain professions provide good examples of closure. Attention to the professions could thus enhance Giddens' own theory of class formation and maintenance. The evidence presented in this book demonstrates, we believe, that professionalism is a method of closure which is of great significance in the understanding of English class structure: it is a crucial avenue of collective social mobility.

Although Giddens, we think neglects the implications of professionalism for class structure, there is no doubt that his contri-bution to the theory of class marks a notable advance. As he says

'when . . . I began a systematic analysis of the literature of fairly recent origin upon the theory of class structure, I was struck by its very sparseness – not in terms of its numerical strength, but in terms of its analytical penetration. Confusion and ambiguity in the use of the term "class" are abundantly evident; but distinctive and considered attempts to revise the *theory* of class upon a broad scale are few indeed' (Giddens 1973:10).

In outlining the characteristics of class, Giddens offers the following definition: 'a class is a large-scale aggregate of individuals comprised of impersonally defined relationships, and nominally "open" in form' (1973:100). In searching for a more positive delimitation of the concept, Giddens examines some of the confusing aspects contained in the literature. He notes that some approaches, such as that of Marx, assume that the number of classes in a given type of society are strictly limited whereas other approaches such as that of Weber, are open to the possibility that there are an indefinite multiplicity of 'market situations' or classes. The problem is reflected in the fact that in everyday speech we can habitually refer either to 'the working class or the working classes' and, similarly, to the 'middle class or classes'. Giddens makes the point that dichotomous models of the class structure, such as that offered by Marx, do not invariably involve a recognition of only a limited number of classes. Whether this is the case or not depends upon the criteria used as a basis for the model. Marx's conception of owner-ship and non-ownership of property is bound to produce a rather simple dichotomised picture of the class structure, but is made more complex by the recognition of the existence of 'transitional classes'. Weber's conception of market situation retains the criterion of ownership of the means of production as a basic element, but he adds also the factor of 'marketable' skill. In this way he is able to differentiate among the class positions of those who are propertyless. Giddens points to the same problem in Dahrendorf's dichotomous model of class which is based upon 'authority'. There are potentially an infinite number of class positions in this model also, essentially because of the possibility that authority can be very widely devolved. A major inadequacy of any model which envisages a dichotomous class structure is that it becomes 'conceptually difficult to recognise the existence of "middle" classes' (1973:101). This is so at least 'in the sense of a class intervening between two others in a single system of classes'. The new middle class in capitalist societies has thus always presented a problem to the Marxian theory. Giddens suggests that the abandonment of some dichotomous models of class have been put forward without giving up a conception of class conflict. It should be noted also that some dichotonomous models of class have been put forward without the idea of conflict being entailed. The most widely used alternative to that of Marx extant in the literature is a model of class based on Weber's conception. For Giddens, this alternative is unsatisfactory, not merely because Weber's ideas about class are not sufficiently worked out, but because he 'does not specify clearly how the potentially very large variety of differing class positions are to be reduced to a number of classes manageable enough for the explication of major components of social structure and processes of social change' (Giddens 1973:102; Parry 1973).

Both Marx and Weber, Giddens points out, share one underlying premise — which is that in a capitalist society *the market is intrinsically a structure of power*, in which the possession of certain attributes advantages some groupings of individuals relative to others' (1973:101-2). Although it is a power structure 'the market is *not a normatively defined system of authority* in which the distribution of power is, *as such,* sanctioned as legitimate'. Property rights, including the sale of labour power, are essential rights of the market system; 'which underpin the system of power, not in spite of, but because of the fact that they are specified in terms of freedom of economic exchange'. The market system operates on general rules, ultimately sanctioned by the state, which define processes of legitimate bargaining and the establishment of contractual ties. Only the general framework and boundaries are so defined, however, leaving wide areas of freedom for individuals participating in economic exchange. The market is composed of 'a system of economic relationships founded upon [the] relative bargaining strengths of different groupings of individuals' (1973:102).

The weakness of Weber's transformation of Marx's original conception of class is, according to Giddens, that it is not radical enough. In other words, Weber seeks through the concept of market situation to explore differences arising among Marx's undifferentiated property-less class. Dahrendorf proposed to invert the Marxian definition of property and subordinate it to what he regarded as the higher order concept authority. Weber was anxious to retain the economic basis of the class concept. Property is best characterised as any set of rights associated with the ownership of physical objects and should not be understood as flowing from any intrinsic characteristics of such objects. Giddens suggests that 'in the market . . . the significance of capital as private property is that it confers certain very definite capacities upon its possessor as compared with those who are "propertyless" – those who do not own their means of production' (Giddens 1973:102). But even the propertyless worker does possess some capacities which he brings to bear when he comes to sell his labour power in the market. Thus, although the bargain struck is an uneven one as between employer and labourer, the employer must make some minimal effort to meet the demands of the worker. The fact that the employer needs the employee is the basis for possible collective action in the withdrawal of labour. Property and labour power are both different forms of market capacity. Giddens defines market capacity as 'all forms of relevant attributes which individuals may bring to the bargaining encounter' (1973:103).

Marx focussed attention particularly upon capitalist society where property is held by a minority and where the vast majority of people are seeking employment in industrial production through the sale of their market capacity. Marx's expectation was that under the conditions of modern technology there would be a de-skilling of the workforce, as man was reduced to the level of servant to the machine. This was the basis for his view that the working class would become an increasingly homogeneous group and was also the reason why he failed to recognise the likely importance of those market capacities which do not arise directly from the ownership of property. Weber, by contrast, incorporated into his analysis the economists' concern with the scarcity value of the capacities individuals bring to the market. He recognised that manual skills and educational qualifications of all kinds are of great importance in shaping market capacity. Since his day, it has often been pointed out that differentiation in the capacities brought to bear on the market can achieve for their owners important economic and non-economic returns over and above income as such. Job security, career prospects and pension rights are examples of these. 'In the market structure of competitive capitalism, *all* those who participate in the exchange process are in a certain sense in conflict with one another for access to scarce returns' (Giddens 1973:104).

Having introduced the term market capacity, Giddens makes us aware that as in the case of Weber's 'market situation', there is a

54

tendency 'to imply the recognition of a cumbersome plurality of classes'. The sociological problem has always been to make the 'theoretical transition from such relationships and conflicts to the identification of classes as structured forms' (1973:104). The problem is shared by Marx and Weber. 'Marx was certainly conscious of the problematic character of the links between class as a latent set of characteristics generated by the capitalist system and class as a historical, dynamic entity, and "historical actor".' He draws the well-known contrast between 'class in itself' and 'class for itself'. The former refers to a set of economic relationships shared by a group in a common situation and the latter refers to their realisation or consciousness of that situation. The manner in which Marx makes the contrast is related very strongly to his desire to understand and promote a revolutionary form of class consciousness within capitalist society. Giddens states that in his view Marx 'gave only little attention to the modes in which classes, founded in a set of economic relationships, take on or "express" themselves in definite social forms' (Giddens 1973:104). Giddens concludes that the problem has been given scant attention by later writers within a general theory of class with perhaps only Dahrendorf excepted from this stricture. The central problems which Giddens articulates for us 'do not so much concern the nature and application of the class concept itself as what, for want of a better word, I shall call the *structuration* of class relationships'. Giddens goes on 'to focus upon the *modes in which* "economic" relationships become translated into non-economic structures' (1973:105). In order to make his position quite clear Giddens tells us what he does *not* mean by class. It is not a specific entity — a bounded social form; such as a business firm or a university. It has no legal standing or even publicly sanctioned identity. Although it is sometimes convenient to speak of classes as if they were acting, this is a verbal usage which is sometimes employed but should be avoided where possible. Neither must class be confused with stratum or class theory with the study of stratification. The latter deals with the ranking of individuals descriptively on a scale and may be decided upon very precisely for example by drawing a line at a particular income level. Giddens says 'the divisions between classes are *never* of this sort; nor, moreover, do they lend themselves to easy visualisation, in terms of any ordinal scale of "higher" and "lower", as strata do — although . . . this sort of imagery cannot be escaped altogether' (1973:106). Finally elite theory and class theory must never be confused. Elite theory was developed as a deliberate counterweight to class analysis by writers such as Pareto and Mosca and represented a repudiation of it.

Turning to the positive consideration of what Giddens calls the structuration of class relationships he distinguishes between the 'mediate' and the 'proximate' aspects of this. He defines the mediate factors as those 'which intervene between the existence of certain given market capacities and the formation of classes as identifiable social groupings, that is to say, which operate as "overall" connecting links between the market, on the one hand, and structured systems of class relationships on the other'. He goes on 'the mediate structuration of class relationships is governed above all by the distribution of mobility chances which pertain within a given society. Mobility has sometimes been treated as if it were in large part separable from the determination of class structure' (Giddens 1973:107). Schumpeter, as we have had occasion to note, uses the analogy of classes as vehicles in which various passengers may be conveyed without the vehicles in any way changing their shape. Similarly, we have seen that Sorokin used the analogy of a building with several floors and individuals passing within it while the building remains rigid. Giddens argues that such analogies, though at first sight compelling, do not withstand closer examination, especially when considered within the conceptual framework he is suggesting. Giddens makes the point that

> 'in general, the greater the degree of "closure" of mobility chances — both intergenerationally and within the career of the individual — the more this facilitates the formation of identifiable classes. For the effect of closure in terms of intergenerational movement is to provide for the *reproduction* of common life experiences over the generations; and this homogenisation of experience is reinforced to the degree to which the individual's movement within the labour market is confined to occupations which generate a similar range of material outcomes. In general we may state that the structuration of classes is facilitated *to the degree to which mobility closure exists in relation to any specified form of market capacity*' (1973:107).

It is clear that the concept of collective social mobility, which we are proposing, is bound up with closure and is rooted in particular types of market capacity. It is also evident that Giddens' reference to the bases of mediate structuration of class relationships is connected to his conception of individual mobility chances. This approach, as we have seen, is customary among students of social mobility in Western countries. It is nevertheless possible to utilise Giddens' concepts of market capacity, structuration and closure in a way which we believe actually strengthens rather than weakens Giddens' theoretical position. The only *caveat* we might wish to make is that the concept of market capacity underplays the degree of occupational *control* over the market which occurs in cases of occupational groups which have been successfully applying techniques of closure. The case we explore is that of the medical profession.

Giddens suggests that there are basically three kinds of market capacity which are relevant to mobility chances or closure in any class structure. These are

> 'ownership of property in the means of production; possession of

educational or technical qualifications; and possession of manual labour-power. In so far as it is the case that these tend to be tied to closed patterns of inter- or intragenerational mobility, this yields the foundation of *a basic three-class system* in capitalist society, an "upper", "middle", and "lower" or "working class" ' (Giddens 1973:107).

It remains true however that there are no legal sanctions or formal prescriptions governing access to social mobility chances. Thus, under capitalism, closure of the class structure can never be complete.

Turning to his second source of class structuration, namely the proximate factors (which refer to 'localised' conditions shaping class formation), he suggests that there are three elements: 'the division of labour within the productive enterprise; the authority relationships within the enterprise; and the influence . . . [of] "distributive groups" ' (1973:108). In Giddens' view, Marx tended to use the concept of the division of labour in a way which encompassed two separable matters, namely market relations on the one hand, and the allocation of occupational tasks within the productive organisation, on the other. Giddens defines division of labour in this second sense and calls this aspect 'para-technical relations'. The division of labour is analytically separated from market relations as a source of class structuration and also influences class consciousness. The division of labour is not always a factor making for the consolidation of class relationships but can also be a basis for fragmentation. Neither does it enhance class formation in so far as it creates groups which overlap and are superimposed upon the same divisions which result from mediate structuration. Giddens does not doubt that the most important element in proximate structuration is the effect of 'technique' such as the introduction of cybernation. He reaffirms the view that it is in this area of the technical aspects of production that the decisive separation between manual and non-manual workers arises. Even the most skilled manual work, he avers, under modern conditions can involve machine minding by sophisticated people. The manual working environment is thus distinct from the world of the administrative employee and this division is merely reinforced by physical separation between the two types of workers; it is accentuated also by the authority structure of the enterprise. Another source of proximate structuration of class relationships arises in the area of consumption rather than production. Marx and Weber both agreed that 'class is a phenomenon of production: relationships established in consumption are therefore quite distinct from, and secondary to, those formed in the context of productive activity' (Giddens 1973:109). Without departing from this view Giddens suggests that consumption patterns are a major influence on class structuration. In particular he points out that Weber's concepts of 'status' and 'status group' . . . 'confuse two separable elements: the formation of groupings in consumption, on the one hand, and formation of types of social differentiation based on some sort of non-economic value providing a scale of "honour" or "prestige" on the other' (Giddens 1973:104). These often coincide but do not necessarily do so. Giddens calls relationships based on common patterns of consumption *distributive groupings* 'regardless of whether the individuals involved make any type of conscious evaluation of their honour . . . relative to others' (1973: 109). Status involves the existence of evaluations and a status group emerges where there is a set of social relationships deriving coherence from their application. Distributive groupings include a tendency towards neighbourhood or community segregation which are often based, not on income as such, but on access to mortgages, etc. or lack of such access.

The three-fold model of class structure which Giddens proposes is, in his view, characteristic of capitalist society, generally, but the way in which the elements of mediate and proximate structuration are combined in any specific case serve to produce a variety of actual class systems in different societies. Thus boundaries between the classes cannot be determined in the abstract and in each case, studies must be undertaken of the strength and application of the class principles. Also, there are in addition 'forms of structuration within the major class divisions' (1973:110). The role of the petty bourgeoisie, the influence of skill differentials within the class of manual labour are both market capacities which influence intra-class structuration.

Moving from a consideration of the purely formal class relationships to the content of behaviour patterns and attitudes, Giddens notes that Weber's concept of 'style of life', which emphasises the way in which 'a status group expresses its claim to distinctiveness', may be further extended where 'there is a marked convergence of the sources of structuration. We may then say that classes tend in these circumstances to manifest common styles of life. It is essential to distinguish between class awareness and class consciousness; class awareness is likely to exist whenever class, as a structured form, involves similar attitudes and beliefs expressed through a common life style among class members. This does not necessarily imply a recognition that other classes exist with different life styles. Class consciousness involves the recognition that other classes and life styles do exist.' The important point Giddens makes is that 'class awareness may take the form of *a denial of the existence or reality of classes*' (Giddens 1973:111). For the middle class, he believes, the ideology of individualism tends to underpin this type of awareness. There is a commonly held view that racial or religious divisions act as obstacles to the formation of coherent classes. Nevertheless 'the tendency to class structuration may receive a considerable impetus *where class coincides with the criteria of status group membership*'. In these circumstances, 'status group membership itself becomes a form of market capacity. Such a situation offers the strongest possible source of class structuration whereby there develop clear-cut differences in attitudes, beliefs and style of life between the classes' (1973:112).

Giddens' theory, particularly the statement just quoted, serves as a basis for our conception of the relationship between professionalism and class structure. We would go further, however, and suggest that it is not merely the *coincidence* of class and status group membership which is central, but the active creation of organisations and associations which themselves serve to implement an occupational strategy which embodies the explicit idea of controlling the market for particular goods and services. Such occupational associations are invariably organised on the basis of the 'work situation'. They are normally associations of peers who share a similar market capacity. Such associations arise in the context of a particular market situation which is broadly shared in common by members of the occupation and the desired aim is to exercise control over the market. This involves collective action and collective control, particularly over the number and type of persons admitted to the occupation and to the market for its services; in short, control over recruitment. Also, it involves the attempt to regulate the market usually by the effort to obtain an officially conferred legal charter. Often the outcome hoped for is the establishment of a legally enforceable monopoly.

The relationship between social class and professionalism must be located in the wider context of class theory and we believe, can be handled by it, provided some additional development of the theory is made. Giddens states, as we have noted above, that professionalism presents no problem for class theory, but he does not explicate the relationship. If Giddens means that professionalism can potentially be accommodated by the development of class theory we believe he is right, and this is the major thesis we are putting forward. If, however, he means that professionalism is peripheral to class theory, we beg to differ from him because we regard the study of professionalism as central to the further advancement of the theory of class. In so far as Giddens makes only scant reference to professionalism he clearly regards it as of marginal relevance, so far as class theory is concerned, and this position is consistent with the earlier literature both in professionalism and class theory.

4. POWER, UNCERTAINTY AND THE FORMATION OF SOCIAL STRUCTURE

The human condition is marked by the confrontation of man with an uncertain world. Human society provides a means for the reduction of uncertainty, both ideologically and socially, but uncertainty cannot be altogether eliminated. If uncertainty is endemic to a greater or lesser degree in all human societies we witness the paradox in the specific case of capitalism that it at once provides unparalleled human control via technology over nature, but at the same time has been regarded by many writers, especially Marxist, as being inherently unstable. Whether or not this diagnosis is correct, capitalism has at least always been associated with cyclical fluctuations in levels of economic activity. This has created considerable economic uncertainty, insecurity and hardship. In the face of uncertainty men have created social institutions and organisations which serve to promote a more certain and predictable future for themselves and their children.

The collective organisation and action of men involves power. Power may be conceived of in terms of the exercise of control (to a variable extent) over defined aspects of the social and physical world. Power often serves as a counterweight to uncertainty, men may derive from institutionalised power a reduction of insecurity, whether economic or otherwise.

Marx realised that power may be used by one group of men to exploit others and that the stability of systems of exploitation invariably rests upon ideological legitimation. It is also dependent upon the relative certainty and predictability of known ways, compared with the uncertainty inherent in radical change. Even a grossly unjust social order is marked by the inertia which springs from familiar and predictable certainties.

Contemporary sociological theories, not least of class and stratification, are rooted in the general sociological engagement with classical economic theory. The origins of modern sociology, it has often been noted, lie in the emergence of industrial society itself. In their different ways the founding fathers of the discipline, particularly such seminal figures as Marx, Durkheim and Weber were obsessed with the causes and effects of the rise of capitalism and of the individualist social philosophy which they regarded as integral to it. Classical economic theory expressed the philosophy of individualism in a highly developed and radical form. It was the social acceptance and application of this philosophy which the founding fathers of sociology regarded as being corrosive of established social institutions. The replacement of various kinds of traditional social relationship by the 'crude cash nexus' of the labour market was regarded as perhaps the most striking phenomenon of capitalism by observers of all political and philosophical viewpoints including sociologists in the nineteenth and early twentieth centuries. The rapid extension of the operations of the market (to the point where market relationships were absolutely predominant compared to earlier forms of social structure) and the creation of a labour market, constituted of free-wage labourers and capitalists were the fundamental elements of the capitalist system.

The doctrine of 'perfect competition' was not only central to economic theory, but entered sociology as a basic conception of market relationships from which the sociologist either made his departure or with which he attempted some accommodation. Writing on this subject W.K. Rothschild makes clear both why the model was attractive to economists and why it has tended to drive out any consideration of the question of power. He wrote that 'perfect competition was at no time – even in the days of nineteenth-century small-scale business – an adequate description of economic reality' (Rothschild 1971:8). There were two reasons why it provided a special attraction for economists. One was that, with the transition to a capitalist market economy, competition became one of the decisive motors of economic develop-ment and of social relationships. The model of perfect competition could thus provide an abstract picture of reality permitting an intensive study of all the corollaries flowing from the working of one very important economic motive force. The second reason was that

> 'the classical economists wanted an optimal development of the
> economic forces set free by the industrial revolution and the
> extension of markets. But this development was everywhere
> hampered by the intervention of powerful vested interests . . .
> who acted directly or via government, and who were aided by
> entrenched commercial monopolies and similar groups'
> (Rothschild 1971:9).

Thus the minimising of state interference became the strategy of the supporters of *laissez faire*.

Rothschild tells us that

> 'from the very beginning . . . the basic model of perfect competi-
> tion was both an abstract analysis of a decisive economic force,
> and the Utopian formulation of a society in which power is so
> widely and thinly distributed that its influence can be neglected.
> In this way, the important social phenomenon of power receded
> into the background as far as the kernel of classical economic
> theory was concerned' (1971:9).

The nub of Rothschild's position is that the neglect of considerations of a sociological nature gave rise to the complete victory of 'perfect competition' as the basic model of economic theorising. The perfect market then, while being an heuristic ideal-type model, had in it major elements of description. Monopoly had only a theoretical interest as the polar type to the free market, and it is significant that economists did not seriously develop an analysis of oligopoly until the twentieth century. The production and consumption of goods and services in a perfect market, and the prices at which these were sold, would be adjusted by the 'unseen hand', the market mechanism; this would miraculously resolve the age-old conflict between the private and public interest. Government activity was to be pared down to a minimum summed up in the phrase 'the night-watchman state'.

Within classical economic and political liberalism, then, power was regarded as dangerous because it was defined in terms of corrupt vested interests. In reply to the more conservative view that only the exercise of power through established social institutions and organisations could protect men from the economic uncertainty and instability, the exponents of economic liberalism urged a belief in the self-equilibrating mechanism of the market. They argued most strongly that provided men had sufficient confidence to dismantle vested interests and political controls, the operations of the market would serve to maximise the welfare of the greatest number.

In the last analysis the concept of the perfect market is the basis of liberal economic theory and by analogy, the individualism of political democracy is also justified. The liberal society is one in which all forms of social control, particularly state control, are minimised. That benign mechanism, the 'unseen hand', operating in the market place, will optimise human welfare both in material terms and by conferring human freedom. This is the expected outcome precisely because it is beyond the corruption stemming from the power of vested interests. As Acton, the nineteenth-century historian, so aptly put this point of view, 'all power corrupts and absolute power corrupts absolutely'.

Durkheim objected in the strongest terms to the individualism inherent in liberal economic theory. His major thesis was that society is created by man and that social control, the external constraint of society, is essential as a means of limiting, channelling and setting bounds to man's insatiable desires. For Durkheim, man's happiness and well being rest fundamentally upon the moral framework provided by established social values in a stable social order. From these values are derived the rules of human conduct which in each society control the day to day activities of man. Society, Durkheim asserts, is essentially a moral and religious phenomenon which gives to man an institutionalised structure within which it is tolerable to live. Without the moral power and the ontological meaning conferred by society man is faced with fearsome uncertainty. Durkheim's criticism of economic liberalism, and its integral doctrine of individualism is that such a philosophy fails to grasp the fundamental *social* nature of man. It is not merely the case that the social world is ignored by economic liberalism but that its existence is denied.

For Durkheim, then, the widespread espousal of individualist doctrines will lead to the destruction of moral order and to the socially dangerous condition of *anomie*. Such a condition of normlessness generates uncertainty and produces the decay of social and moral order which is manifested in increased rates of social pathology. While Durkheim was an admirer of the functional order provided by the Guild system, and particularly by its stress on occupational community as an important basis for social life, he was aware that it would be impossible to reconstruct it under modern conditions. He nevertheless suggested that in the political sphere the liberal conception of individual participation through the franchise and the secret ballot should be replaced, as we have seen earlier, by representation through occupational associations. This, he felt, would help to avert the danger of extreme individualism arising from liberal democracy (Durkheim 1957:1-41).

Unlike Marx and Weber, Durkheim was only peripherally interested in class theory. It seems that he thought of occupational associations as transcending any divisions of interest rooted in differences between, for example, employers and employees. For him, the overriding importance of the impact of individualism was on society taken as a *whole*. This was a much more significant question than the matter of 'structured divisions' on class lines within society. His theory of the consequences of individualism does not really allow the possibility of stabilisation of class interests over a long period. Rather it leads to a fear of the imminent breakdown of social order on the basis of atomised individuals each desperately seeking his own self-interest.

Durkheim sees our salvation in an associational society, in which the occupational association is all important. He does not treat as fundamental the question of class divisions between occupational associations *within* a class society. For Durkheim, power and social control relate to society as a whole. The state cannot function without a basis in communal or associational social order. The power of the state depends upon the quality of social solidarity. The state is therefore secondary to society, and it is in this sense that Durkheim conceives of power, ultimately, in terms of generalised social control stemming from society. The operation of this generalised power in society serves to minimise uncertainty by the creation and maintenance of social structure. Society is external to the individual and constrains him.

Unlike Durkheim, Marx and Weber do not regard power and social control in this generalised sense, as problematic. Neither do they believe that the probable consequence of capitalism is social disorganisation of this general type: for them capitalism is a structured social form. They share with Durkheim the notion that capitalism is defined by a characteristic separation between state and economy. It is from the existence of this separation, which itself is derived from economic liberalism, that two alternative theories of power and control in capitalist society have been developed. Also, as part of this, two distinctive views

63

of the nature of social class have emerged.

In relation to the economic sphere within capitalism the notion of the market has been predominant. Typically the idea of *horizontal* class divisions is offered in which, in the case of Marx, power derives from ownership of property and lack of power relates to non-ownership. In Weber's concept of market situation the notion of 'life chances' is put forward, and in the determination of these all other forms of emoluments are included. Status groups, ultimately depending on shared market situation, are also, for Weber, horizontally organised. Both in the work of Marx and Weber, class is a phenomenon which divides society horizontally. Although Marx is not concerned with the phenomenon of status, both he and Weber share the view that horizontal divisions are characteristic of capitalist society. The idea of a status group — a group characterised by a particular style of life — also incorporates the notion of a degree of monopolisation of a particular market, and hence involves the idea of power as collective control over the market by specified groups. In a very general sense, therefore, both Marx and Weber share a conception of the significance of power based on control of particular markets which produce horizontal divisions in capitalist society. This agreement tends to be overridden, or at least hidden to some extent, by the debate between them concerning other facets of capitalism, particularly over the significance of the state and its relationship to the economy and society.

If the separation of state and economy is a distinctive feature of capitalism, the relations between them have varied historically between the continental European countries compared with Britain and the United States of America. This in turn has influenced theory and research according to the influences on the researcher. For example, both Lockwood and Dahrendorf start their analysis with theory and concepts drawn from both Marx and Weber but develop distinctive theoretical perspectives (Lockwood 1958; Dahrendorf 1959).

Giddens detects an ambiguity in Marx's conception of the nature of the relationship between state and society. The view is put forward by Marx that 'the state is nothing more than the vehicle whereby the interests of the dominant class are realised: the state is merely an agency of class domination'. Yet Marx's writings about the capitalist state contain evidence of a considerable awareness of the administrative significance of the state as a 'supervisor' of the operation of capitalist production (Giddens 1973:51). The fact that Marx was concerned to argue, in this regard, that the administrative functions of the capitalist state are of key importance because they guarantee the working of contractual obligations which underpin the very existence of a free market in labour, suggests that the state might be considered, tacitly at least, as of greater importance in the Marxian scheme than has usually been recognised. The very functioning of capitalism as an economic system is dependent upon the existence of the state to provide a framework of market relationships and therefore for class structure. Giddens pinpoints the ambiguity in the following way. Firstly, there is a conception in Marx's writing 'that the state is, in a direct sense, the *instrument* of class domination, and hence that most of its organisational characteristics are contingent upon the capitalist system of class relationships'; and secondly, 'that the state is a coordinating agency which is responsible for the overall administrative operations of the society *within* which a relationship of class domination pertains in the "separated" economic sphere' (1973:51).

The relative significance accorded to bureaucracy in Marxian and Weberian theories becomes the central issue. For Marx, the state bureaucracy is regarded as a parasitic growth upon society which arises from the class domination of the bourgeoisie and, equally, will disappear with the bourgeois class after the transcendence of class society. It is for this reason, Giddens claims, that the Marxian theory of bureaucracy is somewhat rudimentary. In Weber's theory, the state bureaucracy is the archetypal form of social organisation characteristic of emergent capitalism which determines the form of state bureaucracy, but that bureaucracy is the essential framework of rationalised economic enterprise. The free market, Weber would agree, serves the material interest of capital, but because of the importance of bureaucracy and of state bureaucracy in particular, the abolition of private ownership of property, as such, cannot produce the complete transformation or transcendence of capitalist society which Marx expected. This is because bureaucracy would be carried over into any probable socialist system.

Marx's views about the state derive from the fact that he was caught up in the nineteenth-century tradition of social thought which assumed that the state is subordinate to society. This assumption is found not only in classical political economy but in Saint-Simonianism and tends to suggest that the state is

> 'capable of being "reduced" to [a] condition of dependence upon [society] — in Marx's case, to class relationships. This is why there is in Marx no recognition of the possible existence of the state as an independent force: he comes close to such a recognition only in arguing that, in the phenomenon of "Bonapartism", where there is a "balance" of classes, the state becomes temporarily detached from subservience to the interests of any one class. In contrast, Weber's sociology is concerned with the role of the state as an agency acting upon society' (Giddens 1973:124-5).

Both Marx and Weber believed that the state reflected the character of class interests in a capitalist society. This occurs by the guarantee of the state which insulates the political from the economic sphere and also, under conditions of universal adult suffrage, legitimises and protects access to the political sphere, only on a basis of formal equality. Private property in the economic sphere is protected and legitimated separately: it is shielded from democratic modes of participation by all citizens. In this sense the state acts as an autonomous power. The abolition of private property alone does not itself involve the abolition of the state, but rather the domination by the state of the apparatus of economic life, and thus the entrenchment of bureaucratic power (1973:282). Witness the state socialist societies.

A significant point made by Giddens is that the character of the reaction of peasant and working classes to the introduction of capitalism depends upon the speed and quality of its initial introduction. He points out that revolutions have occured, not as Marx thought they would in societies such as Britain, where capitalism was introduced as a spontaneous development over a comparatively lengthy historical period, but in circumstances such as those which 'obtained where it was fostered rapidly in a backwood economy'. In other words, Giddens is suggesting that the point at which revolutionary consciousness is most likely to be manifested in the working class is at the moment of impact between post-feudalism and capitalism-industrialism. He goes on to say that in his view it is misleading to argue that 'the high point' of capitalist development occurs in the typically *laissez faire* period which follows its rise and that consequently, state intervention and the extension of political democracy, appear as capitalism moves into decline. Not only does this view rest upon the Marxist position that capitalism has a definite life-cycle, but it suggests that 'maturity' is reached rapidly before the decline sets in. Giddens persuasively suggests that only in the recent history of capitalism has something like 'maturity' been reached. Certainly an endemic tendency towards class conflict exists in early capitalist society, and if left unregulated can produce a revolutionary working class movement bent on violent class warfare and the overthrow of the system. The introduction of social democracy and free trade unions dedicated to collective bargaining serve to produce the incorporation of the working class. It is 'the characteristic form in which class conflict expresses itself in developed capitalist society'. Thus 'it is the presence of revolutionary class conflict, rather than its absence', which requires explanation (Giddens 1973:287). The separation of state and economy, which is fundamental to capitalism

> 'also involves at the same time a mutual dependence, and changes in one sphere call into play reciprocal or counter-developments in the other. This is why it is not contradictory to say that the maintenance of the insulation of the "political" and "economic" spheres depends on the existence of definite interconnections between them. State "intervention" − the term is of course itself misleading, but by now conventional − in economic life is in this sense not only compatible with capitalism; it is intrinsic to it' (1973:286).

The relationship between the state and the economy under capitalism has been various. In each of the capitalist countries, even in England where the philosophy of *laissez faire* saw its hey day, the expansion of the role of the state in the economy has developed rapidly. In the mid-twentieth century it is usual to speak of the 'mixed economy', meaning that the intervention of the state in a number of important economic activities has become at least equal to that of private enterprise. In the mixed economy the state has also taken on the task of general management of economic activity. It is now usual in some circles to describe the organisation of western industrial countries as 'state capitalism'. Equally, the industrial countries of eastern Europe and the USSR are frequently described by the term 'state socialism'. Despite the use of the term, state capitalism, there have been, and to some extent still remain, important differences between the relationship of the state and the economy in Britain and the United States compared with the principal countries of western Europe. In France and Germany, the state was far more influential in the development of capitalism than either in England or the United States. Britain was the first new nation in the sense that she was the first to experience an industrial revolution: unplanned and unanticipated by the state. In France, Germany, and Japan and more recently in the USSR, industrialisation has been an object of state policy. As a number of writers have pointed out, this has made a very great difference to the relationship between the state and the economy in the continental European countries, historically speaking, compared with Britain. It is not our intention to go into this matter here but it is important to notice that these differences in the structure of capitalism in different countries have influenced sociological theorisation about power and class, and have sometimes led to considerable divergencies, or at the very least, to differences of emphasis, in sociological studies.

Marx, although himself of German origin, regarded England as the prototype of capitalist society and, as we have noted, had a tendency to think of the state as secondary to the economy. Power is derived, in his view, from the ownership of property, and property owners controlled the state. Class was, for him, fundamentally an economic phenomenon. In the case of Weber the construction of his theory around a debate with Marx, and the influences upon him of British economic ideas, caused him to regard market situation as the essence of class. In a sense, though, his conception of capitalism in terms of division between state and economy caused him to develop a separate theory of the state and arguably an alternative view of capitalism. He spoke of power and authority — and saw these as inhering in the state and deriving from it. The state he defines in terms of its monopolisation of power in a particular territorial area. The theory of legal-rational bureaucracy as the characteristic social form of capitalist society, the very archetype of which is the state, allows the possibility of an alternative theory of class based on authority. Such a theory was subsequently developed by Dahrendorf.

Dahrendorf's analysis of industrial society starts from the state, from legal-rational bureaucratic authority, rather than from market relationships. He draws on that side of Weber's work which conceives of capitalism as a fundamentally political rather than an economic phenomenon. Power, or rather authority, is the lynch-pin of Dahrendorf's analysis. Lockwood, by contrast, founds his analysis on that aspect of Weber's work which starts with market relationships. Dahrendorf tells us that 'neither Weber nor most of the subsequent analysts of bureaucracy were explicitly concerned with developing a theory which might lead to the supersedure of Marx's theory of class in the light of new facts' (Dahrendorf 1959:90-1). It was his ambition to offer such a theory. He posed the problem of the divergence between Marx's predictions and the actual historical developments since his day and confronted them. Unlike Lockwood, he was influenced from the outset by the problem of social stratification in socialist countries. After reading Djilas he focussed on the importance of power as a more embracing concept than property. He argued that private property relations are simply a form of power relations and used the alternative aspect of Weber's work compared to Lockwood: namely Weber's concepts of power and authority. As a matter of fact by doing so he opened himself to a criticism which he levelled against Marx. He charged Marx with adhering to a legalistic conception of property, but because Dahrendorf adopted Weber's definition of authority, he fell into the same trap. The reason for this is that Weber defined power (as opposed to authority) in asocial Hobbesian terms. Only 'authority' inhering in social position was a sociological category. Power was thus defined out of Dahrendorf's theory right from the start. In practice, he only spoke of authority, and because Weber had defined it somewhat legalistically, then so did Dahrendorf. The result is that his insight, which came to him while reading Djilas, was thrown away.

He argued thus: industrial society is characterised by legal-rational authority which itself is manifest in bureaucratic organisation. Authority, he claimed, logically entails the categories of superordination and subordination. Therefore in any association there will be a polarity of groups: one possessing authority, and one lacking it. At once it is possible to see what Dahrendorf's intention was. He simply substituted the notion of 'authority' for the Marxian notion of 'property', and while saving the Marxian theory of the polarity of classes, did so by making the latter just a special case of his own more general theory.

The logic of this argument also enabled him to utilise Marx's concepts of 'class in itself' and 'class for itself', which he called quasi-groups and interest groups respectively. A quasi-group is one in which the people concerned are in a common situation in respect of authority, but are not conscious of sharing this situation in common. An interest group is one that shares a common situation but which is conscious of this, and is organised to pursue its interest on this basis. (For example, a trade union.) Where he differs from Marx is in respect of his belief that conflict in capitalist societies will be increasingly institutionalised by bureaucratic means. This will save such societies from violent revolution.

It is this process which Dahrendorf argued is central to the history of all industrial societies, and here he was developing the views of Max Weber. In support of his thesis he incorporated the view that there has been a managerial revolution in the west which has vitiated the importance of private property. He added that because of the bureaucratisation of socialist societies, and their domination by 'non-owning' bureaucrats, we have entered a stage of 'post-capitalist' society, where property has been superseded by authority as the basis of class, and where, as a result, there has been a convergence between the institutions of industrial countries, both east and west. The whole argument clearly rests on the conception of 'authority' which Dahrendorf employed. Regrettably, because he used Weber's legalistic notion of 'authority' he did not manage to transcend the limits of Marx's equally legalistic definition of property, and thus begged the question to which he had originally addressed himself.

The concept of legal rational authority has as its logical opposite the notion of illegality. But we may need a concept which falls between these two to deal with many situations which are of interest to the sociologist. Lockwood touched upon this point in a footnote when he said

> 'whereas the legitimacy of authority tends to take the form of general principles, acts of authority are always specific, and they are always more specific than the derived rules of authority, no matter how well developed the latter. Thus, the "exploitable" ambiguity surrounding the derivation and interpretation of the legitimacy of specific acts means that authority is never given, but is always contingent upon its exercise. It is precisely with such conflicts arising from within the interstices of institutionalised power that "conflict theory" is concerned, and not simply with the more unusual approximates to "unstructured" power conflicts' (Lockwood 1964: 246-7).

This interesting comment on power remains undeveloped in Lockwood's work and the reason, we suggest, is that any explicit focus on the concept has not been necessary or integral to the major studies which Lockwood has produced. He began, as we noted earlier, with a study of the weakly organised clerical workers using as his primary concepts three drawn from the alternative side of Weber's work; market situation, work situation and status. Deeply influenced by Marx, yet testing the Marxian thesis of false class consciousness (in the case of the clerical worker) against the facts of class identification, he utilised Weberian concepts from that side of the master's work which most closely derived from and developed Marx's own theory.

Bureaucracy figures in Lockwood's analysis as 'the hierarchy of command' which shapes the devolution of authority but, in contrast with Dahrendorf, it is the market situation which is central. The opportunity arises for power to stem from collective control over the market via the trade union. The structural reasons for weak trade unionism and lack of the identifications of white collar workers with the union movement, and indeed with the working class generally, is explored. This thesis has been criticised by G.S. Bain who argues that the intervention of the state, and its encouragement of unionism in the civil service and the nationalised industries, has been the single most important factor in the growing strength of working class unionism in Britain (Bain 1970:187).

In Lockwood's analysis of bureaucratisation it is important to notice that the state is a sufficiently detached entity not to figure too directly in his analysis. We have already observed that Lockwood was able to apply brilliantly the Weberian categories to a case of weak collective organisation to which these concepts were well suited. He had no need to deal with the phenomenon of collective control through the occupational association (especially professionalism) among the middle class, but it is for this reason that his theoretical scheme tends to preclude any full understanding of that class.

In our view, then, both Marx and Lockwood fail, for different reasons to grasp the significance of the occupational association, and in particular professionalism, in capitalist society. Marx because of his overriding concern with the emerging polarity of classes, and his insistence that class must only be defined in terms of property relationships. Lockwood, basically because his focus of attention is on a weakly organised middle class group. Nevertheless, they both share the belief that class is fundamental to capitalism and therefore agree on the significance of *horizontal* class divisions in society as a potential basis of power and of collective action. This is by no means a conception absent in Weber, but the alternative of centralised authority inhering in the state and devolving vertically down the structure, each layer controlled by the one above, has been the context in which 'power' is discussed in his theory and in developments of it. Our contention is that the existence of formally free, private occupational associations and their significance for class theory has been neglected except for the case of the trade union. These associations arise from *horizontal* market relationships. Market control is the source of their power but their relationship with the state is also of the greatest importance. Market capacity is frequently influenced directly or indirectly by the nature and terms of that relationship.

Power has in some respects been very inadequately treated in sociology. Sociologists have often been willing to allow the matter to be treated by specialists in the neighbouring discipline of politics. Power in the generalised sense of 'constraint' arising from the very existence of a social system reappears in a number of sociological guises. The Marxian notion that power stems from the unequal possession of resources (property) has also been extremely influential as indeed have the dual notions of power, contained in Weber. These form another important strand in sociological theorisation. Weber offered a micro-definition, the quintessential element of which was the ability of one party to get another to do something against his will. But at the macro level in his definition of authority, for example legal-rational authority, Weber was concerned with the principle of imperative coordination.

In a recent analytical essay, Lukes examines the concept of power as it has been used in political and sociological studies. (Lukes 1974). He suggests that we may distinguish between the essentially one-dimensional point of view, such as that of Dahl, which focusses on the process of decision-making, and the two-dimensional approach which additionally includes the study of non decision-making, that is, a process by which latent or manifest challenges to the decision-maker are thwarted. The one-dimensional perspective is criticised by Lukes as being overtly behavioural and subject to the problems of methodological individualism. These defects, he suggests, are only partially overcome by the two-dimensional view which treats non decision-making as itself a form of decision-making and 'allows for consideration of the ways in which *decisions* are prevented from being taken on *potential issues* over which there is an observable *conflict* of [subjective] interests, seen as embodied in express policy preferences and sub-political grievances' (Lukes 1974:20). The work of Bachrach and Baratz is used as an example (Bachrach, Baratz 1962, 1970).

Lukes asserts that a radical three-dimensional view is necessary because 'the bias of the system can be mobilised, recreated and reinforced in ways which are neither consciously chosen nor the intended results of particular individuals' (1974:21). It is interesting to notice that Lukes does not wish to exclude the elements of decision-making or non decision-making contained in the first two approaches but adds a third systemic dimension. Probably this derives from Lukes detailed analysis of the concept of constraint in his brilliant study of Durkheim (Lukes 1973). The bias of a particular social system 'is not sustained simply by a series of individually chosen acts, but also, most importantly, by the socially structured and culturally patterned behaviour of groups, and practices of institutions, which may indeed be manifested by individuals' inaction' (1974:21-2). He argues that Bachrach and Baratz pursue the same path as the pluralists in that their conception of power remains too much bounded by methodological individualism. Both the one-dimensional and two-dimensional views of power Lukes shows

'follow in the steps of Max Weber, for whom power was the probability of *individuals realising their wills* despite the resistance of others, whereas the power to control the agenda of politics and exclude potential issues cannot be adequately analysed unless it is seen as a function of collective forces and social forces' (Lukes 1974:22).

He distinguishes between two cases

'first, there is the phenomenon of collective action, where the policy or action of a collectivity (whether a group, e.g. a class, or an institution, e.g. a political party or an industrial corporation) is manifest, but not attributable to particular individuals' decisions or behaviour. Second, there is the phenomenon of "systemic" or organisational effects, where mobilisation of bias results, as Schattschneider put it, from the form of organisation. Of course, such collectivities and organisations are made up of individuals — but the power they exercise cannot be simply conceptualised in terms of individuals' decisions or behaviour. As Marx succinctly put it, "Men make their own history but they do not make it just as they please; they do not make it under circumstances chosen by themselves, but under circumstances directly encountered, given and transmitted from the past" ' (1974:22).

It is interesting to note that Lukes, following Gramsci (Gramsci 1971) draws a distinction between studying the action of groups in normal and abnormal times. In abnormal times it is possible to see how groups act when certain existing structural constraints are removed or attenuated. 'It signifies that the social group in question may indeed have its own conception of the world, even if embryonic; a conception which manifests itself in action, but occasionally and in flashes — when, that is, the group is acting as an organic totality' (1971:327). Gramsci distinguishes between the autonomous activity of a group under abnormal conditions contrasting with their submissiveness and subordination in normal times. Such a conception has to do with circumstances where the apparatus of power is relaxed or asserted. The study of power in normal times concerns the question of 'how people react to opportunities — or, more precisely, perceived opportunities — when these occur, to escape from subordinate positions in hierarchical systems. In this connection data about rates of social mobility can acquire a new and striking theoretical significance' (Lukes 1974:48).

We trust that the study of collective social mobility, which is represented by our book, is precisely such a contribution, although Lukes, like other writers whose work we have described uses as an example the case of the Sanskritizing caste seeking upward social mobility through upward assimilation within the Indian caste system. He makes the valuable point that although this is usually taken to be a genuine case of value consensus, yet there is in fact 'a gap between thought and action, since the adoption of the Brahminic way of life by a low caste is theoretically forbidden and in general caste position is held to be ascriptive, hereditary, and unchangeable' (Lukes 1974:49).

72

On the other hand, various 'ways out' have been taken by the outcastes from the insufferable consequences of the oppressive caste principle. The adoption by large numbers of untouchables at various historical times of more egalitarian religions, such as Christianity, Islam and Buddhism which offer an opportunity for escape from caste discrimination, have been well documented.

Lukes is well aware of the 'difficulty . . . of attributing an exercise of power to collectivities, such as groups, classes and institutions'. (This difficulty has often been put forward to us in seminar situations where we have presented our thesis of collective social mobility.) 'The problem is: [says Lukes] when can social causation be characterised as an exercise of power, or, more precisely, how and where is a line to be drawn between structural determination, on the one hand, and an exercise of power, on the other?' (1974:52). The debate has been couched, particularly in the history of Marxist thought, between determinism and voluntarism and recently has been explicitly argued 'between the Althusserian, Nicos Poulantzas, and . . . Ralph Miliband'. Lukes rejects

'Poulantzas' implied dichotomy between structural determinism and methodological individualism . . . These are not the only two possibilities. It is not a question of sociological research "leading finally" *either* to the study of "objective co-ordinates" *or* to that of "motivations of conduct of individual actors". Such research must clearly examine the complex inter-relations between the two' (1974:54).

Regrettably, Poulantzas stipulatively redefines power in terms of structural determination.

'To use the vocabulary of power in the context of social relationships is to speak of human agents, separately or together, in groups or organisations, through action or inaction, significantly affecting the thoughts or actions of others (specifically, in a manner contrary to their interests). In speaking thus, one assumes that, although the agents operate within structurally determined limits, they nonetheless . . . could have acted differently. The future, though it is not entirely open, is not entirely closed either (and, indeed, the degree of openness is itself structurally determined). In short, within a system characterised by total structural determinism, there would be no place for power' (1974:54-5).

The nub of Lukes claim

'is that to identify a given process as an "exercise of power", rather than as a case of structural determination, is to assume that it is *in the exerciser's, or the exercisers' power* to act differently. In the case of a collective exercise of power, on the part of a group, or institution, etc., this is to imply that the members of the group or institution could have combined or organised to act

73

differently' (1974:55).

Such an approach to the concept of power is clearly germane to our study of collective social mobility, and has in general terms a great deal in common with the approach adopted in a paper written as a preliminary to writing this book (Parry 1973). Under the heading 'Power and Uncertainty', the senior author wrote:

'I assert that men are everywhere and always to a greater or lesser degree faced by uncertainties in their relations with each other and with nature. In their attempts to control these uncertainties, men exercise power. Power in my definition is therefore an activity of obtaining control or maintaining control over individuals, institutions, and organisations that the actor believes are the source of uncertainty or are likely to be. This activity itself involves the creation and change of social structure, the modification and the transformation of social institutions and organisations. Power and uncertainty are therefore indissolubly wedded.

The exercise of power involves an actor in:

a) a definition of the content of a situation and its boundaries, including options for action through time.

b) a definition of interests.

c) a strategy or policy designed to achieve the objects specified as fulfilling these interests.

d) the day to day tactics conceived to be useful in implementing the strategy.

e) the mobilisation of such resources as are defined as relevant and available for the strategic or tactical purpose.

It should be noted that while human activity is conceived as purposive, it is not suggested that this is self-consciously so all the time, or that the pursuit of interests does not have unanticipated consequences. On the contrary both of these factors play an important part in generating uncertainty. In the social world, men and associations are often at cross purposes to say the least.

Power in a capitalist society typically depends upon the extent to which a group can control its market situation. This is so because, as is generally recognised, the market is the most important social institution of capitalism. The model of the market offered by classical economists, as we have seen, eschewed power, and as a matter of historical fact, was not self-equilibrating at its optimum. In practice the operations of the market diverged dramatically from the model and in any case men had to make the best of their relationship to the market as they found it. It is for this reason I contend, that private occupational strategies are generated in the attempt to reduce uncertainty and obtain a high degree of control over market forces. The market is the mechanism of the unequal distribution of the means of life itself or as Weber said, of life chances. The majority of people participate in it directly through their work. It is not surprising therefore that the work situation is the locus in which collective efforts to control the market situation of a group are most often made. It is usually the foundation both for private strategies, often embodied in occupational associations, or in the linking of these to public strategies embodied in the activities of pressure groups or political parties in their efforts to influence state action' (Parry 1973:14-5).

5. COLLECTIVE SOCIAL MOBILITY AND SOCIAL STRUCTURE

Giddens' excellent analysis of the significance of the relationships between state and economy within capitalism helps greatly to clarify the problem. On the other hand, his concept of market capacity seems to us to reflect the Weberian notion, drawn from classical economic theory, of the market as a 'natural' rather than a 'social' phenomenon. We feel that he is not perhaps radical enough in synthesising the analytically separated elements of class and status. Like Weber, Giddens stresses the fact that status is a concept which refers to style of life, that is to a set of shared normative and value components which serve to identify a group of people to themselves and at the same time distinguish them from others. He articulates, as we have seen, the key problem of contemporary class theory which is how to conceptualise and explain the relationship between shared market capacity and class as a structured form. Where class and status coincide, Giddens rightly observes, status itself (as we have had occasion to note) can be transformed into a market capacity (Giddens 1973:112). The use of the word 'coincide' does however suggest that where the coincidence of class and status occurs, it is the outcome of an 'accidental' rather than a political process. We wish to take an additional step and argue that market capacity is itself partly the outcome of a political process, a power struggle, in which the principal social form (especially in the Anglo-Saxon countries) has been the free occupational association. This may take the shape of the free trade union, the professional association or the association of businessmen. Among these associations there are many variations but professional associations, trade unions and business associations are fundamentally rooted in the market even if in different market situations. The latter are the foundation upon which men may, under appropriate conditions, create occupational associations, one of the most important objectives of which is the definition and control of particular markets. Occupational associations are typically formed on the basis of a particular market capacity. Using Giddens' typology of market capacities we can see that occupational associations may be formed on the basis of each of them: capital; skill and education; or manual labour power.

In the most general terms, then, there are three characteristic types of occupational association. Associations of businessmen use capital as a resource for the manipulation of labour and also markets for specific ranges of goods and services. Professional associations are concerned with the manipulation of education and skill with the objective of control of markets for specific forms of service. Trade Unions are engaged in the manipulation of labour power with the aim of regulating specific labour markets, most frequently through the process of collective bargaining with the employer. In practice unionism and professionalism, as occupational strategies, overlap and often compete within particular occupational groups. These different strategies are reflected in the formation of separate occupational associations within a single occupation. There is room for contradiction, ambiguity and conflict, and thus for a failure of solidarity in particular cases. The effort of occupational associations is directed towards the creation of an identity between a *likeness of interest* (class) and a *likeness of kind* (status) (Newman 1974:2, 11).

The occupational association is thus a major link between the market and status. In the long run, as Weber said, status follows the market (Gerth and Wright Mills 1948:187). Increased income can follow from some measure of occupational control over the market for specific goods and services. Thus occupational control can help to stabilise income through time and allows the possibility of raising the status of the occupation in society. Control of the labour market of a particular occupation provides at least the conditions in which selective recruitment is possible. Persons from higher status families may be attracted by the enhanced income and will thus readily apply for education or training: in short they will seek entry to the occupation. In the longer run, selective recruitment of persons from high status backgrounds reinforces the status of the occupation and confirms its position in the class structure. The barriers erected by higher status occupations are in themselves an important element in the establishment and continuation of class division. Behind this barrier a homogeneity of 'kind' is created and sustained by a shared style of life. This includes similarity of family and educational background, shared normative assumptions and expectations as well as relational patterns in which members typically participate. The predominance of 'endogamous' marriage and shared educational experience, participation in clubs and leisure groups shared in common, similar neighbourhoods containing houses within an accepted range of taste and price, all serve constantly to create and recreate a social world, a style of life typifying and identifying a class/status group both to itself and to outsiders. The basis is however almost always a market capacity which is to an important degree controlled and shaped by the activities of key occupational associations. Similarities in the level of remuneration, which are an outcome of market capacity and the degree of market control, provide a basis for similarities of consumption essential to a shared lifestyle.

Occupational associations then are typically organised, on the basis of similar work situations and in relation to specific broadly-shared market capacities. They are also guided by the espousal, whether self-consciously or not, of ideological positions which are expressed as occupational strategies. Associations of employers, professional associations and trade unions are based on the manipulation of specific market capacities namely, capital, education and labour respectively. It is not possible within the confines of this book to deal with the occupational strategies of capital owners so we must be content to study professionalism, with which we are mostly concerned, and to a lesser extent, unionism. These we will examine in relation to our major theme: collective social mobility.

In order to understand the process of collective social mobility, it is important to refer to the conditions for its existence in capitalist society. Firstly, under capitalism sociologists usually agree that there are no legal or formal sanctions against social mobility as such, whereas in the earlier estate systems there were. Secondly, collective action directed towards social mobility is typically based upon occupation, because occupation is itself rooted in market relationships. Thirdly, a threat to an occupation (particularly of an invasion of newcomers whose arrival may swamp existing occupational opportunities, and thus tend to depress the price of labour secured by that occupation in the market place) usually evokes awareness, consciousness and the formation of associations directed towards the closure of occupational opportunities against outsiders. Several occupational strategies are possible.

Their implementation involves collective efforts to close the occupation off to newcomers. Nevertheless, control of an occupation's existing position within the class structure need not necessarily be connected with a process of upward social mobility. For example, the pursuit of the strategy of unionism tends to militate against such a possibility. There are, on the other hand, occupational strategies, particularly professionalism, which have been typically associated with efforts to assimilate an occupational grouping quite deliberately into a higher social class or to a higher status position within a class. Collective social mobility involves the closure of an occupation against entry of newcomers from below and selective recruitment with a view to creating and maintaining a common identity of background between a parvenu group and a group of those already established. This requires, if it is to be successful, the breaking open or removal of existing barriers which have previously functioned to defend established groups.

Social and economic threats are an important stimulus to the development of occupational associations. These tend to enhance the articulation of the collective consciousness which the group has of itself. An occupational association typically proposes a strategy and tactics designed to defend the group from such threats or to secure for it an improved position. It should be noted that although several strategies are possible only some, for example professionalism, tie up with the sufficient condition for upward collective social mobility, *viz.* the desire on the part of particular groups to assimilate with other groups regarded as higher in the class/status structure than they are themselves. Upward collective social mobility therefore requires a group to breach any barriers erected by those above it and at the same time construct defensible barriers against those aspiring to move up from below.

The sociological criteria which are most useful to analyse this process are adopted by us from Lockwood and Goldthorpe's study. The latter suggest that for assimilation to take place between one class and another three conditions have to be met. Firstly, there has to be 'economic' identity, what Giddens calls similarity of market capacity; secondly, there also has to be some assimilation in the 'normative' sphere, that is, in terms of values; thirdly, it is necessary for there to develop some identity of 'relational' patterns, specifically familial and friendship networks, including patterns of visiting and entertaining (Goldthorpe *et al* 1969:24). All of these together make for the emergence and maintenance of a common lifestyle. Our contention is that occupational associations perform a key role in class formation and maintenance, not least in regard to collective social mobility. *Unionism* and *professionalism* may be considered as alternative occupational strategies which typify the approaches to market and status control of numerous occupational associations based on particular types of market capacity.

Unionism has been regarded essentially as a product of class society. Itself primarily a creation of the working class, it has indisputably played a key role in the structuration of that class. Professionalism and unionism are both varieties of collective action but there has been disagreement about the extent to which they should be thought of as fundamentally similar or different forms of association. Some writers have claimed that professions are nothing more than middle class trade unions, whereas others have argued that they are characteristically different, particularly in that they espouse a code of ethics and standards of behaviour in relation to practice which have an element of 'altruism', of service to the community, an element allegedly not to be found among trade unions.

We regard professionalism as an occupational strategy whih is chiefly directed towards the achievement of upward collective social mobility and, once achieved, it is concerned with the maintenance of superior remuneration and status (Parry 1973:18-20). Haug and Sussman briefly mention the idea that professionalisation is associated with the upward movement of occupational groups but they are incorrect in suggesting that unionism is normally directed at upward collective social mobility (Haug, Sussman 1973:89). On the contrary, unionism, it is generally conceded, is centered on the process of collective bargaining but it has not usually been associated with a drive towards collective social mobility across class boundaries. Also, in the case of craft unionism, the strategy is to maintain a top position within the working class. Studies of the *embourgeoisement* thesis have offered evidence that there is little sign of a desire among highly unionised affluent workers to become middle class. Nor is there evidence that trade unions have set such an aspiration as their goal. Quite the contrary, the mobilisation of union solidarity in working class occupations tends to preclude the espousal of middle class aspirations either by the individual unionist or especially by unionists collectively. In these circumstances there is little prospect of assimilation via unionism, as such, into the middle class. None of this is in any way contrary to the aim of unions or union leaders to maximise money income for their members. But as several studies have shown, affluence does not of itself make for assimilation of unionised workers into the middle class (Goldthorpe *et al* 1968-9).

Weber pointed out in his 'ideal type' of the market economy that where the cash nexus is the principal criterion of value, invidious distinctions of status are irrelevant. Goldthorpe and Lockwood found an approximation to this in the ideology of the affluent worker who saw society in terms of a 'money model', an ideology which discounted the pretensions of status. Sociologists have researched the idea that in western countries two differing conceptions of class structure exist side by side associated with the middle class and the working class respectively. The middle class are said to hold to a hierarchical status model and the working class to a dichotomous view of society characterised in terms of 'them and us'. Goldthorpe and Lockwood focussed their research on the class boundary between routine white-collar and affluent manual workers. They found that their

> 'respondents' own images of the social order were rarely structured in terms of class oppositions or status hierarchies, and [noted rather] the prevalence of largely destructured "money" models, [which] would appear to show quite strikingly the extent to which the "civilisation of individual consumers" was indeed represented in their social consciousness — inhibiting their awareness of the inequalities of power and forms of exploitation upon which the existing order rests' (Goldthorpe *et al* 1969:180).

The existence of 'middle class' aspirations among working class people in regard to education and jobs were also investigated, especially the aspirations held by parents for their children. But, the authors concluded, 'in attempting to account for such aspirations, the hypothesis of vicarious status striving is neither the most economical nor the best supported one' (1969:134). They argued that the relevant factor was not the failure of affluent workers to achieve white-collar status, but the existence for them of a 'distinctively working class dilemma . . . namely, that of having to choose between work which provided them with some degree of intrinsic satisfaction and work which afforded the highest going rate of economic return' (Goldthorpe *et al* 1969:133).

If this is granted, then it seems logical for the workers and their wives who find themselves in this situation, to desire for their children entry to occupations which maximise both the satisfaction of the job *and* economic returns. Here, then, for working people, are 'adequate reasons for seeing many "middle-class" occupations as highly desirable for their children' (1969:134). There is no necessity to invoke the hypothesis of vicarious status emulation.

In spite of the fact that middle class aspirations exist to some extent among affluent manual workers it appears that their knowledge is often vague as to what elements are appropriate for these aspirations to be actualised. This must affect their judgement. For example, mistaken ideas exist about the subjects which their children should study at school if they are eventually to qualify successfully for specific occupations. Parental hopes are high, but their expectations that these hopes will be translated into real career chances for their own children are weak. Indeed, the performance of the children at school is itself lower than would be expected.

Another factor which acts as a barrier to the espousal and pursuit of middle class values, aspirations and life styles among the working class is the response of affluent workers to the idea of promotion or of starting their own businesses. This 'brings out well both the way in which certain aspirations may be held with relatively little conviction as to their plausibility and, more importantly, the way in which aspirations can thus be weakened, or indeed inhibited altogether, by the severity of the objective barriers to advancement that the individual faces'. The contrast between white-collar and manual attitudes towards promotion, and also towards the whole middle class package of a career containing the concept of 'getting on', should be emphasised. These ideas can be of little relevance in relation to the 'typical life-chances of largely unqualified rank-and-file industrial workers employed in modern, large scale plants' (Goldthorpe *et al* 1969:123).

Goldthorpe and Lockwood point out that the trade union is itself both an expression of, and a reinforcement for, these workers' attitudes. In the traditional working class perspective

> 'a prime value is that set on mutual aid and group solidarity in the face of the vicissitudes of life and the domination which "they" seek to impose. This value in turn confirms the shared, communal nature of social life and constitutes a further restraint on attempts by individuals to make themselves "a cut above the rest" ' (1969:119).

The view that the trade union movement is in decline and that the unions are losing their function in society was not one which Goldthorpe and Lockwood were inclined to share, given their theoretical standpoint, nor one which was subsequently supported in the light of their own research evidence. The frequently iterated view that apathy is the predominant characteristic of contemporary union members, a view based on attendance figures at branch meetings, is put into a different

perspective when it is known that a high level of interest and participation at shopfloor level is reported. In any case, since the publication
of the *Affluent Worker* series there has been a sharp change in the
economic and political climate. The 1970s in Britain are not the same
as the early 1960s. Confrontations between government and unions,
not to mention employers, have exposed any doubters to a barrage of
media coverage which suggests that the unions, far from withering away
by erosion at the grass-roots, or through lack of a function, are in fact
sometimes themselves goaded to take strong action by pressure arising
through rank and file militancy in an era of inflation. It is now
commonly stated in the media that the unions are too powerful and too
important to be left to police themselves.

The trade unions of craftsmen or skilled manual workers are often
thought to share important characteristics with professional associations.
Their reliance on the use of specific methods of occupational closure,
their insistence on differentials in pay and conditions, their claims to
superior status over unskilled workers and the training required for
entry to the job, all these are regarded as similar to the features typical
of professional associations. In fact there is considerable historical
evidence suggesting a common origin for each of the types of
occupational association which we have distinguished. Associations of
small businessmen and those of skilled craftsmen had a great deal in
common, not merely in formal structure, as they emerged from the
decay of the guild system. The early modern professional associations
have also grown from the same common root and most of them were at
one time simply associations of small businessmen or craftsmen (Reader
1966).

The gradual emergence of a division between those who owned and
manipulated capital on the one hand and those, on the other, who
specialised in offering their skills to a capitalist employer in return for
wages, was the basis for the development of associations of employers
and of trade unions respectively. The early unions could by no means
be solely defined by the activity of 'collective bargaining' which today
is regarded by most writers as the very core of unionism. Early unions
of skilled workers behaved more like associations of small masters.
They would set an agreed price among members below which no
unionist would sell his labour (Phelps Brown 1959:116-18). Collective
bargaining has gradually emerged as the dominant form of relationship
between employers and unions. Early professional associations, too,
were concerned to set up tariffs pricing the services of members in
order to prevent undercutting. What has distinguished the professional
association from the trade union and the employers association is the
use of education as a key resource for the manipulation of the market
and control over entry to it. Specialised education, including the
establishment of qualifying associations and examinations for
membership, provides a means of control over recruitment and hence

over the numbers entering certain markets and supplying a particular service (Millerson 1964). It is a form of monopolisation leading towards closure. Scarcity in the supply of a service in the face of excess demand will raise the price. An increased price will improve the remuneration of practitioners and this can be the foundation for enhanced standards of living and for higher status. It is the basis for professionalism as an important form of collective social mobility.

Professionalism, in our definition is a strategy for controlling an occupation in which colleagues, who are in a formal sense equal, set up a system of self-government. It involves restriction of entry to an occupation through the control of education, training and the process of qualification. Another aspect is the exercise of formal and informal management of members' conduct in respects which are defined as relevant to the collective interests of the occupation. Occupational solidarity and closure are used to regulate the supply of services to the market. This serves also to provide a basis for the domination of institutions, organisations, and other occupations associated with these. Finally, there is the reinforcement of this situation by the acquisition of state support in order to obtain, if possible, a legal monopoly backed by legal sanctions. Where this is not possible, at least the tacit acquiescence of the state is required. In so far as an occupation is organised to practise all or most of these things it will be exercising the power of professionalism. This conception of professionalism has been particularly important in the British and American context where 'free' or 'autonomous' professional associations have flourished.

In the contrast to this, there is the notion of the professional expert who is employed either by government or in private industry. The distinction between these two ideas is particularly marked in the German case. As Hughes puts it 'the concept of *freier Beruf* (free or liberal profession) once stood for something like a complete philosophy. A man in such a profession was self-employed, learned, devoted to his work, full of the sense of honour of an historic estate (*Stand*), courageously indifferent to pressures from outside, politically neutral (yet, on the whole, *Kaisertreu*). But at the same time there was developed in Germany a model and philosophy of the *öffentlichen Beamten* (civil servant). While all civil servants were to do their work competently and loyally, the higher officials were to be – and were – men of learning, of high professional conscience, and of great prestige. But they were, even more than the men in the liberal professions, to be at once politically neutral and loyal to authority. It was a loyalty which sometimes showed itself in a sort of condescension to those ephemeral and erratic creatures who headed governments and made childishly unwise and impractical policies. There were thus, in German culture, two images of the professional man, one *frei* (self-employed) and one *beamtet* (secure in a bureaucratic position)' (Hughes 1971:370).

In the British case, the ideology of independent professionalism has

83

continued to have a much more powerful influence than it has in Germany, if only because the prestige of the state and of state employment as well as the levels of remuneration accruing, have been higher in the German case. Detailed state regulation of the professions, particularly of modes of qualification, have also been greater in the German situation and in France. In any study of the professions an examination of the changing relationships between the state and the professions is crucial and we focus on this because it has been an important structural consideration for our case studies of doctors and teachers in England (Parry 1974:160-85).

Professionalism as an occupational strategy must be understood in relation to the development and maintenance of class structure. Historically, as we have seen, the fluctuations of a capitalist market economy have given rise to uncertainty and insecurity, in the face of which men have discovered over and again that individually they are to a great extent powerless. Collective action has been used to achieve the necessary degree of organised power to minimise uncertainty arising from the market and to maximise control over present and future conditions of life. The basis of such action is typically in the occupational context, but communal and political action are also frequently developed. Nevertheless, the political party and the communal response are often closely related to the operation of the free, private occupational association. Certainly this is true of the English experience. The occupational association has thus become a fundamental social institution which men have constructed and reconstructed in their search for a means of achieving some measure of control over the market in a capitalist society. Through it they have striven to reduce the uncertainties inherent in a market economy. The occupational association, as a social institution, has provided a measure of security through structuration in an uncertain world. It is an important theoretical problem to conceptualise and understand the significance of the occupational association in class theory.

Giddens, in our view, offers the most sophisticated formulation of class theory to date. In many respects it is closer to the position which we wish to espouse than the theories of other writers who deal with the concept of class. Nevertheless a weak link in his argument, we suggest, is his failure to treat adequately the central role of the occupational association. It is true that like other writers he links unionism with the development of the working class, but he touches upon professionalism only to tell us that it is not a problem for class theory (Giddens 1973:186). In this sense he does not move beyond the position of earlier writers treating of class and of professionalism, who, as we have seen, do not make the theoretical connection between these two phenomena. Having articulated the key issue of contemporary class theory, namely, the problem of making the transition from market capacity to class as a structured form, he then fails to offer a satisfactory account of the *processes* by which closure is achieved. He identifies closure as a fundamental concept in class theory but does not appear to understand the full *general* theoretical importance of 'occupational association' in the process of closure, and thus in class formation and maintenance.

Giddens deals with the bases of social class under capitalism, an understanding of which should lead to the possibility of determining the nature of class boundaries (Giddens 1973:99-112). He proposes three basic criteria upon which the class systems of capitalist societies are founded. These are property, skill *and* education, and manual labour. Thus there are potentially three basic social classes in modern Western societies. In practice, it is necessary in each case to determine empirically the variations which occur. Giddens suggests that market capacity is related to class structuration through opportunities for *individual* social mobility on the one hand, and the processes of *closure* of class boundaries on the other. We believe that Giddens is working on the right lines but, for our purpose, his theoretical position is insufficiently developed. The reason is that he fails to deal adequately with the question of closure. Having alluded to the concept and noted its importance he passes quickly on without undertaking any development of the idea. The fact that he pays attention only to individual social mobility and seems unaware of the significance of collective social mobility (which we regard as fundamentally based on closure), makes it more difficult for him to take the analysis further in this direction. There is a hesitation on the part of Giddens to come to grips fully with this central problem of class theory which he poses. Marx and Weber were, as we have seen, both convinced that under capitalism the market was a determining feature of other institutional structures. The concept of closure, of which Weber was aware, would suggest the possibility of some groups dominating and controlling the market for the services they provide. Giddens' concept of market capacity is presumably intended to go some way towards regarding 'control', through closure, as an important influence in the distribution of economic and honorific rewards. Market capacity, as a concept, however, seems to us to err on the cautious side. It suggests that 'natural' economic forces always have the major causal role and that the influence of closure is relatively marginal. The point is reinforced, as we have noted, by Giddens' failure to pursue the concept of closure in more detail as a key element in class structuration. In our view, his valuable concept of class structuration requires the support of such further analysis. There is a gap between Giddens high-level and abstract theoretical model of the threefold class structure, and a consideration of the mechanisms causing variation. He does not succeed, for example, in deriving from his theoretical scheme the actual class boundary between non-manual and skilled manual workers, which has constantly been demonstrated empirically, to be a fundamental division. This division cuts right across that suggested by his theoretical model, particularly his postulate that one important basis of market capacity in such societies is skill and education. He attempts to cope with this division by reference to a criterion external to his theory, namely authority. He follows Goldthorpe and Lockwood, as well as other writers, in arguing that the reason for the occurrence of the manual non-manual class division lies in the closeness of even the most junior routinised grades to authority. They have a different structural position in the hierarchy of command from skilled manual workers.

Certainly Giddens spells out the crucial prerequisites for class formation through his analysis of the 'mediate' and 'proximate' factors but we feel the breath of life never enters his analytical framework. The crucial *process* by which closure is achieved escapes him altogether. In view of this it is not perhaps surprising that Giddens neglects the significance of professionalism which is in fact an exceptionally interesting case of the process of closure, both theoretically and empirically. The specific study of professionalism, we believe, can lead forward to a detailed analysis of the social processes through which class and status are linked and thus to a realisation of the significance of the relationship between occupational closure and class structuration. Such an analysis requires that we focus on professionalism as an important occupational strategy which, in circumstances where it can be pursued successfully by specific occupational associations, results in tight occupational closure. Such a process is essential to the development of class theory and to our understanding of upward collective social mobility.

Collective mobility downwards is equally a phenomenon of great importance in class formation and relates to the distinction between manual and non-manual work, and between unionism and professionalism. It is not enough to infer (for example on the basis of evidence obtainable from surveys or community studies) that certain class boundaries, such as the one between manual and non-manual groups actually exist. It is necessary also to show how they become established and are maintained or modified. Collective social mobility does not necessarily only involve the transfer of an occupational group across a class boundary and its assimilation into another class, it is often related to modifications of the class structure itself. The process of class structuration can thus be influenced by collective social mobility both upwards and downwards.

The failure by Giddens to develop adequately the concept of closure, which he rightly identified as central to the theory of stratification, has recently been rectified in a short conceptual paper by Parkin (Parkin 1974:1-18) 'By social closure', Parkin reminds us, 'Weber means the process by which social collectivities seek to maximize rewards by restricting access to rewards and opportunities to a limited circle of eligibles' (1974:3). Closure is concerned with the exclusion of outsiders usually from specific economic opportunities which the eligibles wish to keep to themselves (Weber 1968:342). The argument advanced by Parkin

> 'is that the basic line of cleavage in the stratification system is that resulting from the opposition between two contrasting modes of social closure, exclusion and solidarism. This suggests that the distinction between, for example, bourgeoisie and proletariat may be conceptualised in terms of contrary principles of social action, rather than as differences in the formal attributes of collectivities. The concept of closure refers to the *processual* features of class, thereby directing attention to the principles underlying class formation' (1974:12).

Clearly professionalism, in terms of our definition, is a specific form of Parkin's more general category of exclusion, and unionism is an important example of his concept of solidarism. Parkin defines solidarism as 'a generic term designating the closure attempts of excluded groups, whether of a class or communal nature' (1974:9).

The relationship between the relative success of exclusion practices and the reaction of the excluded is fundamental to an understanding of collective social mobility. Upward collective social mobility is dependent both upon the existence of appropriate aspirations in an excluded group, and their ability to organise themselves for the purpose of breaking into and assimilating with a higher status group from which they are excluded. (In the second part of this book we deal in some historical depth with the rise of the surgeon-apothecary in nineteenth-century England as an example of this process.) Speaking of the 'crucial distinction between the two modes of closure', Parkin asserts that the 'techniques of exclusion exert political pressure downwards . . . in that group advantages are secured at the expense of collectivities that can be successfully defined as inferior; whereas strategies of solidarism direct pressure upwards in so far as claims upon resources threaten to diminish the share of more privileged strata' (1974:5).

The terms exclusion and solidarism have the advantage of generality but, in our view, they may not be the most appropriate terms, though this is a minor *caveat* in so far as we can discern a class fit between the views we have advanced on collective social mobility, professionalism and unionism, and those of Parkin (Parry 1973). The reason is that although solidarism is the *only* resource available for those who lack market capacities with attributes upon which exclusion can be built (unskilled manual labour) it is not exclusive to them. Solidarity can be built-up and used effectively among those who also have other resources with which to follow strategies of exclusion and closure such as those of a credentialist kind, and as a matter of fact, has been. It should not be assumed that solidarist strategies are always based in communal action such as that proposed by the term 'traditional orientation' in regard to working class unionism as used by Goldthorpe

(Goldthorpe *et al* 1968b: 74-6). The occupational association has been of fundamental importance in class formation throughout the history of capitalist society.

The close affinity in the origins of the middle class and the modern working class are generally agreed in so far as they originated in the emerging urban context of the late medieval period. There is less agreement on precisely how and when the class distinctions grew up *between* these two classes and the attention of historians and sociologists has been focussed upon the emergence of a dividing line between artisans, who were referred to in the nineteenth century as the aristocracy of labour, and the petty bourgeoisie who were increasingly regarded as on the other side of a class boundary. Alongside the bourgeois businessmen, were to be found the clerical workers and the emerging professions. According to Gray, (Gray 1974:24-6) whose research in Edinburgh was designed to explore the existence of class divisions among working men, it is not merely the case that a well-developed class division existed in the nineteenth century, between the skilled artisan on the one hand and the semi-skilled and unskilled worker on the other, but also that the boundary between the artisan and the lower middle class was blurred compared to the situation today. The process of formation and structuration of the modern working class, the division between non-manual workers and manual workers was only fully developed during the second half of the nineteenth century, although in the early decades, the process of class structuration which produced this division was emerging at an increasingly rapid pace. Non-manual workers were beginning to define themselves as separate from craftsmen and were becoming aware of themselves as in a different class/status position. This involved, in some cases, the sloughing off of any elements of manual work in which they may have previously been engaged but always there was a vital process of attenuation in their relational connections with manual workers. This was justified by a set of normative or cultural values which connected them with the 'gentleman ideal' as a mark of their aspiration to be regarded as members of a higher class. In our view therefore, the concept of the aristocracy of labour, which was actually used in the nineteenth century, was a term which indicated that people included in that category had until recently been part of a 'middle stratum' made up of those who were involved in urban as opposed to rural life, and among whom there had previously been little differentiation or recognised division. The concept of the aristocracy of labour represented a social recognition of the former standing of a group which was being downgraded in class/status terms. This process of downward social mobility had its origins much earlier. In one sense the term reflects a nostalgia for the former standing in society of the craftsman which was expressed in literature and politics throughout the nineteenth century.

The separation and eventual division between masters and men appears to have been a long drawn-out process. Chances for skilled workers to become masters had been diminishing over several centuries but eventually the decay of the Guild system destroyed even the pretence of a continuing common interest and produced the notion of separate interests. The impact of the new industrial technology sharply accentuated and confirmed an existing trend. It provided a powerful stimulus to class formation. Asa Briggs tells us that 'the concept of "social class" with all its attendant terminology was a product of the large-scale economic and social changes of the late eighteenth and early nineteenth centuries' (Briggs 1967:43). Before modern industry made its impact, the usual terminology was of 'ranks', 'orders' and 'degrees' when the 'interests' of economic and status groupings were being described. By the mid-1820s in England, the word 'class' was already established as a social label. In 1834 John Stuart Mill wrote of the three classes of landlords, labourers and capitalists and proposed as a 'subject of inquiry, what changes the relations of those classes to one another are likely to undergo in the progress of society' (*Monthly Repository* 1834:320). The question of class became a predominant one in socialist writings, not least in the work of Marx. Although 'there was no dearth of social conflicts in pre-industrial society, they were not conceived of at the time in straight class terms. The change in nomenclature in the eighteenth and early nineteenth centuries reflected a basic change not only in men's ways of seeing society but in society itself' (Briggs 1967:44).

The distinction between labouring people who rely on manual work for their living and those who could afford not to do so had long been established in English society. The difference between lord and peasant in the feudal system or between the gentry and the tenantry and farm labourers in the eighteenth century was accentuated by the fact that the gentry could afford not to do any of their own manual work. Likewise in the case of trade, those who were not actually involved in the manual aspects of the shop or the movement of goods, but whose activities were exclusively concerned with the planning and profit-making activities, were similarly distinguished by the fact that others undertook the manual labour of merchant enterprises on their behalf. In the developing class system, which depended on the application of machinery in types of work which had been traditionally the monopoly of the craftsmen, the distinction between manual and non-manual elements were peculiarly difficult to make. Craft work embodies the highest manual skills and was often associated with the ownership of one's tools and even of a small business enterprise on a 'craft shop' basis. Nevertheless, even before the industrial revolution, the division between owners and craftsmen, that is the emergence of a class of skilled artisans depending solely on wages, was underway. The use of powered machinery simply stimulated and accentuated this process.

Writers of the period, such as Cobbett and Southey, drew attention to what they regarded as the social disintegration which stemmed from the rise of factory production. Cobbett thought that the 'chain of connection' was being broken between rich and poor and Southey described the breakdown of the 'bond of attachment' (Briggs 1967:45) between social ranks. In 1833, John Wade wrote about the impact of 'a vast and overtopping superstructure of manufacturing wealth and population'. He regarded this as 'an extraordinary revolution' (Wade 1842: preface 1) and spoke of the growth of an opulent commercial class as well as a restless and intelligent operative class. The factory system substituted for the bond of attachment the 'cash payment which was becoming the "sole nexus" between man and man' (Carlyle 1967:205). This phrase used first in 1829, was soon shortened to 'the cash nexus', a term subsequently much used by Marx and the socialist writers. This process was a powerful force in the development of trade unionism, not only at the local level, but also in stimulating the cry for a general union. Cobbett was aware of the manner in which combinations of masters and workmen respectively would be likely to produce conflict and turmoil. The model of society based on cleavage became widely accepted not only by Marx and Engels but also by Conservatives like Disraeli.

On the basis of the census data of 1801, Colquhoun estimated that the 25,000 manufacturers enumerated had an aggregate income of £20 million, a figure ten times greater than that of the shipowners as a group and considerably more than that of merchants (Lewis and Maude 1949:47). Such an estimate even if it is wide of the mark gives an indication of the significance of the new industrial wealth. Many of the new manufacturers had themselves been craftsmen. Halévy draws our attention to the fact that quite often the newly-built factory was in danger of being burned or looted by the artisans or workmen of the neighbourhood at the first sign of an economic recession. The owner might often have to defend it under arms by day and night and in some instances he was forced to give way and build his factory in another district (Halévy 1927:88). It was both possible and frequent for factory owners to become rapidly wealthy but it seems that the maxim governing the attitude of industrial employers was that labour should be bought as cheaply as possible and that no obligation was owed to the workman beyond his cash wages or, in some instances, goods in lieu. The position is put graphically in the following words:

'success in business meant turning a blind eye to the miseries of one's fellowmen. In the eighteenth century masters could rise to eminence without watching the degradation of their fellows, and even in the early nineteenth century to start a factory in a small town did not necessarily imply worsening the lot of one's hired hands. But as factory production spread, the status of the craftsmen worsened and his lot grew harder. As the northern towns grew, without services or government, the middle classes prospered at the cost of suppressing their "humanity", of refusing to see what went on about them. When the towns became too unsanitary, they built suburbs for themselves and cultivated the suburban values which go with them' (Lewis and Maude 1949:48-9).

Engels description of Manchester in 1844 was perhaps not widely known to the middle class which benefited from the prosperity generated by industrial wealth and improved the status of that class in society.

By comparison with the division between the middle class and working class in the northern towns and cities, it is probably true to say that the commercial cities such as London or Edinburgh had not proceeded so rapidly towards a polar division. In the 1850s Bulwer Lytton was still suggesting that the middle class 'cannot be called a class, because it comprises all classes, from the educated gentleman to the skilled artisan' (Christie 1927:67). Gray, examining the evidence for mid-nineteenth-century Edinburgh, gives some evidence for this view. He points out that industry depended greatly on the skills and initiative of the artisan who was often engaged in the direction of semi-skilled and unskilled labour in ways which today have been taken over by managers. The artisan often enjoyed considerable autonomy in his work situation, strengthened by traditional craft norms. The higher stratum of skilled working men was composed of persons of some culture, accustomed to read in political and social history and with a well developed sense of self-respect. They were better housed and belonged to voluntary associations, participation in which they shared with small business and white-collar groups with whom there was also some degree of intermarriage (Gray 1974).

Compared with the mid-nineteenth century the evidence for the middle decades of the twentieth century suggests the emergence of considerable structuration of the boundary between non-manual and manual workers, that is between the middle and working class. It is only necessary for us briefly to refer back to our earlier discussion of the *Affluent Worker Studies* to support this claim. It seems safe to conclude that the institutionalisation of the manual/non-manual class division has been associated with the relative downward social mobility of skilled workers, taken collectively, and this in turn rests on the deeply entrenched normative belief that manual labour is demeaning and that non-manual work, by being associated with the long standing, if now attenuated concept of the 'gentleman', retains a status-conferring capacity.

Class is not however the only feature of social structure which is influential in structuration. Generally speaking there has been a marked tendency in sociology to treat the problem of class structure as a distinct and separable problem from that of social structure. The reasons for this are embedded in the history of sociological thought itself and most particularly derive from the fact that sociology grew up as a response to the impact of capitalism and industrialism in Western societies. Capitalism as a term denoting a particular type of social structure has always implied that economic activity is both a fundamental and separable element in social life. Fundamental in the sense that classical economic theory and Marxism both take the position that other social forms and social institutions are rooted in economic relationships. Marx, for example, argued that the relations of production constitute an economic base from which a superstructure composed of all non-economic institutions and organisations are derived. Changes in the economic base therefore produce changes in the superstructure, and not *vice versa*.

The question of sexual divisions, which we regard as an extremely important element in social structure and in social structuration, is treated by Marxist writers as ultimately reducible to the theory of class and class exploitation in capitalist society. Lockwood's analysis, while, not straightforwardly Marxian, being admixed with Weberian theory and concepts, does contain evidence of the impact of feminisation on clerical work but sexual divisions are not incorporated as an integral feature of his theoretical scheme. Goldthorpe and Lockwood did not regard sexual divisions as of sufficient importance in their study of *embourgeoisement* to consider sampling women workers in their own right; rather, they enter the study only as wives of their male sample of affluent workers. Sexual divisions have been typically treated as an *ad hoc* element to be referred to only as occasion requires. The matter is not conceived of as a fundamental structural element like class itself. It is often the case that the matter is treated under headings like 'the woman question' which in turn is frequently located within the specialised 'sociology of the family', which itself starts from different ideological and theoretical postulates than 'class theory'. Giddens' notion of structuration can and should be used more widely than he suggests. Structuration, we consider, should properly be related to the concept of social structure, in which class is *one* among several structural elements. Although the concept of structuration lends itself to such a venture, Giddens chooses to confine his book to class structure. This makes it impossible for him to undertake an analysis of 'social structure' within its limits. The treatment by Giddens of the position of women conforms with the current state of theoretical development in sociology rather than transcending it in that he refers to the situation of women within the class structure, especially in relation to occupation.

We regard sexual divisions as an independent structural element cutting across class divisions in capitalist societies and we demonstrate the importance of this aspect of social structure in relation to class. Giddens rightly points out that although some writers consider it to be the case that religious or racial differences tend to blurr class boundaries, it is an open empirical question as to whether they do so or not. We examine the extent to which institutional religion has been influential in facilitating or inhibiting collective social mobility.

In 1974 the theme of the British Sociological Association Annual Conference was 'Sexual Divisions in Society'. This was important precisely because it marked an effort to move away from the notion that sexual issues could be treated by sociologists only in terms of the situation of women. It had been possible ten years earlier for J.A. and O. Banks to point out that 'sociologists have, on the whole, been remarkably uninterested in feminism . . . yet, changes in the status of women have occurred in all countries where there are sociologists, and feminist organizations have been and often still continue to be associated with the movement towards emancipation' (Banks 1964:547). Other social movements, such as those of socialism or trade unionism, have received massive attention, but not feminism. They suggested that the existence of a readily identifiable and separate movement consciously established, with appropriate organisations, which have set out to foster the rights of women and which has directly observable consequences, made feminism a relatively easy moment to study. They contended that because 'organized feminist movements, if they continue at all today, can only be counted alongside vegetarianism and nudism as bordering on the cult . . . make the task of the sociologist in studying them much easier because their influence is now spent' (1964:548). Clearly the rise of a qualitatively different and quantitively massive movement seeking for the liberation of women in the second half of the 1960s was not anticipated.

The Banks did point out however that sociologists of the family have developed a considerable literature on the social position of women which simply confirms women in their traditional role — the role of wives and mothers. Parsons, a leading structural functionalist, is also a 'reproductive determinist'. This is to some extent disguised within his treatment of the modern household in which he sees the nuclear unit as typical and in which differentiation occurs between the sex roles along 'instrumental-expressive' lines. Such differentiation is grounded for Parsons in the bearing and early nursing of children which establishes 'a strong presumptive primacy of the relation of mother to the small child and this in turn establishes a presumption that the man who is exempted from these biological functions should specialize in the alternative instrumental direction' (Parsons 1955:23). The Banks pointed out that this is precisely the type of argument which the organised feminist movement sought to combat

> 'asserting that some women would never become mothers, and that others would be obliged to combine the role of mother with that of income-earner, and that *for these women* it was absurd to deny them occupational opportunities on the ground that they

ought to be in the home. In effect, what the feminists asserted was that the simple Victorian identification of role differentiation within the household with biological differentiation between the sexes was nothing more than ideology, a negative reaction to the everyday demonstration that women were quite obviously filling instrumental roles on behalf of the family' (Banks 1964:565). Thus the writing of structural functionalists appears to be couched mainly in conservative terms and fails to translate the social position of women into an important problem of social structure seen from the perspective of social change. The failure to explain social change has been regarded by a number of writers as a weakness in the theory of structural functionalism.

The Banks also argued that the influence of Marxism in sociology and in social history has weakened the consideration of feminism as a significant force in social change because of the predominant 'interpretation of history which sees all struggles for power in economic terms' (1964:548).

Juliet Mitchell elaborated this point when she wrote about women in socialist theory. She showed that all the great socialist thinkers of the nineteenth century recognised the fact that women were subordinated in society and accepted the claim for their liberation. Marx himself, moved 'from generalised philosophical formulations about women in the early writings to specific historical comments on the family in the later texts. There is a serious disjunction between the two. The common framework of both was Marx' analysis of the economy, and of the evolution of property' (Mitchell 1971:78). Engels believed that 'the emancipation of women becomes possible only when women are enabled to take part in production on a large, social scale, and when domestic duties require their attention only to a minor degree' (1971:79). He underlined the point by claiming that the entire female sex ought to be involved in public industry and when that happened the individual family would have been abolished as the economic unit of society. Juliet Mitchell cryptically summed up by saying, 'the position of women, then, in the work of Marx and Engels remains dissociated from, or subsidiary to, a discussion of the family, which in its turn is subordinated as merely a precondition of private property. Their solutions retain this overly economist stress, [and] enters the realm of dislocated speculation' (1971:80). She made the further point that the socialist writers do not specify any mechanism by which the liberation of women will be accomplished in the transition to a socialist society. Rather they simply assume that the liberation of women would be an automatic by-product of the liberation of the working class when the capitalist order is transcended.

Middleton in an interesting paper attempted a development of the Marxist analysis of sexual inequality (Middleton 1974). He argues that 'Marxism has been theoretically deficient in integrating the problem of sexual divisions into Marxist theory. He also argues cogently that the Women's Liberation literature has generally not been very theoretical, and he agrees with the view we have offered that the academic writers of a liberal persuasion have tended to demonstrate discrete inequalities between men and women in a number of respects, without demonstrating that they can be explained in systematic theoretical terms. His chief complaint about Marxism is that women have been seen as an oppressed but marginal group of citizens. For example, he accuses the New Left's view of being entirely concerned with the woman in the context of the family, where she is taken to be consumption-oriented and non-productive. In an interesting section, Middleton shows the striking similarities between the Marxist and functionalist analyses of the family, and the position of women within it. In his own concluding section he suggests that Marxist theory can be fully extended to cover the role of women in society. This is done by examining the way in which domestic labour for the proletarian class, which is typically performed by the labourer's wife, is a major cost in the production and reproduction of labour power. Marx himself, says Middleton, failed to make the point that domestic labour "is therefore of the utmost productive importance to the capitalist economy". The nub of Middleton's argument is that the relationship between the sexes in a capitalist society is governed by the process of production. Our criticism of this view is firstly that both in theoretical and empirical terms sexual divisions are of such great importance that it would be an abdication from sociological understanding simply to reduce them to a dependent relationship upon economic class divisions. Secondly we contend that the similarity in the analysis of both New Left and liberal functionalist perspectives which Middleton so shrewdly points out, is caused by the fact that both types of theory start from a debate over the nature and importance of the market ideology. Our position, which proposes the existence of two ideologies, which are articulated through sexual divisions, would undoubtedly not find favour in a Marxist analysis. From a Marxist point of view, the familial ideology would merely be indicative of the existence of false consciousness masking the "real" productive economic basis of the relationship between the sexes. Our contention is that economic class divisions *are* of fundamental importance, but so too is the structural factor of sexual divisions which cuts across the former. It is our belief that the exclusive emphasis in the Marxist theory upon economic class divisions causes the neglect of sexual divisions in theoretical terms which Middleton himself argues is characteristic of the Marxist treatment of the women question.

'The problem with Middleton's own suggestion that proletarian women must be seen as fully productive labourers within the capitalist system, supporting the workforce through their domestic labour and reproducing workers for the next generation, is that it operates entirely within the limits of the ideological terrain of Marxism and the market ideology. Middleton begs the question which he posed at the beginning of his paper, namely, why was it that Marxists had virtually disregarded, both in theory and in practice, "the subjugation of those women who are not employed in the market sectors of the economy". His failure lies in the fact that by pressing the Marxist argument further than Marx himself took it, he ends up by saying that women as domestic labourers are simply incorporated in the market and in that respect are neither more nor less oppressed by the capitalist system than are men. Hence any discussion of sexual divisions becomes theoretically quite superfluous' (Parry, Johnson 1974:21-3).

In the paper quoted above the point is also made that the divisions within sociology between for example the sociology of social class on the one hand, and the sociology of the family on the other, make it very difficult to provide a unitary perspective for sociology. Both of these sub-disciplines themselves tend to be informed by different ideological positions. The structural functional position has rested very much on the familial ideology whereas the sociology of class and stratification has rested on the market ideology or its Marxian critique. Nevertheless, there is one standpoint which has been predominant in examining the position of women, and which treats seriously the question of inequalities between the sexes: it is, liberalism. For example, Young and Willmott have written about the 'symmetrical family' (Young, Willmott 1973).

'They take the view that where men and women both participate on an equal basis in the market and also in domestic duties, the problem of sexual conflict will be avoided. The implication is that where people adopt the liberal ideology, the woman in particular will become dissatisfied with the relative "unfairness" of her position compared with the man, and it is this sense of "unfairness" which is the basis for sexual conflict. Equality and role-sharing between men and women at home and at work is, for Willmott and Young, both a moral and practical solution to the problem. Fogarty and the Rapoports adopt a similar perspective. They envisage a time when the battle over crude discrimination against women will be won, and there will be no more need for what they call "a women's trade union approach". At that stage, they envisage a shift ". . . towards the idea of a joint enterprise on the part of men and women to revise work and family roles to the advantage of both". They are careful to avoid suggesting their own solution of the dual-career family as the only possible replacement for traditionally segregated sex roles, but they abandon the sociological perspective when they return to the moral stance of the liberal by saying that "each married couple may select the pattern best suited to its own circumstances" [Rapoport 1971:511]. Writers on the family and especially on the "women" question have most frequently taken a liberal stance, and themselves represent the moral motive force for change which they are studying in society. We take the view that liberalism has been the most powerful ideological driving force behind the women question in the last one hundred years, so that legislation on the franchise, on equal pay, on sexual discrimination, are all fundamentally of a piece because they attempt to dismantle special constraints on one group of citizens, namely women, constraints which are not experienced by other citizens (namely men). For the liberal, a person's sex is irrelevant as a criterion for participation in any sphere of social life. For him also, the moral recommendation that each individual ought to have freedom of choice is basic. Whether or not one agrees with this moral principle, one cannot fail to note that writers adopting this liberal position propose a future in which the structural constraints which are fundamental to a sociological perspective are simply waived' (Parry, Johnson 1974:20-21).

The Women's Liberation movement marks a break with liberalism. It has turned instead to more radical social philosophies, such as Marxism. Juliet Mitchell found that the Marxist position did not in her view contain the theoretical apparatus to sustain the critique of society and of women's position in it which she would wish to make. Juliet Mitchell asked,

'is the feminist concept of woman as the most fundamentally oppressed people and hence potentially the most revolutionary to be counterposed to the Marxist position on the working class as *the* revolutionary class under capitalism? If so, with what consequences? What is the relationship between class struggle, and the struggles of the oppressed' (Mitchell 1971:14-15).

These considerations pose a problem for the sociologist. Hitherto the divisions within sociology between branches such as that of class stratification on the one hand, and the family on the other, made it extraordinarily difficult to consider the question of sexual divisions because this particular structural element was reduced to the narrow 'woman question' and this in turn was reduced to an aspect of the sociology of the family. Marxist writers, we have suggested, tend ultimately to reduce the question of sexual inequality exclusively to inequalities of class. Even sophisticated theorists like Giddens find it difficult to break out of this perspective. His recent book may perhaps be interpreted as an attempt to do precisely that. But like most sociological writers, the relationship between sexual divisions and class divisions is treated on the basis of the *ad hoc* introduction of the issue rather than the incorporation of sexual divisions in theoretical terms. The influence of the Marxist position on Giddens' conception is indicated in the following quotation:

> 'given that women still have to await their liberation from the family, it remains the case in the capitalist societies that female workers are largely peripheral to the class system, or, expressed differently, *women are in a sense the "underclass" of the white-collar sector.* They tend to monopolise occupations which not only have a low economic return, but which are lacking in subsidiary economic benefits, have limited security of tenure, and offer little in the way of chances of promotion' (Giddens 1973:288).

The point which we regard as crucial, as we have previously indicated, is that theorists of class tend to abstract class structure from social structure. This is done for excellent heuristic reasons, principally because of the undoubted importance of class as a determining factor within capitalist societies. There is a tendency then to forget that this abstraction has been made and that structural divisions, other that is than those of class, are necessary for a full understanding of the social structure. Our contention is that sexual divisions must be treated as a structural element which stands independently of class divisions but which nevertheless cross-cuts the latter and interacts with it. This interaction is mediated through ideological conceptions including religious ones, particularly those articulated by social movements, and also through the state.

In our study of collective social mobility we attempt to demonstrate the way in which sexual divisions have played an important role in relative success or failure. We would propose that where Giddens speaks of class structure we would wish to extend the concept by introducing the term social structuration. In other words, it is our contention that social structuration is the result of the interaction of more than one structural element. We would not wish in this sense to remain within the narrower limits imposed by the sociology of class and stratification. For example the concept of market capacity, which for Giddens is rooted in property, education and skill and manual labour respectively, is deeply influenced also by the sexual division. The argument about ownership and control in relation to property is sometimes conducted in a manner which leaves aside the idea that women owners are seldom if ever controllers. Within the market for education and skill it is ordinarily the case that equal possession of skill does not confer equal market capacity and even in the context of manual labour, male manual labour is 'more equal' than that of female, irrespective of the fact that among the unskilled there is a fundamental equality shared by all those who lack skill or training, whether men or women, but which is cut through by the sexual

98

division which produces conventionally defined inequalities between the sexes.

Juliet Mitchell recognises that only by reconciling in some way, or transcending the conflicting viewpoints of feminists and Marxist-socialists will it be possible to provide a theoretical basis for the abolition of structured sexual inequalities (Mitchell 1971). We might add to Giddens' contention, *pace* Weber, that legal rational bureaucracy has been, and will remain, the important force in the state socialist societies, the further proposition that sexual divisions have been, and will be a continuing feature of such societies, as they are of ours, and that they will be peculiarly difficult to eradicate (Parry, Johnson 1974). This points up the weakness of Marxian theory as an explanation of sexual divisions and sexual inequalities.

Religion is important to our study because religious ideologies and organised religious groups, particularly churches and denominations, have been influential in the formation of occupations, and have affected occupational strategies and in some cases have hindered or fostered collective social mobility. The religious organisations and their ideological assertions have, under some conditions, been a reinforcement of class divisions and at other times in other ways have cut across them. Religion is relevant to the understanding of class, but within sociology the emergence of increasingly separate sociologies of social class and stratification on the one hand and of religion on the other, both with rather different concerns and foci of interest, has tended to inhibit a thorough theoretical and socio-historical analysis of their relationships. Similarly, sexual divisions in society are recognised to have been powerfully affected by religious prescriptions particularly regarding the role of women. However, the systematic relationship between class divisions, sexual divisions and religion have not, we believe, been given the attention they warrant.

For many years the concept of 'secularisation' was paramount in the sociology of religion. It was asserted that religion was in decline in the Western world and that this decline would be likely to spread over the globe under the impact of industrialisation and urbanisation. A 'secular' trend was discerned in both senses of the word. Today this thesis is coming increasingly under attack and the current view is that while church-orientated religion has been pushed to the periphery of modern society it is being replaced by new religious phenomena. Luckmann is one among those who propose such a revised thesis. He refers to the 'invisible religion' and sums up his position succinctly when he says,

'the social form of religion emerging in modern industrial societies is characterised by the direct accessibility of an assortment of religious representations to potential consumers. The sacred cosmos is mediated neither through a specialized domain of religious institutions nor through other primary public institutions. It is the direct accessibility of the sacred cosmos, more precisely, of an assortment of religious themes, which makes religion today essentially a phenomenon of the "private sphere". The emerging form of religion thus differs significantly from older social forms of religion which were characterized either by the diffusion of the sacred cosmos through the institutional structure of society or through institutional specialization of religion' (Luckmann 1967:103).

From our point of view, however, the change in the 'reach' of institutional or 'church' religion is of great importance because our study is not only sociological but historical, and historically the role of churches and denominations has been very influential. Religious organisations cannot simply be ignored. Like Luckmann, we would reject the view that religious phenomena can be reduced without residue to the economic level, or simply to propositions about 'material interests'. Religion is not just epiphenomenal, a mere 'opium of the people', neither is religion a substitute for cognitive or scientific knowledge. Its role in human society and human history is more than to fill-in while we await the triumph of 'positive science', of cognitive rationality which, it has been asserted, confers upon man not only the power to explain the world but also to control it. Religion has always been, is and will remain an important social force, though its social forms have in our era undergone considerable change.

The relationship between religion and social structure is very different in the West from that which obtains in India. According to Dumont, power and wealth are subordinated in Indian society to the all pervasive religious domination of Hinduism (Dumont 1972). By contrast in Europe, even in the medieval period at a time when Christendom meant more than 'country', the incipient conflict between secular and ecclesiastical power was present. At the Reformation, the conflict was institutionalised in England by the determination of Henry VIII to subordinate the church to the state and church property was sequestered. The dissolution of the monasteries and access to landed property and power and even to positions in the church itself were monopolised by the monarchy and its supporters. This embraced also the key educational institutions. The Catholic church in some parts of Europe, for example in Italy, remained independent of the state and has even retained a rump of temporal power in a restricted territory, the Vatican. Concordats continued to be signed between the Church and various states up until the 1930s.

In England, however, the fragmentation of the theological cosmos produced religious conflict both between Catholic and Protestant groups, and subsequently among Protestants themselves. Catholics were outsiders from the Anglican establishment and so too, subsequently, were those who dissented in a more radically protestant direction from the prevailing orthodoxy. Under these circumstances the process of fragmentation of the 'sacred cosmos' characterised by the concept of

'Christendom' was set in train. Religion had become a divisive force in society willy nilly. The religious conflict between established insiders and outsiders became also, to a great extent, a class conflict. There is evidence that even before the Reformation the small but growing middle class of traders and craftsmen were anxious as much to evade the control of the church as of the state. They began for example to found schools free from ecclesiastical control just as they sought to minimise the control of the crown and of the aristocracy in civic affairs (Gretton 1919). Weber argued that Protestantism in its Calvinist form was particularly powerful as a stimulus to capital accumulation among the *mittelstand* not only in Germany but also in Britain and the United States.

Hill has paid particular attention to the Halévy thesis (Hill 1973:183-203). This suggests that Methodism in the eighteenth and early nineteenth centuries was class based, but because of the fact that it was an 'enthusiastic' and actively proselytising form of Anglicanism, which had been pushed out of a moribund established church, it retained and further developed a role as mediator between the state plus the established landed order and the great mass of ordinary people. It provided a link between the governing class and the politically excluded middle and working classes. Also, among the sympathisers with Methodism who remained within the Anglican Communion there was formed the nucleus of the Evangelical movement. This served to produce among the governing class a degree of acceptance and even of legitimation of Methodism. Eventually, by extension, the process of legitimation came to include other dissenting groups, and even Catholics. The political movement leading to the Reform Bill of 1834 involved not only an attack by Protestants outside the Anglican Communion upon a state apparatus which they regarded as corrupt and unrepresentative, but an attack also on the corrupt and moribund Anglican Church. The Evangelical revival however was able to secure rapid progress from within Anglicanism itself towards the reform of the Church in the late 1830s. This matched the reforms introduced in the political sphere by the Reform Bill of 1834. The struggle between the Anglican Church and Nonconformity was quickly reduced to a battle principally in the sphere of education. Keeping or extending control over the hearts and minds of the young was regarded as absolutely crucial to the maintenance and extension of Church or Nonconformist influence in the future. It was regarded as the important base which must at all costs be secured. Hence, the teachers found themselves at the forefront of religious and class struggles. On the other hand supervisory and licencing functions in medicine had passed from the control of the church in the early eighteenth century. The reach of the church had already contracted.

Halévy regards the mediating influence of Methodism and of the Evangelicals as crucial in explaining why there was no revolution in

England in the late eighteenth century or even in the difficult years of the early nineteenth century. He had in mind the contrast with France after 1789. Hill reports that Halévy also poses the possibility that religious affiliation was important in providing avenues for social mobility, a question which has not really been researched historically (Hill 1973:186). Certainly, the Marxian dictum that 'religion is the opium of the people' takes on a different interpretation from that provided by a crude materialist reductionism when it is seen in the context of the religious history of a period which Marx, like Halévy, studied intensively.

After 1834 there was an important sense in which the Anglican Church was no longer established 'in fact' even if it remained so in name. The Nonconformist and Catholic vote, Nonconformist personalities and policies especially in Whig (Liberal) administrations, forced governments, even Tory governments, to become more even-handed in their approach to the religious question. It could no longer be a case of the Anglican ascendency right or wrong. The importance of Methodism and Nonconformity in the early Trade Union movement is stressed by Halévy. The continuing predominance of Anglicanism in much of rural England was also bound to find political expression. The rise of a labour element in the Liberal party and eventually the emergence of the Labour party itself also brought a religious articulation to class divisions.

In England in the twentieth century the decline in the 'reach' of religious organisations has quickened, particularly in the decades since the Second World War. More especially, the fact that the state has directly taken over much of the educational work of the churches and denominations which, in the nineteenth century, had been given increasing financial help from the state, has reinforced the tendency for the churches and denominations to be pushed to the periphery of society. The shift from the central place of the Church of England in the national life which it had retained even in the late nineteenth century to the minor place it occupies today, is charted by a decline in the number of ordinands coming forward to be trained as priests. Also the fall in social status of ordinands, as measured by occupation of father, has been considerable (Coxon 1964). The supply of those coming from public schools has virtually dried up and the Church has been forced to accept a debasement in the 'coinage of status' so far as its recruits are concerned. Late vocations were tapped as a source after the Second World War, and the acceptance of women for ordination has been more insistently pressed for during the last decade. It is a solution which other sects and denominations have long tried, some on theological grounds, but others as a matter of sheer survival. Sexual divisions are thus bound up with organised religion.

Class variations in church attendance have long been confirmed by a number of studies, but the fact is that the working class are not merely unchurched because of the failure of the churches, such as the Church of England, to adapt its age-old parish system to an urban environment (with the consequence that even today the distribution of ministers and churches favours rural areas), but that as the working class participate in all types of association far less than the middle class, there is little likelihood of a revival by the established church. Sectarian movements particularly of a millenarian kind, are usually found among the dispossessed, the lower classes of society. Currently, such religious movements are not a major force in English society. In Northern Ireland, however, the religious division does interact explosively with the class division and has been a major factor in sectarian power struggles with specifically political objectives. In this case the Marxian argument that 'religion' is epiphenominal (part of the superstructure of society) and class the phenominal element (the economic base), seems to oversimplify the problem of the relationship between class and religion.

The fact is that religion, where it is institutionalised and where its latent power is harnessed in religious organisations, can and does influence market capacity. Opportunities in relation to the ownership and control of property, education and skill as well as manual labour can be markedly influenced by religion. It has frequently been an important element in social structuration, and was particularly important in the development of the modern teaching occupations.

We have now reached the point where the major theoretical and conceptual approach of our study of collective social mobility and social structure is concluded. In the next part, we turn to the study of a particular case, that of the doctors, which we have chosen as a test of our theory and concepts. The case of the medical profession affords us material by means of which we can examine the process of occupational closure and collective social mobility in relation to facilitating and constraining elements of social structure, and allows us the better to understand the efforts of men and women to influence and control collectively the social worlds in which they act out their lives.

6. FROM APOTHECARY TO GENERAL PRACTITIONER: A SUCCESSFUL STRUGGLE FOR UPWARD ASSIMILATION AND OCCUPATIONAL CLOSURE, 1790–1858

The historical context: class and status divisions

In 1800 the medical profession consisted of three separate orders; physicians, surgeons, and apothecaries. In theory the three orders exemplified a system of closed status groups inherited from the earlier estate type of social structure. Each had its own function defined in law and maintained by legal sanctions; its own forms of education, tests of competence and its own corporate body. These were respectively the Royal College of Physicians, the Royal College of Surgeons and the Worshipful Company of Apothecaries. Only gradually was the rigid distinction between the ranks broken down. At first this happened between the apothecaries and surgeons, though it was still the case in the late eighteenth century that an apothecary would have to give up his membership of Apothecaries' Hall before he could obtain the licence of the Surgeons' Company. Even as late as the 1830s surgeons and apothecaries were still required to give up membership of their own qualifying bodies before they could be admitted as licentiates of the Royal College of Physicians.

In practice the system of 'orders' was itself breaking down as part of the general decay of guild control over occupations. By the latter years of the eighteenth century the doctrines of *laissez faire* were becoming increasingly influential in English society. The industrial revolution, the growth of commerce and the development of transport were creating a national orientation which burst asunder the remnants of the ancient but highly localised guild system and transformed also the balance between town and country, metropolis and provinces. These factors, together with the rapid growth in population and a shift in the centre of gravity, both of population and industry to the new and dynamic cities of the North and the Midlands, were of enormous importance. The effects on medical practice were several; the gradual breakdown of the control exercised by the traditional orders was matched by the rise of a new phenomenon, the general practitioner, who defied the compartmentalised structure represented by the system of orders. The expansion of the middle class and the growth of their incomes produced a massive increase in the market for medical care which was the basis for this development (Franklin 1950:1-2).

Nevertheless the market for medical services in England during this period continued to be dominated at the higher end, as it had traditionally been, by fellows of the Royal College of Physicians. They were normally graduates and typically recruited from among the second sons of the gentry, or the sons of clergy. Physicians managed to exercise a virtual monopoly in the market for the medical care of the rich. In fact the number of physicians, recognised by the Royal College in London was very small, just a few hundred in a population of about eight and a quarter million. These men practised almost exclusively in the big cities, chiefly in London. The fees that could be charged were high — fifty guineas for a visit to the country was not out of the way — and successful practitioners could amass large fortunes. The Royal College of Physicians was not only exclusive but judged by some to be moribund. The physicians themselves were divided into two grades, the fellows and the mere licentiates. Few of the latter could make a living by giving advice alone. By 1834 there were thought to be about 120 physicians in London and an equal number in various parts of England and Wales who were sufficiently secure financially to limit their practice to giving advice and writing prescriptions only (Holloway 1964:307). There were many persons with university degrees practising in the provinces whose work was largely comprised of surgery, midwifery and even pharmacy. This was especially true in Northern England because of the number of physicians with Scottish degrees who were in general practice.

The clash between physicians educated in Scotland and the Royal College of Physicians in London was already a source of conflict in the eighteenth century. The continued pressure from this quarter contributed to the breakdown of the traditional medical orders in England. In Scotland the universities, unlike those in England, already had flourishing centres engaged in the development of scientific medicine. The influence of new developments emanating from the continent, at first from Leydon and later from Paris, were important in creating a new type of physician who had trained not only in medicine, but also in surgery and pharmacy. During the second half of the eighteenth century increasing numbers of physicians who had qualified in Scotland began to come to England in order to find suitable locations for practice. Some Englishmen who sought a good medical education went to Scotland to train, although most subsequently returned to practise in England. Edinburgh did not simply offer a good medical education; it offered a medical education of a type quite new in Britain involving the integration of a wide range of medical and allied subjects. As early as 1739 'students at Edinburgh were given instruction not only in all the main branches of medicine, but also in anatomy and surgery, botany, chemistry as applied to pharmacy, and midwifery' (Waddington 1973:14). These well-trained doctors could by no means secure an adequate livelihood simply by treating the wealthy. They began to enter general practice based principally on the market offered by the rising middle class, though they also gave their services to those rather less well off, through the mechanism of the differential fee. The better off patients were expected to pay higher fees than the poor, and for this purpose the doctor attempted to make some assessment of the ability of each individual patient or family to pay. Scottish physicians were not however formally recognised in England. Nevertheless the fact that there was a chaotic lack of organisation or control of medical practice enabled Scotsmen to settle and practice in England without undue interference. Many of them were concentrated in the North but some were to be found in every part of the country. Those who came to London often tried to obtain the recognition of the Royal College of Physicians or the Company of Surgeons. Both of these colleges were themselves internally divided on a hierarchical basis. We have already noted that during the development of the Royal College of Physicians a distinction had grown up between the fellows on the one hand and the lower status members on the other. Political offices and decision-making functions within the College were monopolised by the fellows, almost all of whom were graduates of Oxford and Cambridge. These alone were allowed to vote at elections. The licentiates had none of these privileges but held only a licence to practise medicine in an area, seven miles around London. Waddington provides evidence that the conflict between the licentiates and fellows became particularly acute in 1767-71 and can be seen as the first sign of 'a long series of movements [among] general practitioners to achieve a recognised and respectable position within the profession'. It is not the case that, at this time, the increasing number of graduates who were licentiates actually saw themselves as general practitioners. They aimed to get themselves incorporated as fully-fledged fellows of the Royal College in London. First and foremost they wanted to be accepted as physicians. In fact, however, they were already engaged in general practice whether they were conscious of it or not and their origins in the Scottish situation, where little distinction was made between physician and surgeon, was a basis for this new mode of practice. Waddington suggests that 'general practitioner consciousness' was not a product of the eighteenth century but rather of the nineteenth. He argues that it was not merely the development of the general practitioner as such which was the cause of the internal struggle in the Colleges but also the wider political attack on privilege which was an essential part of the radical movement in the late eighteenth century; a movement which was directed at the institutions of the state and the church. What the licentiates were demanding was essentially full membership of their professional community just as the radicals demanded full membership of the political community.

This was to be the subsequent basis for the reform movement in medicine which centred around the increasing consciousness and organisation of the general practitioner. The Scottish practitioners formed an important and somewhat militant element among those who wished to reform the Royal College in London. The Scottish combination of good educational facilities in medicine, which was in such sharp contrast to the English case, was combined with a relative ease of access to training and also a lack of distinction between the traditional ranks in medicine. These factors made a medical career very attractive as an avenue of individual social mobility in Scotland. It is paradoxical that a high standard of education existed along-side the opportunity to obtain a degree in a rather lax manner. It was still possible, for example, simply to buy a degree from the University of Glasgow without the drudgery of study. While it was still the case therefore that a Scottish degree did not guarantee competence, yet in most cases Scottish physicians who had attended university, were usually much better educated in medical terms than their exclusive English counterparts.

In the rise of the modern professions during the nineteenth century, tensions between the metropolis and the provinces were a key factor. The guild system had been organised on the basis of local commercial and trading ties, whereas increasingly the nation was becoming the theatre of operations for commerce, industry and the professions. The Colleges in London and the Society of Apothecaries were institutions moulded in the guild tradition and were essentially local in the scope of their legal powers. The decay of earlier forms of licensing in the provinces was the principal reason for the chaotic situation which obtained in 1800. During the nineteenth century the movement towards a national system of control often sprang from the tensions generated by the metropolitan-provincial axis. In the case of the apothecaries, some movements for reform had their origins in London and some sprang up in the provincial context. The English/Scottish differences also played a key role. In spite of antipathies between reform movements which had their origins in London or the provinces, the development of national systems of occupational control required, at some stage, that there would be the co-operation or acquiescence of one or other of the parties involved.

At the beginning of the nineteenth century the main problems of the apothecaries flowed from the breakdown of licensing and regulation by local guilds and societies. Medical practice, particularly in the provinces, was almost completely unorganised. The three London medical corporations 'were merely guilds with powers to regulate their members resident in London'. In practice even such powers as they possessed were ineffective and little used. As Holloway puts it 'administrative difficulties, partly the result of the sudden growth of the new industrial towns, and a doctrinaire belief in the efficacy of free competition to ensure the interest of the consumer, led to the decay of these guilds and of the mediaeval system of local regulation' (Holloway 1966:114). Yet it was widely believed that these corporations had significant power to regulate the medical occupations if they chose to use it. In fact the Society of Apothecaries, as Champney pointed out (Champney

1797:123), did not even have the monopoly of title; anyone in England could quite legally call himself an apothecary and also prescribe if he chose to do so.

It was under these circumstances that the General Pharmaceutical Association was founded in 1794. It was the creation of several leading London apothecaries and it began at a meeting in the Crown and Anchor in the Strand. The meeting was attended by some 200 people. They were concerned with the hardships currently suffered by the apothecaries, including the problems of taxation and rent, as well as the increase in the price of the materials which formed the basis of medicines. The fear was expressed at the meeting that the trade of apothecary was being threatened by the competition of the chemist and druggist. The importance of the gathering was 'that it was the first expression of the growing group-consciousness of the new general practitioner in England. For the first time town and country apothecaries co-operated in defending their common interests. Moreover by appealing to the legislature to protect those interests, they anticipated future movements' (Holloway 1966:111). Holloway argues that the General Pharmaceutical Association was a reactionary body in that it looked to the past in the hope of reasserting the monopoly in the sale of drugs which historically had been the exclusive preserve of the Society of Apothecaries. It was, however, the comparative neglect of dispensing by the apothecaries themselves which was the main reason for the emergence of the druggist and chemist. Rather than helping in re-establishing their former privileges the attack by the apothecaries caused a reaction among the druggists who began in turn a movement for their own protection. This was to lead eventually to the creation of the Royal Pharmaceutical Society (1841). The apothecaries' future lay in the general practice of medicine and not in pharmacy. It was a trend which was already clearly discernible by the late eighteenth century.

In terms of status the apothecaries were the lowest of the medical orders. It is for this reason that it is more difficult to find out the background from which they were recruited. As Newman says, 'the humble apothecary was not so biographied as his more conspicuous colleague (the physician)' (Newman 1957:21). Dickens, in *Martin Chuzzlewit,* wrote that 'no medical practitioner was actually resident in the village but a poor apothecary who was also a grocer and a general dealer'. The novel of the period, as both Holloway and Newman recognise, is one of the best sources for understanding the situation of the apothecary. Observations about the medical men of the day and their circumstances are contained in the works of Trollope and Jane Austen, and are confirmed by Thackeray, George Elliot and Mrs Gaskell. Drawing on his study of these writers Newman says that 'the apothecary by and large, came from the stratum of society from which a fundamentally shopkeeping order would have come, the shopkeepers and other lower middle class groups, combined with the rather higher stratum of what might be called the depressed middle class, the younger sons, the sons of curates or of village schoolteachers' (1957:21). He goes on to say that some came from good families and that others were the sons of respectable craftsmen. Newman also suggests that the aristocracy and the gentry still preferred their medical attendants to be on a footing with servants. As a humble shopkeeper the apothecary would sell toothbrushes, hairbrushes, perfumery as well as drugs. His education was practical and the method of training him was naturally the same as in other mercantile trades: apprenticeship. This was designed to teach the apprentice 'the trade, the art, the mystery or business [no nonsense about 'profession' be it noted] of a Surgeon Apothecary and Man-Midwife' (Newman 1957:22-3).

The aim of an apothecary's education was wholly practical even in the matter of learning some Latin, for this enabled him to read the prescriptions written by the physician. His was a lower place; he was neither expected to be much learned nor in any way to trespass upon the prerogatives of the physician. The position of the apothecary in the provision of medical services was flanked by the physician on the one side and by the new pretenders, the druggists and chemists on the other. An important stimulus in the efforts of the apothecaries to control their situation arose from the threat of unqualified practice from below.

One contemporary observer wrote 'within the last thirty-five years, a new order, the dispensing druggist or chemist has arisen, which is very similar to what the apothecary was a century and a half ago' (Gray 1818). He also says that they do not scruple to advise, prescribe or manage cases where they 'inadvertently' have been called in. Gray noted that chemists' and druggists' shops 'are in general confounded with those of apothecaries'. The only noticeable difference was that the contemporary apothecary specialised more in medical practice, whereas the chemist or druggist was principally engaged in the retail and dispensing side of the business. Although prescribing across the counter was widespread it was generally confined to that location. Certainly the latter part of the eighteenth century was a golden age for quackery. What was objected to by qualified practitioners was the evasion of a long and expensive education. It has been said that at the time there had been so little useful medicine in a doctor's training that its absence was of minor importance and at bottom, 'a charlatan was not one who has been insufficiently taught, but one who is not sufficiently scrupulous' (Newman 1957:58). Nevertheless unqualified pretenders were said to exceed the qualified in the proportion of nine to one. The threat from this quarter to the livelihood of regular apothecaries was a great stimulus to the reform of medical education.

In 1806 Harrison reported specifically that diplomas were rather freely given away and that a great many men were too easily becoming doctors. It was the view of many apothecaries 'that the profession was overcrowded [and] that the emoluments of doctors were reduced by dilution' (Newman 1957:58). In addition there were the effects of the Napoleonic wars; the needs of the Army and Navy for medical men were not met as they were in France by increasing the facilities for medical education but by 'mobilising the half qualified'. It was felt that dangerous imposters were sharing the rightful medical market of the qualified practitioners and that quantities of empirical medicines were being sold without reference to the apothecary. 'Thus the apothecaries, the largest order of medical practitioners, began to feel themselves encroached on from below. The result was that when unqualified practice grew to sufficient proportions the apothecaries felt that something should be done' (1957:58).

Whereas the physicians were in the main concentrated in London, the apothecaries were spreading throughout the country and local societies or associations were set up for benevolent or study purposes. The significance of these local societies was to be considerable. By the beginning of the nineteenth century, the Royal College of Physicians, comprehending the problem and fearing the rise of the new 'general practitioners', put forward a proposal to extend its powers of control over all types of medical practice in England and Wales (1806). The suggested Bill covered not merely physicians, surgeons and apothecaries but also chemists and druggists. It was intended to assert the control of the Royal College of Physicians throughout England and Wales and over all the various grades of medical practitioner. The intention was to strengthen and even extend the system of antiquated hierarchical orders in the face of the disintegration which had become increasingly apparent during the course of the previous half century. Legislation was intended which could form the basis for appropriate administrative action to stop, what the College regarded, as the 'decay of authority'. Although the Bill was soon put aside, 'the ideas behind it endured and guided the policy of the College throughout the agitation [which led up to] the Apothecaries' Act' (Holloway 1966:115).

Among the apothecaries the plans of the Associated Faculty are of great interest because they so clearly envisage collective social mobility as an object of policy. They looked forward to the reservation of places in the profession to 'youths of reputable birth, and liberal education' and sought to prevent the admission of 'mean and low persons'. Harrison, in particular, was concerned that 'since admission into the faculties of divinity and law have been regulated with greater circumspection young men of humble birth and little wealth have been drawn into the medical profession to its great detriment' (Harrison 1810:28-43). It was his hope that in the case of physicians none but those with the resources to qualify at a university would be admitted to practice, and even then not before attaining the age of twenty-four.

Harrison drafted a bill which did not receive much encouragement from the existing licensing authorities. Indeed those in Scotland and Ireland were positively hostile. A revised version (1808) contained provision for a medical register listing the names of all those qualified as physicians, surgeons, apothecaries, midwives, veterinary practitioners, chemists, druggists and vendors of medicines. Each registered person was to pay an annual fee and none other than they would be allowed to practice. The notions of merit and self-help were (interestingly) very much to the fore. As against the virtually impermeable estate-like divisions of the 'orders' a central place was given to the concept of freedom to move from one grade of practice to another, subject only to passing the appropriate examinations. As Holloway wryly remarks 'such a concept was the very reverse of the ideas which informed the College of Physicians' Bill of 1806' (Holloway 1966:118). It was thus not unnatural that the College stated that the bill was 'highly objectionable' and that they would oppose it. As they put it 'the real design and tendency of Dr Harrison's proposal are less directed towards the amelioration of medical practice than to the subversion of the existing authorities in Physic, and the depression of the rights, the rank, and the importance of the Physician'. Worn down by the implacable opposition of the College, Harrison in 1811 gave up his attempt to reform the profession.

In 1812 a meeting of London apothecaries was held to protest against the new tax on glass bottles. Another Edinburgh graduate, Anthony Todd Thomson, who had a large general practice in London, turned the attention of the meeting to the subject of medical reform. An association of apothecaries and surgeon-apothecaries was set up which tapped the same grievances as the former General Pharmaceutical Association. In its first report threats from unlicensed practitioners as well as from druggists were mentioned as well as 'the degradation of the apothecary from a gentleman to a tradesman by the mode in which he is remunerated'. A Bill was drafted in 1813 which was, in effect, a compromise between the College of Physicians' and Harrison's Bills respectively. None of the established medical corporations would have anything to do with the proposed Bill. But the Association pressed forward and obtained a first reading in the House of Commons. At once the masks dropped from the faces of the Royal Colleges: they opposed the Bill. Similarly, the chemists and druggists, aroused by the fear of medical control which the Bill threatened — from the direction of Apothecaries' Hall — did likewise. The Associated Apothecaries then quickly dropped the clause referring to control over the chemists and druggists; they also bought off the surgeons by agreeing that all surgeon-apothecaries must obtain the membership of the Royal College of Surgeons before practising surgery. In addition they withdrew the proposal that general practitioners would sit on the superintending body which the Bill proposed as the regulatory organ of the profession. Informed of the changes, the apothecaries said they could not contemplate action except in concert with the College of Physicians. It was at this stage that the physicians decided to act. Fearing the passage

111

of a Bill inimical to their interests, they worked quickly in conjunction with the Apothecaries' Company. The latter was so subservient in its attitude to the physicians that it offered not merely to bring in a Bill designed to accord with the physicians' interests but, in the event, introduced it with a set of clauses drafted by the Royal College itself. After further delays and considerable manoeuvering a final Bill was introduced (1815) which simply confirmed, with minor amendments, the original patent of James I. This had separated the Apothecaries' Company from the grocers and from the standpoint of the nineteenth century it was very retrogressive. The one major innovation was the extension of the power of the Apothecaries' Company from London only to the whole of England and Wales. This applied both to its right of search of apothecaries' shops (although not the shops of chemists and druggists) and also its important function as a qualifying association. A significant proviso was that the Act was in no way to affect the existing privileges of the Royal Colleges or of the universities of Oxford and Cambridge.

The Apothecaries' Act has been regarded by some commentators as an important reform to which may be attributed the rapid improvement in the standards of medical education and practice during the first half of the nineteenth century. Newman went so far as to argue that it could more properly be ranked with the series of great reforming Acts which followed on after the watershed of the Reform Bill itself (1832). He regards it, in this sense, as curiously misplaced coming as it did in that earlier period. We accept the alternative view which has been most cogently argued by Holloway. He notes that the reaction of those in the medical reform movement itself to the 1815 Act 'was not one of triumph but of dismay' (Holloway 1966:127); it represented a profound setback to the reform movement and a considerable victory to the College of Physicians. Although the attempts of the latter to gain complete control over the medical profession in England had failed in 1806 yet, it remained either aloof or hostile to the reform movement from below. The rapid change of position at the end of 1813 was caused by the fear that the reformers would achieve their objectives in spite of the medical corporations. It was for this reason that instead of opposing the 1815 Bill, it decided 'to mould it into compliance with the principles held by the College' (Holloway 1966:127). If the college itself could not institute its direct control throughout England and Wales, it would work to maintain the shackles of the outdated Charter of King James upon general practitioners throughout the country. To this end it negotiated with and used the Society of Apothecaries, even utilising sections of their charter *verbatim*. Holloway suggests that this charter which 'separated the apothecaries from the grocers had three aspects which appealed to the College of Physicians. It emphasised the humble origins of the Apothecaries' Society; it stressed both the guild and trading activities of the Company; and, above all, it placed the Society under the tutelage of the College of Physicians' (1966:127). Not content with this, the College further insisted that the Act should make it an offence for apothecaries to refuse to compound physicians' prescriptions. By drawing attention to the retail aspects of the apothecaries' work it challenged their pretensions to the status of a learned profession and this was reinforced by the insistence on the retention of a five-year apprenticeship which was a very controversial matter. Apprenticeship after all was 'the time-honoured qualification for membership of a trade of craft guild' (1966:128). It remained the central element in the apothecaries' education.

> 'The general practitioners' demand for an Act of Parliament to further their advancement was so skilfully manipulated by the College of Physicians that the Act ultimately passed tended to degrade rather than to elevate the rank and file of the profession. The general practitioner was subjected to the direct control of a London mercantile company, still largely engaged in the whole-sale drug trade, and to the indirect supervision of the College of Physicians, whose policy was to make permanent the subordinate and inferior status of the apothecary' (Holloway 1966:128).

As we have noted there are two distinctly opposing views about the consequences of the Apothecaries' Act. Several distinguished writers have judged the Act to be an important reforming measure and a major cause of the rapid improvement in medical education. Holloway, on the contrary, argues that the Act and its consequences were retrogressive. He suggests too that the connection between this measure and the reform of medical education was much slighter than has been supposed. In his view, the powerful influence of the Royal College of Physicians caused the Act to have a much closer 'affinity to a Stuart patent of monopoly than to a statute in the age of *laissez faire*'. The achievement of the physicians was to maintain 'the ancient hierarchical structure of the medical profession, and the apothecary's inferior status within it' (1966:221). Far from being hungry to gain additional powers the Apothecaries' Company were unprepared for the extension of privileges and duties thrust upon them. The hasty passage of the Bill based on the sudden move of the Royal College of Physicians from opposition to sponsorship meant that a number of clauses were loosely drawn and their subsequent meaning was left to be decided in the courts of law. Even the functions of the apothecary were not clearly stipulated and it was only in 1834 that Justice Cresswell defined an apothecary as 'one who professes to judge of internal disease by its symptoms and applies himself to cure that disease by medicine' (1966:222). The major effect of the Act was that general practitioners whether they be physicians, surgeons or apothecaries would henceforth be required by law to take the examinations of the Company of Apothecaries. It was only the elite of physicians and surgeons, who were able to make a living simply by giving advice or specialising in surgery alone, who were exempt from this obligation. All but a few medical practitioners in England Wales would henceforth be obliged to be licentiates of the Apothecaries' Company. Scottish physicians were by now, as we have observed, practising in considerable numbers in England. They were equally obliged if they were practising generally (as most were) to obtain the Apothecaries' Licence. This point was made in 1831 by the Report of the Royal Commission of Inquiry into the state of the universities of Scotland (Royal Commission 1831:66). There is considerable evidence that great resentment was aroused by this requirement of the Apothecaries' Act among the majority of medical practitioners. One writer made the point in the following way: 'it does not seem quite so reasonable that, because the apothecaries have ceased to be grocers, that they should be forthwith invested with the entire regulation of the practice of medicine in England.' He goes on 'a mercantile company originally instituted for the sale of certain commodities, and whose chief business that still continues to be, would not seem to be the fittest authority in which to confide the superintendence of one of the liberal professions, and the power of saying who shall, and who shall not, be permitted to enter it'. There was a particular dislike among general practitioners of the fact that the connection with the mercantile company implied 'that the general practitioner was a tradesman, not a member of a learned profession' (Holloway 1966:224). They objected to the statutory obligation to enter a five-year apprenticeship and thought of this as a hindrance to a more appropriate course of secondary education which would include classical and general knowledge. Such a course was regarded as more appropriate to a gentleman than apprenticeship which involved service behind the counter of a shop from the age of fourteen or fifteen. Secondary education on the other hand would continue full time until about eighteen or nineteen years of age. The apprenticeship clause was, as we have noted, particularly hard on the Scottish-trained physicians who by law would have to submit themselves to five-year apprenticeships. This created an important grievance for such practitioners, especially as the statute was not left in abeyance where they were concerned. In 1833 a court ruling specifically found that a qualification from a Scottish university to practice as a physician did not exempt a man from the relevant clauses of the Apothecaries' Act. Letters were issued from Apothecaries' Hall to Scottish licentiates making this point. Equally, qualified surgeons found themselves in a similar position after a judgement of 1828. This was reinforced by a judgement of 1843 which stipulated that in cases of internal disease, where surgical treatment was not required, a surgeon had no legal right to administer medicines. Holloway concludes that 'the Apothecaries' Act proved a major obstacle to the improvement of the general practitioner's status'. He goes on

'this was precisely the result foreseen by the Royal College of Physicians when they agreed to the introduction of the Act, and when later they resolutely insisted upon the inclusion of the apprenticeship clause despite the desire of the Apothecaries' Company and the House of Commons to delete it. The [Royal] College of Physicians had successfully diverted a movement, which sought to advance the general practitioner, into an Act which chained him to the lowest order of the medical profession' (Holloway 1966:227).

The avowed intention of the Act was to prevent unqualified practice which was a danger to the King's subjects, but judged in those terms it was a peculiarly ineffective piece of legislation. The provisions of the Act applied only to England and Wales and not to Scotland or Ireland but those persons who could demonstrate that they were practising prior to its introduction were exempt from its provisions. From the outset it was clearly anomolous that well-qualified graduates from Scotland or Ireland or members of the College of Surgeons were excluded from practice in England and Wales but were freely permitted to exercise their skills elsewhere in the King's domains. Such men could serve in the East India Company, or in the Army and Navy, where their qualifications were recognised. Perhaps even more surprisingly chemists and druggists, whose practices were not clearly distinguishable from those of apothecaries, were also exempt because of the pressure this group had brought to bear prior to the passage of the measure through the House. It was not until 1841 that a chemist was convicted for attending the sick and providing them with medicines, which was then interpreted as contrary to the legislation of 1815. Much later, in the 1870s, it was decided in a court of law that a chemist who prescribed medicine in his shop and sold it to customers was also infringing the provisions of the Apothecaries' Act. Holloway's conclusion is that while the Act deterred many highly qualified medical men from working as general practitioners, yet it failed to prevent the unqualified from flourishing. It was not merely that the Apothecaries' Company seemed dilatory in its policy of prosecutions of the unqualified, but that it was most difficult to prove a case in the courts. The two factors may not have been unrelated.

A major problem for the practitioner in establishing his professional status was that as an apothecary the law allowed him to charge for medicines only and not for attendance. He was thus 'considered a tradesman in an age when trade was regarded as a debased occupation' (Holloway 1966:230). Prior to the Act it had been an object of the medical reform movement to change this situation; it did not do so. Only in 1829 was a legal decision given which stated that an apothecary could choose to charge for medicines or for attendance but not for both. A year later, in another case, the decision made it possible for an apothecary to recover fees for attendance as well as charges for medicines. The *Lancet* was eulogistic about this judgement, 'general practitioners have been raised a thousand degrees in the scale of professional usefulness and respectability, and ten thousand degrees in the estimation of society' (*Lancet* 1830:538). The decision was reaffirmed in the result of another case in 1838 but Scottish trained medical graduates and also surgeons still remained unaffected by these decisions. Holloway's overall conclusion is that contemporary opinion may be more valid in this case than the retrospective judgement of twentieth-century historians. In summing up the position he says:

> 'the 1815 Act sought to perpetuate the obsolete hierarchical structure of the medical profession; it placed the general practitioner under the supervision of a London mercantile company and tied him to a system of education more suited to a trade than to a liberal profession; it failed to protect him from the competition of the unqualified and did nothing to change the degrading system by which he was remunerated; above all, it deterred many of the more highly qualified members of the profession from acting as general practitioners' (Holloway 1966:232).

Finally, Holloway affirms that simply because the reform of medical education took place after the Apothecaries' Act, this in itself is no reason to conclude, without further study, that the Act was the cause of educational reform in medicine. In fact it has been overrated in that regard. The system of apprenticeship frustrated efforts to provide a sound secondary education for surgeon-apothecaries and only with the regulations drawn up in 1835 was it the case that the apothecaries' examination became most comprehensive in London, comparing favourably even with the Scottish universities. Certainly, the Society may rightly claim that its examinations were very well run on a modern basis after that date, but the College of Surgeons obtained 'an even higher standard in its inspection and recognition of hospitals and medical schools' (1966:233-4). There remained great weaknesses in the apothecary's curriculum. For example, they were not empowered to examine in midwifery, a subject essential to the work of every general practitioner. The Society went as far as they could in modifying the apprenticeship rule which was enjoined on them by the 1815 Act; they allowed time spent in hospital training to count towards the total period spent in apprenticeship.

The Royal College of Surgeons must have at least an equal claim to recognition in the matter of the advance of medical education. The number of candidates taking their examination between 1823-33 was only slightly fewer than those taking the examinations of Apothecaries' Hall. This situation obtained in spite of the fact that there was no legal requirement for practitioners to become members of the College of Surgeons whereas such a requirement was mandatory in the case of the apothecaries. The College of Surgeons had no monopoly or power to prosecute but its diploma carried the signatures of many leading surgeons in London and established itself a *sine qua non* for all those who had serious intentions of entering reputable medical practice. Holloway suggests that 'it would be equally legitimate to argue that the medical schools which were organised in the period after 1815 were established to prepare candidates for the examinations of the College of Surgeons as for those of the Apothecaries' Society' (Holloway 1966:235). While recognising the significance of his interpretation, it might be considered that Holloway places too little importance upon one consequence of the 1815 Act. The College of Surgeons may well have been stimulated to reform their own examination requirements by the competition and example deriving from Apothecaries' Hall. Reader makes the point in the following way: 'by 1834 the Apothecaries' system ... [had] no doubt reacted sharply on the Surgeons, who also set about tightening up their educational requirements and examinations' (Reader 1966:53).

The Doctors' Registration Movement

It was during the 1820s that Thomas Wakley, the leading member of this movement, together with his co-worker in Parliament, Mr Warburton, generated a new conception of a unified and self-governing profession which would include the general practitioner and would involve the destruction of the ancient medical corporations which symbolised the conception of medical practice divided into hierarchical orders: physicians, surgeons and apothecaries (Sprigge 1899). These activities took place in the same social climate as the wider reform movement which led to the great Reform Bill of 1832 and to the simultaneous attacks upon the established church and legal institutions. The idea of self-governing professionalism was at the same time being vigorously pressed in other occupations. 'The engineer and the surveyor, the accountant and actuary, the manager and administrator were all developing pretensions to rank with the older professions, and in varying degrees were making good their claim' (Holloway 1964:321). In great part the doctors' registration movement was an attempt to remove the subordination of the rising general practitioner to the 'superior' high status physician. Although Wakley specifically set out to destroy the medical corporations the mass of ordinary medical practitioners wanted only to acquire an acknowledged rank in society equal to that of the fellows of the Royal College of Physicians. But the destruction of the hierarchy of rank which was represented by the medical corporations was to the reformers, a prerequisite to this. The connection between the craft of surgery and the lower status of the craftsmen in society generally precluded the surgeon from being fully recognised as a gentleman. This was a central issue.

Similarly the connection of the apothecary with trade prevented the new practitioners from being fully acknowledged as 'gentleman'. Unlike the agitation which led to the reform of Parliament or the movement to reform or even to disestablish the Church of England, the issue of the reform of the medical corporations was not one which had any immediate impact on the public. Even the better informed middle class was simply ignorant of conditions obtaining in, for example, medical education. It was for this reason that Wakley and Warburton engineered the establishment of the Select Committee on Medical Education of the House of Commons (1832). The Committee decided to publish an account of their proceedings in full, precisely so that the whole background would become available publicly. The representatives of the medical corporations condemned themselves out of their own mouths in so much as they were forced under questioning to agree at one and the same time that there was a great deal wrong in the existing state of affairs, but equally that no better system could be devised. They put themselves in a position where they were forced to take the posture of reactionaries defending an indefensible *status quo*. Wakley used the journal of which he was editor (the *Lancet*) as a platform from which to launch vigorous attacks upon the medical establishment. After the publication of the Report of the Select Committee, he became a well-known radical reforming figure and on the strength of this was himself elected to Parliament in 1835. He and the reformers devoted all their energies in the decade of the 1830s to raising the consciousness of both the public and medical men about the abuses inherent in the system of medical corporations.

In 1840 the first Bill for medical registration was introduced. It contained clauses not only for the registration of all medical practitioners based upon examinations (numerous existing qualifying associations were listed as well as others which did not yet have the privilege) but also set out to establish a College of Medicine 'enabling the Fellows of that College to practise medicine in all or any of its branches and hold any medical appointment in the United Kingdom' (Newman 1957:155). The Bill failed because it raised the opposition of each of the medical corporations who were opposed to the very idea of a unified profession in which all practitioners would have a formally equal status before the law. Seventeen years were to pass and seventeen bills were to be presented to the House before a Medical Act was passed in 1858. The political process, by which the medical registration movement was finally successful, was complex, but it involved a gradual process of compromise in which the extreme views of Wakley were moderated by the inhibitory strength of the medical corporations. As Newman puts it 'they may have been inert and incapable of movement, but their power of inertia was still formidable' (Newman 1957:155).

In 1841 another Bill was introduced to the House by Mr Hawes, the first one having been opposed by the medical corporations who feared that Wakley's concept of the College of Medicine would come to supersede them altogether, for the Bill appeared to imply that their existing powers, as well as certain additional ones, would be vested in it. The new (1841) Bill provided for a single register in each of the three countries namely England and Wales, Scotland and Ireland. In this case, compared with the first Bill, extreme democracy in the government of the profession was to be ensured by a postal ballot of all registered practitioners. It also proposed that the new governing body of the profession should publish a pharmacopoeia. This was a provision included in the subsequently successful 1858 Act. The fact that a proposed Senate would make by-laws on the education of students, whether medical or druggist and also regulate examinations 'had the effect of so frightening the chemists and druggists that they came together [to create the new] Pharmaceutical Society, so as to ensure regulation by themselves of their own affairs'. Newman, himself a doctor, regards this as 'a very happy provision which prevented later a further upsurge of doctors of another origin from below' (1957:157). This Bill also met opposition from the medical corporations; the Society of Apothecaries in particular petitioned against it. As Newman suggests (confirming Holloway's position) the Apothecaries' Society when it wanted legislation appealed to the College of Physicians as 'the natural guardians of the public health'. He goes on 'in other words the Apothecaries, so far from entertaining revolutionary antagonisms against the predominance of the Physicians, actually thought it right and natural' (1957:157).

The third Bill was identical with the second save that because the second one had failed due to the opposition of the chemists and druggists, the revised Bill dropped any reference to them. The major innovation was the introduction of the notion that each National Council should offer its own general qualification instead of those already in being associated with University, College or Hall. This idea which has been termed 'the single portal of entry' had the virtue of simplicity and administrative tidiness, but it was bound to meet opposition from the existing medical corporations and universities which had a vested interest in maintaining their own individual powers to award qualifications.

The spurt of activity on the subject of medical reform and registration appears to have exhausted itself and certainly the political climate was less favourable in the later stages of Melbourne's last administration. Peel's government of 1841 included as Home Secretary Sir James Graham, who in 1842 contacted the Society of Apothecaries about a Bill he was preparing. This contained once again the concept of a Central Council and the Society immediately objected that it was assigned no place in this administrative body. Sir James begged to differ and thought, that it would improve the position of 'the Company', as he chose to call it, in relation to the whole body of medical practitioners. He also refused to outlaw unqualified practice on the grounds that members of the public would always choose a more highly qualified practitioner. There was some delay in the introduction of the Bill to the House but it was brought in on 7 August 1844. It was the fourth of the reform Bills and proposed a Council of Health and Medical Education comprising a principal Secretary of State, five Regius Professors of Medicine and Surgery, one representative from each of the College of Physicians and Surgeons in each one of the three countries as well as six crown nominees. An important innovation was the idea of a single register for the whole of the United Kingdom and one registration fee only to be paid at the time of registration. Nevertheless, within this settlement 'the orders' were not only to be maintained but increasingly distinguished by differential examination requirements and official designations of the ages at which practitioners could qualify for practice, for example a physician could only start at a minimum age of twenty-four years. In another respect, though, it did provide for a unified profession internally divided by differential levels of education as expressed in qualifying examinations. This allowed a place for the more highly qualified type of practitioner who had begun to supersede the apothecary, and thus to blur the distinction between 'the orders'. The Bill contained another innovation, namely conjoint examination rather than the simpler, but politically untenable proposal of a single portal of entry. It thus placated the medical corporations. In many respects it was very similar to the Bill which ultimately succeeded in 1858.

Unfortunately it was too late in the session to proceed with the Bill and in any case the apothecaries opposed it (as we have already noted). This was principally because, while Sir James made it clear that he was against apprenticeship, he wished to obtain advantages for the qualified, and in any case, he did not believe that unqualified practice could simply be abolished by law. Sir James also hinted that he was thinking of depriving the apothecaries of the right to grant licences (in this sense he seems to anticipate Holloway's doubts about the way in which the apothecaries had used their powers under the 1815 Act.) It is certainly the case that the Apothecaries' Society had made 'themselves very unpopular by such silly actions as prosecuting members of the College of Surgeons for dispensing' (Newman 1957:161). Mr Hawes representing the general practitioners' interests, thought that the Council of Health ought to contain representatives of all branches of practice, but this was a Whig view. It could not be expected in a Tory measure and it was the corporations (other than the Apothecaries') who were to constitute the membership of the governing body of the profession. Wakley, as one would expect, opposed the Bill because it gave no power to the ordinary members of the colleges. In any case his *animus* against the Council of the College of Surgeons could not be satisfied by a Bill which made no proposal to interfere with them. The Society of Apothecaries naturally opposed the Bill by all means available giving as its reason that it deprived the general practitioner of all control over the education or examination of practitioners.

During the parliamentary recess discussions took place which formed the basis of a new Bill, the fifth. Under its terms registration would be common to all doctors but the 'orders' would, Sir James hoped, be maintained if only by tradition rather than by legislation. Moreover he was forced to concede that the older universities be exempted from the provisions of the Bill, thus maintaining their exclusive privileges. It was also proposed to repeal the Apothecaries' Act of 1815 while leaving to the Society its right to enforce penalties against those pretending to be qualified. The Bill gave due importance to the College of Physicians' views that entry to medicine should be through a university education. On the other hand the suggestion that a college of general practitioners should be created was not proceeded with. The argument given was that it was better to retain the attachment of general practitioners to the Royal College of Surgeons. More than a hundred years were to pass before a College of General Practitioners became an established institution among the medical corporations.

Newman suggests that if Sir James Graham's Bill (his first) had been carried through it might well have become law but that the recess, together with the additional time for debate prior to the introduction of his second Bill, allowed the proliferation of dissension among the interested parties. It was for this reason that his amended Bill failed in the House. Wakley, in particular, was able to argue, following his usual hobby-horse, that the differences between the Royal College of Surgeons and the general practitioners were irreconcilable. Sir James argued that if general practitioners were enfranchised the College of Surgeons would come under their control, a consequence which he wished to avoid because he said pure surgeons in London would thus come under the virtual domination of Apothecaries' Hall. One of the suggested amendments was for the establishment of a College of General Practitioners and also of a Joint Board of Physicians, Surgeons and General Practitioners which would conduct the preliminary examination of candidates for each college, but the conduct of the final examination should be carried out by the separate Colleges each in its own particular field. The effect of this would have been to establish general practice as a specialism in its own right a hundred years before this actually took place. Moreover, the conception of orders would have been clarified on a functional basis.

Another variation which was introduced at the committee stage was that all physicians and surgeons would first have to pass the examinations of the College of General Practitioners before those of the Physician and Surgeon's. In this new form, to become a member of the profession a novice would have first to register as a general practitioner before becoming a specialist. This anticipated the basic concept of the modern medical qualification. After 1858 the aim of undergraduate education was to train all doctors as 'safe general practitioners' before they could proceed to qualify as specialist physicians or surgeons. Interesting as these proposals were, they were stillborn.

Newman says that after the printing of the Bill nothing more was heard of it, presumably because of the conflicts among the reformers themselves. Sir James Graham had attempted a large scale reform of the government of the medical profession but for the time being his efforts were in vain. Wakley and Warburton introduced another Bill in August 1846 which was an attempt to cut through the complexities of the previous debate by simply providing for a register in each of the three countries making up the United Kindom. This too was dropped due to the opposition of the College of Physicians and to the fact that time was limited because the parliamentary session was near its end.

Outside Parliament negotiations were taking place between the Royal College of Surgeons and the Apothecaries' Society in an effort to harmonise their educational programmes. A conference was held and the results were so promising that the College of Physicians also joined in. Somewhat surprisingly three general practitioners were invited to participate, at the suggestion of Apothecaries' Hall, and a draft constitution for a Royal College of General Practitioners of England was prepared. The introduction of a new Bill, the seventh, cut across this initiative which as a result went no further. The Bill was to be the last with which Wakley was involved.

It returned to the concept of separate registers for each of the three countries of the United Kingdom. The idea of a General Council was dropped and the role of the state was enlarged by the proposal that examining bodies would submit schemes for courses of study to the Secretary of State. The Home Office was to be charged with the responsibility of ensuring uniformity in educational courses and examinations. The Secretary of State was at his discretion to depute a qualified practitioner to undertake the inspection of such courses and examinations, as well as making sure that any Orders in Council were duly observed. Surprisingly, after the first reading, objections were received even from the National Institution of General Practitioners. Newman suggests that the most likely reason was that they wanted their own Royal College, though in other respects they had everything to gain from the Bill. More predictably the College of Physicians stood out against it and Wakley found, once again, that in spite of his express wish, the second reading of the Bill was postponed. Wakley and Hume objected to what they regarded as 'back-stairs methods' but judging the opposition to be too strong, Wakley moved, on the 13 May 1847, for the formation of another Select Committee on Registration and the Practice of Medicine and Surgery. The Home Secretary was pleased at this opportunity to side-step the immediate problems of the Bill and it was agreed that a Select Committee be appointed and the Bill withdrawn. The members of the Committee included Macaulay, Sir James Graham, Sir Robert Inglis and Thomas Wakley. The latter had been unable to sit on the 1834 Committee because he was not yet an MP. He had spent twenty-five years of his life campaigning against the great medical corporations using his journal, the *Lancet,* as a vehicle for his views. His knowledge of the corporations was unrivalled and was clearly much greater than that of the men who were temporarily the officers of the Colleges. He took the opportunity to direct the line of questioning of those who were brought to give evidence to the Committee and had the satisfaction of demonstrating that precisely those defects and corruptions which he had always argued existed, were in fact true. He made his case out of the very mouths of those whose function was to defend the *status quo*. The Committee of 1847 proved to be his triumph and at this moment he showed his generosity to individuals while damning institutions. Following the precedent of 1834, the Committee published its proceedings and all its evidence in full. It proved to be the strongest possible basis for the view that reform was urgent.

Nevertheless, paradoxically the deliberations of the Select Committee put an end to discussions between the two Royal Colleges and the Society of Apothecaries which might well have led to reform. Discussions were terminated because legislation was thought to be impending. 'Enthusiasm for reform [thus] had the effect of postponing reform' (Newman 1957:171). A further round of discussions and conferences took place on the possibility of founding a College of General Practitioners. It was the refusal of the College of Surgeons to concede that such a proposed college should have the right to examine in surgery, together with the refusal of the National Association of General Practitioners to consider a Charter which did not contain this right, which brought the negotiations to deadlock in March 1850. In any case, the Society of Apothecaries decided against relinquishing its existing powers under the 1815 Act. Permission was obtained by Mr Wyld to introduce a Bill into the House of Commons to incorporate the general practitioners, but in the state of political deadlock on the medical reform question nothing more was done. By now, governments tended to be understandably chary of medical reform but nevertheless the pressure groups for this cause continued to seek for a satisfactory legislative outcome.

It was during the early 1850s that the Provincial Medical and Surgical Association, soon afterwards renamed the British Medical Association, began to exert its own pressure for medical legislation. Under the chairmanship of its founder, Sir Charles Hastings, the Association's Medical Reform Committee brought forward a draft medical Bill in 1854. The situation was complex in that at least two Bills were in existence and the subsequent political activity has been aptly described by Newman as 'the period of confusion'. By the time the House had considered its eleventh Bill on the subject the 'whole issue of medical reform [was] in a muddle' (Newman 1957:179). It was hoped that referral to a Select Committee would enable the problem to be sorted out. After a period of initial disagreement the Committee finally reached a surprising degree of unanimity. A Bill was drafted

123

proposing a Council of Medical Education. There were to be no representative members of the Council, but the corporations were to be represented, as were the universities of Oxford, Cambridge and London and also the Society of Apothecaries, at least until 1865, after which time it would lose its membership. Naturally this Bill was opposed by those reformers who had for so long fought to establish representation of general practitioners on the Council. As subsequent Bills were introduced it became evident that at least two irreconcilable camps had emerged among the reformers. One group led by Mr Headlam 'wanted a representative independent Medical Council, a preservation of "the orders" and examinations by Colleges and Universities' (Newman 1957:182). The other led by Lord Elcho 'wanted a nominated Council answerable to the House of Commons and a single portal of entry to the profession', leaving it optional for individuals to take the examinations of the colleges or universities. Another group led by Mr Duncombe, who was the radical successor to Wakley, wanted to overturn the medical corporations and make all doctors equal. It was at this time that Lord Elcho remarked that as Sir Robert Peel had once said hardly a session passed without a Salmon Bill and it now seemed to be the case that the same was true of Medical Bills. In spite of the unanimity of views in the Select Committee, the production of different Bills by different interests produced what Newman calls a 'whole congeries of Bills' (1957:183). In the subsequent debate arguments were put forward for free trade in medicine and those supporting this view were asked by their opponents whether they would equally like free trade in the professions or the church or the law.

It was in December 1857 that Mr W.F. Cowper announced his intention to introduce a Bill. He was President of the Board of Health, and had only recently been chairman of the Select Committee. Interestingly he was in addition, at the same time, Vice-President of the Privy Council's Committee for Education. John Simon, who was Medical Officer to the Board of Health, assisted Cowper by suggesting that 'what was wanted was the definition of a qualified medical practitioner, an accurate register, the application of privileges to the registered and penalties to those who pretended to be registered and the removal of territorial restrictions'. He made these points by the way of an office memorandum to Cowper, who set out to use his political experience to implement them. By this time, there appears to have been general agreement among all but a few medical reformers on the desired content of a medical Act, except on the vexed question of a representative or nominated General Medical Council. Even the question of the medical orders was not such a stumbling block as it had been. It was tacitly agreed that they could not be maintained and that before the law, for the sake of simplicity, a uniform status of medical practitioner would have to be accepted.

Although a new government in which Lord Derby was Prime Minister took office in 1858, Mr Cowper nevertheless introduced his Bill in March of that year. This, the sixteenth Bill, contained detailed provisions which were by now generally accepted and also a compromise, namely, that a 'General Council of Medical Education and Registration' should be established 'in a form both representative and nominated'. The profession was to govern itself and all the members of the Council would be doctors. The new Home Secretary, Mr Spencer Walpole, had suggested a device by which the Medical Council would be responsible directly to the Privy Council rather than being presided over by a Minister and answerable to the House of Commons. In the twentieth century, this device was to be employed to provide for the freedom and independence of both the Medical Research Council, and the University Grants Committee.

The General Council of Medical Education and Registration was empowered to make orders and regulations which would be approved by the Privy Council. There were four principal duties laid upon it. The establishment and maintenance of a register; the definition of any degrees, diplomas or any other qualifications judged suitable to admit candidates to the register; the right to require the co-operation of examining bodies, where this was thought necessary and to appoint examiners. Rather than independent Councils in England, Scotland and Ireland, three branch Councils were set up, one for each country. A single alphabetical register of qualified medical practitioners was instituted instead of, as had been proposed in an earlier Bill of Mr Headlam's the recognition of higher and lower classes of physicians and surgeons respectively. This would have been by means of an A and B roll, a proposal of the type which was to be so vexatious among schoolteachers. The Royal College of Physicians had fought for a separate register. The more radical reformers were disappointed with the Bill on a number of grounds especially in that it failed to abolish the medical corporations and did nothing to introduce the single portal of entry or, as the general practitioners wished, to place heavy penalties on unqualified practice. The British Medical Association, which was now such a powerful influence on behalf of the general practitioner, would ideally have liked a Bill containing these provisions, together with the radicals' other major concern — 'a council made up wholly of the elected representatives of the profession' but the BMA appeared more willing to compromise. Mr Duncombe brought in another radical Bill — the seventeenth, which was intended simply to block Mr Cowper's. The tactic was however unsuccessful and after trying to stop it in committee Duncombe was defeated and the Bill passed the House of Commons. Thus, in the end, it was Cowper's Bill, the sixteenth, which became law, with some small amendments from the Upper House among which the most important was the institution of a fixed single registration fee rather than an annual one.

It had taken thirty years of protracted political struggle to get a Medical Act on the Statute Book. As we have noted, Wakley and the radicals were disappointed in that they thought the Act compromised too much with the medical corporations. On the other hand the Royal College of Physicians was also against it on the ground that they expected that the equalisation of entry qualifications to the profession would produce greater homogeneity, but only at the expense of pulling down the status and privileges of the physician. In the event, the development of the consulting physician or surgeon proved to be the factor which inhibited homogenisation of the medical profession. In any case, the status of physician and surgeon was strongly entrenched by custom and would not have disappeared overnight. One important feature of the Act was the abolition of regional licences which was an inheritance from mediaeval times and had stemmed from the local nature of the old guild system. Perhaps the most important outcome of the Act was that it provided the basis for the unification of the medical profession through the concept of the equal recognition of all registered practitioners before the law. Moreover the profession was now not simply unified but also self-governing and licensed to be so by the state.

The British Medical Association and the Reform Movement

The Provincial Medical and Surgical Association was founded in 1832, the year of the first great Reform Bill. Its founder was Charles Hastings, the son of a clergyman who was secretary of the Association until he was elected president in 1843. In its first years it was a self-consciously provincial association having been founded at Worcester. There were already several associations of medical men in London and others were started in the provinces. The Provincial Medical and Surgical Association was distinguished by its ambition to cover the whole kingdom, excepting only the capital. It claimed to speak on behalf of the whole profession and for this reason stated as one of its explicit objectives 'the maintenance of the honour and respectability of the profession generally in the provinces' (Little 1932:31). In the earliest days the journal of the association *Transactions* was not greatly different in content from others, such as those of the Medical Society of London or in the provincial cities. But the Association soon became involved in the advocacy of medical reform and espoused several medico-political objectives. Indeed, it was bound to do so if it was jealousy to guard and improve the honour and respectability of the profession in the provinces.

There appear to have been some rival medical associations in existence during the 1830s and 1840s. In 1841, for example, a meeting was convened in London by an organisation known as the British Medical Association which claimed to speak for medical practitioners throughout the United Kingdom. The delegates of twelve medical associations, including the Provincial Association, were present. Subsequently the Provincial Association was to take over the title of the by then defunct British Medical Association. For a time however this London-based association appears to have been a serious rival. The movement which gave birth to the first British Medical Association had its origins among practitioners in Camberwell and Southwark. It was supported at its inauguration in 1836 by Wakley and the *Lancet*. The opportunity to attack the Provincial Association was taken in the *Lancet* where it was referred to rather disparagingly as 'the migratory Provincial Club', a reference to the fact that it held its annual meetings in different locations each year. In this respect it was similar to the early trade unions. Dr George Webster was chairman of the first British Medical Association throughout its relatively brief existence and it undoubtedly had influential support at its inception. Webster urged immediate action for reform of the medical corporations and the creation of 'one great Faculty of Medicine for the whole United Kingdom, which should control medical education and practice and put down quackery' (Little 1932:33). Petitions to parliament were agreed seeking these objectives, and also asking for an enquiry into Poor-Law Medical Practice. In Little's view the failure of the original British Medical Association was precisely that it tried to do too much too quickly. It generated a great deal of opposition to its radical programme. The Provincial Association under Hasting's leadership 'while as anxious for reform, wished to obtain it by changes from within the corporations and by moderation and reasonableness' (1932:33).

The provincial and London-based associations fell out with each other. Dr Webster and his London colleagues expected the provincials simply to endorse London policies and tactics. The provincial delegates resigned. Hastings came in for some personal abuse from Wakley in the *Lancet*. The involvement of the tempestuous Wakley with the London Association caused it to lead an 'Israelitish existence' which was undoubtedly a key element in its downfall. It ended finally bereft of members. The situation was graphically described in the *Medical Times* report as follows:

> 'The British Medical Association, suffering a resurrection under the galvanic agency of the new Bill, met in the person of Dr George Webster on September 28th (1844). The Secretary was absent, and the resolutions appear to have been moved by the President, seconded by the President, put to the vote by the President and carried by the President. He was the whole meeting' (1932:34).

The association continued a shadow existence for several more years before becoming extinct.

The Provincial Medical and Surgical Association has been regarded by many writers as essentially a general practitioners' organisation. Certainly the bulk of its members were general practitioners which is perhaps unsurprising as they constituted the majority of the profession. But the evidence suggests that it was reasonably representative of the profession as a whole in the provinces. The membership included physicians and surgeons attached to provincial hospitals and infirmaries. These men were as much consultants as those practising in London hospitals. At the very first meeting of the Provincial Association, in the Board-room of the Worcester Infirmary on 19 July 1832, the Regius Professor of Physic at Oxford University, Dr Kidd, was present as well as physicians and surgeons from Bath, Bristol, Birmingham, Cheltenham, Warwick, Hereford and elsewhere (1932:24).

By contrast the National Association of General Practitioners in Medicine, Surgery and Midwifery, which was active in the mid-1840s, had a membership confined mainly to those in general practice. George Ross, a London general practitioner, was its secretary. There is a report of a meeting in 1846 at which seven hundred people were present and it was proposed that a National Institute of Medicine should be established as a licensing body. It was probably intended as a counter to Wakley's College of Medicine. There is a record of a joint deputation composed of members of the Society of Apothecaries and the General Practitioners' Association which had an interview with the Home Secretary, but the meeting was apparently abortive (1932:36). The Minutes of the Royal College of Surgeons of England contain a record of negotiations between that College, the Apothecaries' Society, the Royal College of Physicians and the National Association of General Practitioners. The meeting took place in February 1848. On the subject of medical legislation those present agreed upon the appointment of a General Council, the registration of practitioners and students and reciprocity of practice between members of the three medical corporations. It was further resolved 'that a charter of incorporation should be granted to the Surgeon Apothecaries of this country under the title of "The Royal College of General Practitioners" ' (Little 1932:63). The proposal came to nothing.

Meanwhile the Provincial Medical and Surgical Association was going from strength to strength. New branches were being formed year by year (1932:41-60). It provided a great deal of active backing to the movement for medical reform and medical registration. In 1837 it had set up its own Medical Reform Committee which was very active in the reform movement. The radicals, especially Wakley and his friends, wanted the 'abrogation' of the privileges of the corporations and the substitution in their place of a State Examining Board, whose licence should constitute the sole qualification to practice. The Provincial Association took a more cautious view. In 1841 it adopted the following resolution: 'That in the opinion of this meeting, it is expedient that existing institutions be respected, provided their existence can be rendered compatible with uniformity of qualification, equality of privilege to practise medicine, and a fair system of representative government' (1932:62). Little records the view that 'the Act of 1858 was almost entirely the work of the Association' (1932:65) but it should be remembered that he was writing as the Association's official historian. A fair historical assessment would require considerable detailed research similar to that carried out on the Apothecaries' Act by Holloway (1964).

Undoubtedly, however, the Association did play an important part. There were several matters which it regarded as of vital concern which were not secured by the 1858 Act.

> 'The Act did not attempt to suppress unqualified practice, except in the service of the State, and the representative principle in the selection of the members of the Council was practically disregarded for in the selection of representatives of the Universities and Medical Corporations the great body of graduates and licensees had no direct and but very little indirect influence. The representatives sent to the Council by the various Colleges were naturally more concerned with the reputations and pecuniary resources of the institutions which they represented, than with the suppression of quackery'

and status of their licensees (Little 1932:65). It was for these reasons that the Medical Reform Committee was not dissolved in 1858 but was simply renamed, being known as the Committee on Medical Legislation. Its object now was the amendment of the Medical Act. In 1870 a Bill was introduced with the purpose of getting direct representation of the profession (meaning the general practitioners) on the General Medical Council. It failed. Partly this was due to the split in opinion within the medical profession itself. There were those who continued in the tradition of Wakley (he had given up his seat in Parliament in 1852) (Sprigge 1899:348), who wanted the abrogation of the powers of the medical corporations, particularly their independent authority to licence doctors. They wanted to put an end to what they regarded as the 'disgraceful competition (between the licensing bodies) which has for so long existed'. The reformers desired to see a single portal of entry rather than the confirmation of 'the privileges possessed by certain mediaeval Corporations [and rather than] to dignify those bodies by the title of "Medical Authorities", and seemingly to fasten them about the necks [sic] of the profession for ever' (Little 1932:66-7). If the intention in opposing the Bill was that another and better one would soon be obtained the outcome must have been a disappointment. In 1881 a Royal Commission was established, but in the intervening years some 'twenty amending medical Bills had been brought into Parliament, besides three Government ones' without success (1932:69).

The Provincial Medical and Surgical Association, which had changed its name to the British Medical Association in 1856, adopted for itself a new 'representative' constitution which was to earn its General Meeting the sobriquet 'Doctors Commons'. The determination to make the institutions of the profession responsible to the constituency of medical men was instanced by the efforts of the British Medical Association to reform the Royal College of Surgeons. A system of personal voting then still obtained which effectively excluded those fellows who lived outside London. The British Medical Association pressed for the introduction of voting by ballot papers, but the Council of the College declined to seek the necessary legislation to alter their Charter. The British Medical Association sent a delegation to see the Home Secretary with yet another proposal to amend the Medical Act in that respect. It also noted 'with regret in 1876 that in filling three vacancies on the General Medical Council neither the Association nor the . . . body of general practitioners had been recognised' (Little 1932:67).

During this period a new solution of conjoint examinations between the several medical corporations was being canvassed. Some such reform was very necessary because it was still possible for a person to be licensed to practice without being examined in all three crucial subjects, medicine, surgery and midwifery. In 1884 the General Medical Council at last adopted a proposal that every candidate should be examined in all three subjects by one or more licensing bodies. Also, it approved the introduction of conjoint examinations by the Colleges of Physicians and Surgeons in London and similar arrangements were made in Scotland. The British Medical Association agreed to drop its demand for State Boards rather than lose the Bill. In the words of the Association's historian, it was 'beaten owing to the strength of the Corporations. The General Medical Council was timid and loath to act' (1932:71). Writing in 1932 Little said 'the representation of the licensing bodies on the Council so far from being diminished, has been increased. Owing to the creation of English and Irish Universities there are now twenty-eight representatives of those bodies, while the number of direct representatives of the profession remains fixed at six' (Little 1932:72).

7. PROFESSIONAL CONSOLIDATION AND STATUS
1858 – 1911

The Medical Registration Act (1858) was the major landmark in the rise
of the apothecary and of the surgeon from their lowly status of tradesmen and craftsmen and their assimilation into a unified medical
profession with the higher status physicians. The Act marked a legal
closure of the profession against parvenu outsiders, but in one important
sense the process of assimilation was only beginning. The reform of
medical education had been initiated long before that date, but the
newly established General Medical Council quickly realised that if a truly
unified and homogeneous profession was to be created it would require
more than legal closure; it would require efforts at homogenisation based
on selective recruitment of new entrants from appropriate social backgrounds and with suitable preliminary education. The position was put
clearly by the Council in 1870 when they said:

'prior to 1858, although the education, both general and
professional of . . . the higher walks of the profession was such as
secured the supply of a certain number of well-educated gentlemen
and accomplished practitioners, yet the strictly professional
education of even those was in many respects seriously defective.
But as regards the main bulk of the profession . . . the education
was so defective that the profession was in danger of being overrun
with illiterate and incompetent men' (Newman 1957:197).

In the early days after its establishment the General Medical Council was
thus concerned with raising the general educational level of the
profession not least in terms of assimilating the newly joined lower
branch through an education of new members which stressed character
and the cult of the gentleman. Examining this issue, Ashe wrote

'the question is, are we a profession or a trade, are we gentlemen or
are we not . . . it is of no avail to say that if a man is within the
ranks of the profession he thereby becomes a gentleman; for the
question is evidently not in what light do we look upon ourselves
or upon each other but in what light are we looked upon by the
external world. It is admittedly desirable that medical
practitioners, the members of a learned and liberal profession,
should be gentlemen, that is to say that they should be held the
equals of gentlemen in education and position [and] as the equals
of the members of the other learned professions.'

Ashe goes on to tell us

'as regards *position* we may remark that the gentry look upon the
clergy as their social equals, that they look upon members of the
Bar as their social equals, nay more that they regard a certain pro-

131

portion of our profession in the same light. Which portion then? and why not all of our members. That portion, we reply, which regards our profession as a profession strictly and not as a compound of a profession and a trade; and those of our body are excluded from such a status who accept the compromise and add the business of a trade, the sale of medicines to the practice of their profession. For this is a point of which society is very tenacious; a gentleman must not engage in *retail trade*' (Ashe 1868:146).

The desirable preliminary education for medicine increasingly became the public school with its focus upon the production of the Christian gentleman. Entry to the profession via the public school became an established tradition which has continued in the twentieth century and has been one of the social bases of the tendency towards self-recruitment in medicine. In the nineteenth century the sons of the clergy provided perhaps the most important numerical contribution to the ranks of the medical profession in its period of consolidation but this has been subsequently replaced by self-recruitment from among the sons of doctors themselves.

As early as 1859 the first Committee on Education set up by the General Medical Council stated in its report that 'no person should enter the medical or surgical profession who has not received an education in general knowledge such as will be equal, at least, to that required by the national educational bodies'. Newman points out that they were speaking of universities and 'were expressing the opinion that surgeons and apothecaries ought to be as worthily educated as were physicians' (Newman 1957:197).

The position of apprenticeship was greatly affected by the development of new forms of education and qualification in the profession. This was bound to reflect on the activities and status of the Society of Apothecaries. 'We cannot', says Ashe,

'but deeply regret but that an old trade monopoly should not only appertain to, but be actively maintained by one of the Corporations belonging to the medical profession; and whose licences are now accepted by the Army, Navy, and Poor Law Boards as constituting a sufficient title to practise medicine. There has been a struggle regarding the admission of the Corporation referred to into the practising ranks of the profession; that struggle is now passed.'

'But', he goes on to say, 'it is highly derogatory to her sister Corporations' (Ashe 1868:147). Apprenticeship was already in decline but the process was speeded up after 1858. The medical reformers were all opposed to it but the Society of Apothecaries were constrained by the Act of 1815 and tended to 'threaten fire and sword' to anyone who proposed to evade it as, for instance, in their threat to prosecute the first member of the College of Surgeons who dared to dispense medicines without going through it. The first breach in apprenticeship had occured a hundred years before because of an Act of 1749 which allowed officers of the Armed Forces who had practised while in the services to set up in trade without being bound to apprenticeship. After 1860 apprenticeship was not merely frequently combined with attendance at lectures and practical experience in a recognised hospital medical school but the two together were made compulsory, as a condition of qualification by Apothecaries' Hall. An Act of 1874 amended the original Apothecaries Act of 1815 and allowed the requirements of apprenticeship to be bypassed. In 1907 the Society of Apothecaries was at last empowered to give a complete medical qualification. There is no doubt that the status factor, the effort to dissociate the united medical profession from trade, is crucial to an understanding of the extraordinary disfavour into which apprenticeship had fallen by the 1870s.

In summary, it is possible to say that the first objective of the General Medical Council after its foundation was the incorporation into the newly unified profession of the large majority of general practitioners. Newman points out that 'they were not thinking about the physicians (the physicians were already highly educated, civilised men) but about those who had been the apothecaries and were now about to become the general practitioners among the new "registered medical practitioners"'. Technically, the emphasis was now on the 'safe general practitioner' because the elite of the profession, whom Newman describes as eighteenth-century minded, were condescendingly obsessed with the idea that 'inferior practitioners', unlike themselves, might be a danger to the public.

> 'They were worried about the lamentable state of the majority of medical students as they remembered them; what they wanted to do was to see to it that the profession should, in future, be recruited from a better sort, that its members, in other words, should constitute a "profession", purged of the remnants of commercialism inherent in the old, trade-derived apothecary' (Newman 1957:194-5).

The reforms in medical education were but a part, even if an important part, of education reform in the nineteenth century. Within this Newman tells us,

> 'the reform of professional education was a general movement of self-regulation among the professions as a whole, not a reform of the medical profession in isolation. Professional reform was part of the movement elevating the status of all professions, ensuring that if the most interesting occupations were to be reserved for the most intelligent, and rewarded by the highest remuneration, they should involve the obligation of an efficient and thorough education, rigid tests of admission, and adherence to a strict professional ethical code' (1957:112).

The success of the lower branch of the medical profession in creating a unified profession in 1858 did not abolish important conflicts and divisions within the newly closed profession. By the late 1860s certain accusations against consultants, many of whom were merely superior general practitioners, began to be voiced. They were accused of taking over patients referred to them, or at least making no enquiries as to whether they already had a medical adviser or not. The British Medical Journal after dealing with this issue on several occasions over a number of years, began to suggest in the late 1870s, that a consultant should always be a specialist. He ought never to see a patient unless attending with a general practitioner or without first receiving a referral and after-wards reporting back his opinion. Indeed, some went so far as to say that there should be a distinction between the upper and lower branches of the medical profession (the general practitioners and consultants respectively) as there was in law between solicitors and barristers. One proposal was to create a group of consultants equivalent to the Queen's Council (QC) or 'silk', who would only come in where a third opinion was required, and never appear without a 'junior'. General consultants or even specialists had existed prior to 1858. But the creation of a unified profession, and the increasing propensity of medical men to qualify as physicians greatly exacerbated the problem. There was simply not enough consulting practice to go round. All this was an ironic reversal since general practitioners were now complaining about consultants poaching on their territory in the guise of higher class general practitioners, when hitherto it had been this kind of man (the physician) who had done his utmost through the Royal College of Physicians to keep the general practitioner out altogether.

What we can see happening here is a blurring of the distinction between the general practitioner and the consultant. This was due to the fact that their work situations were not very distinct during this period. Both practised from home, saw patients at certain hours of the day, visited, gave opinions and prescribed but did not dispense. Only with the increasing influence of hospital practice did the situation of the consultant and the general practitioner once again become separated. The 1858 Act had defined the boundaries around the profession but this brought into sharper focus a marked degree of intra-professional uncertainty and conflict. The struggle of the general practitioners to become part of the profession was over; the question now became what should be the proper relationship between the consultant and the general practitioner. The issue was partly precipitated by the growth of effective demand for doctors' services associated with the expansion and greater affluence of the middle class, but also by the fact that patients themselves were less clear about distinctions between different doctor's functions in a unified profession. There was a tendency for patients not to distinguish so clearly as before between grades of practitioner and consequently they no longer confined themselves to consultation with one kind of doctor. This was the reason practitioners began to criticise, not merely the behaviour of consultants and their assistants in the out-patient departments of hospitals, but also the alleged unethical behaviour of consultants in their own private practices. They were said to be accepting smaller than usual fees, not more than a guinea or two for a visit or consultation, thus cutting out the general practitioner altogether.

In terms of remuneration, the profession was divided. There were those who were earning what in some instances amounted to considerable fortunes as top consultants, but these were relatively few. There were general practitioners in a good way of business (these were an increasing number), and finally there was a large group of doctors who 'were extremely poorly paid and worked under degrading conditions'. In these circumstances, 'competitive undercutting, fee-splitting, canvassing for patients and other unethical practices were widespread' (Titmuss 1958:172). It was during this period that the British Medical Association sought urgently for the introduction of more ordered market relationships within the profession itself. Out of this struggle grew up the referral system between consultants and general practitioners as we know it today. In addition, the British Medical Association condemned advertising by medical practitioners. This form of intra-professional competition was reduced, and in the end almost eliminated by the efforts of the British Medical Association. Pressure was put on the General Medical Council which began to use its powers to examine cases of infringement of professional ethics and in particular to strike off the register practitioners who advertised themselves. Even so it was a long time before the policy really began to bite.

This issue points up the fact that professional ethics have much more to do with the regulation of relationships between professionals themselves than between professional and clients — a fact which is central to our conception of professionalism. The harsh effects of open competition between practitioners were minimised by these means. A greater degree of professional control began to be exercised over the medical market place. Fluctuations in the remuneration of practitioners due to market forces were considerably reduced and the status and honour of the profession was enhanced. The governing ethic regulating relationships between professionals became that which should obtain between gentlemen.

The threat to the general practitioner from the consultant had been an unanticipated consequence of the creation of a unified profession. Nevertheless, by following the strategy of professionalism, with its stress on occupational control through the manipulation of education, the general practitioner found that a golden opportunity was given to the prestigious Royal Colleges to reform themselves and to regain control of the commanding heights of the profession. The General Medical Council itself, as we have noted, did not accommodate directly elected representatives of the profession. In particular, the largest constituency in the profession, the general practitioners, had no such representation. The Royal Colleges, the Universities and the Crown members composed the Council. It was natural that the Royal Colleges, the Society of Apothecaries and the Universities should play a key role in the General Medical Council because it was they, in the persons of their most distinguished members, who were responsible for the education and qualification of the profession. The intending general practitioner was the biggest consumer of medical education but those in general practice were allowed least say in shaping it. Whether the education of doctors was done well or badly, it is the case that the general practitioner had little control over it. The reason for this, of course, was the rise of hospital-based medical education. This had three consequences. It introduced a new type of doctor-patient relationship (Waddington 1973). It provided the vehicle for the re-establishment of the Royal Colleges, and it reaffirmed the superior position of the consultant over the general practitioner within the profession.

The Medical Profession and the Hospital

At the beginning of the nineteenth century the hospital in England was not a significant institution in society. A few hospitals had existed for centuries and a number of additional ones were added during the eighteenth century, but they played a very small part in the treatment of the sick. In this respect, there was a sharp contrast between England and France. In 1800 there were probably only about 3,000 patients when the population of England and Wales stood at nearly eight million, and in 1851, when hospitals were first enumerated in the census, there were only 7,619 patients in a population approaching eighteen million. The voluntary hospitals were concentrated in the principal cities of London, Edinburgh and Dublin. The nineteenth century was to see a transformation in the number and significance of hospitals in society (Abel-Smith 1964:1). In the early years of the century the state of medical knowledge was such that little effective treatment could be obtained in hospital. In any case the risk of cross-infection made it preferable to be treated at home. At the end of the century the hospital was an important institution. By then Florence Nightingale's first requirement of a hospital 'that it should do the sick no harm' had probably on balance been achieved although it has recently been argued, on historical evidence, that hospitals were not so bad prior to the Nightingale reforms as has often been made out (Woodward 1974). Among the voluntary hospitals, the more venerable foundations had been created by Royal, aristocratic or civic initiative. Most founders were persons of superior social standing. Many members of the House of Lords and of the Royal Family were governors of voluntary hospitals, and it was therefore a mark of superior social status much sought after, especially by the parvenu rich and other persons with social aspirations. Some hospitals, such as St Thomas's and St Bartholomew's, could be run on the income from their endowments. The mixing of wealth and status was a potent source of charitable funds for the hospitals, and the mixture was widely used also to support other deserving causes. In some cases the charitable purpose merely masked an interest in status-seeking, but in others a very concrete material interest. Certain hospitals stipulated that purchases on their behalf should be made from those tradesmen who were subscribers. Even governors sometimes had this kind of financial stake. Usually subscribers had the right to nominate beneficiaries of medical charity, for example by writing letters of introduction for prospective patients. In this way employees, servants or even family members could all be treated for the price of a single subscription. In the main however, these institutions took in the sick-poor and they were neither intended for, nor used by, the middle or upper classes.

The significance of a hospital appointment for the physician or surgeon lay not in the paltry honorarium received, but in the prestige which such an appointment conferred upon him. This was especially the case in London where the appointment connected him to the aristocratic and Royal patrons of the hospital. They would call upon his services in time of need and recommend him to other members of their family as well as friends and acquaintances. By this means a consultant could be assured of a lucrative private practice among those in the highest social circles.

The fact that the older hospitals had failed, through inertia, to revise their scales of payment over the years in line with current money values was ironically a positive advantage to the consultant. It allowed him to demonstrate an especially patrician quality, that of providing his services to the poor, gratis. The duties of the honorary medical staff were not strenuous, and any gaps in attendance were filled by junior men. Later in the century they were supported by well-trained matrons and nurses. In some hospitals an apothecary was employed in a subordinate position and was paid for his services.

The rise of the hospitals was one of the most important elements in the re-affirmation of the Royal Colleges' control of the upper end of the medical market. The development of surgery had enabled the craftsman-surgeon to establish himself alongside the physician in the hospital setting. The concentration of medical education in the hospital gave the consultant physician and surgeon the chance to obtain high remuneration from private practice — from this his juniors were excluded. He also had the opportunity to secure fees from students over whose future he had much control through the examination system, and through patronage of appointment to medical posts. Junior hospital doctors today complain about low remuneration, but this system has its roots in a custom which continued even in the 1860s. The practice was that junior appointments up to registrarships were secured by making a payment to the consultant. Although apprenticeship has long since disappeared it has however left its mark.

Quite early on the consultant began to control admission of patients to the hospital. He acquired the right first in cases of accident, and then through the introduction of a general policy of accepting only 'curable cases'. The policy of excluding all but the acute sick to the voluntary hospitals was a triumph of the 'honorary doctors' over the charitable public, who would have been content to see pain relieved in the chronic sick also. The doctors naturally wanted to demonstrate success in terms of the number of cases cured.

The honorary status of the consultant gave him the advantage that the hospital administration and the governors of the hospital did not have any direct financial control over him. As hospitals became larger, governors began to appoint sub-committees to look after day-to-day management in which the doctors themselves participated so far as decision-making was concerned. Hospital secretaries were offered posts on a salaried basis, and this was the beginning of hospital administration by full-time lay administrators. The doctors had a free hand on the medical side, and started to gain control of hospital policy through the organisation of their own medical committees. It is not perhaps surprising that honorary medical staff passed on their posts to close relatives or sold them to their successors. This was entirely consistent with the practice of patronage in the Church, the Armed Forces and the Civil Service at the time. Family influence and money were important ingredients of success, but there was not much room at the top. Even in 1860, out of 15,000 registered practitioners fewer than 1,200 were working in 117 of the larger voluntary hospitals. Of these, only 579 were classified as 'physicians and surgeons who have charge of in-patients'; the rest were assistants and junior housemen (Abel-Smith 1964:19-20).

Control over the ladder to success has always been a characteristic of the established consultant's position in the hospital. At the beginning of the nineteenth century the chance of promotion for the aspirant was small. Progress on the career ladder was slow for those who wanted to reach the rank of honorary physician or surgeon. Then, as now, these posts had a high monopoly value and there was little incentive for incumbents to recommend the creation of new posts. Moreover, the good opinion of existing senior staff was essential for promotion, and juniors were often prepared to be blatantly exploited for the chance of preferment. This was the basis for a system which continues to exist today. The exploitation of junior by senior medical men is dependent upon the fact that the junior knows that his chance of promotion to consultancy, and therefore the opportunity of obtaining access to the lucrative private market, depends upon his civility to the present incumbent without whose goodwill he will not be promoted at all. On the other hand, his work situation is also characterised by stiff competition with his peers as he strives to outshine them. For the most part junior hospital doctors were content to accept exploitation, rather as at public school they would have accepted fagging, on the under-standing that one day they would be exploiters themselves. Those who did not succeed were often, as we shall see, forced to go out and start new lines of medical enterprise. Some of them were founders of the special hospitals, and others took over the senior posts in the Poor Law hospitals.

The hospital was becoming the bastion from which the consultant surgeons and physicians could reach out to dominate the profession as a whole, as well as the auxiliary or para-medical occupations. The domination of the profession was centred in the manipulation of the educational process. In the early nineteenth century the hospital, with its rich source of case material, became of vital importance to the new medical education. Private anatomy schools could only be a supplement to the hospital so far as live subjects were concerned. In hospital, large classes could attend demonstrations and the supply of more or less willing subjects to be prodded and shown-off was assured. Charity patients, unlike those who paid, were in no position to object. This system had several advantages over apprenticeship, not least that the student was able to see all kinds of cases by 'walking the wards', and did not have to wait on the chance of seeing a particular type of case in private practice. At first 'walking the wards' was a rather casual business, and only much later was it incorporated in an organised teaching programme. Indeed it was only gradually that apprenticeship to an apothecary of the majority of medical men was replaced by a hospital medical school training. But once the trainee apothecary entered the medical school he soon fell under the control of the consultant. Admittedly, while the Society of Apothecaries continued to provide a main examination for entry to general practice the hold was not complete. When eventually the Royal College of Physicians, with the Royal College of Surgeons, became the most important examining bodies, the control of the education process by the honorary doctors in the teaching hospitals (who were also the key men in the Royal Colleges) was finalised. The process was a self-reinforcing one, because teaching itself was profitable particularly during the era when fees went entirely into the teachers' pockets. In addition it was an investment because former pupils would later send wealthy patients for private consultation. Through this process private patients learnt that hospital staff possessed the most up-to-date knowledge, for were they not the teachers of the profession? In this way a consultant post in a charity hospital became the recognised apex of the profession. It conferred both fame and fortune. Control over recruitment to the profession, and over teaching and examining, were rapidly consolidated in the hands of the consultants. It was they who determined curricula, syllabi and examinations: in other words they controlled the process of defining professional competence. This gave them an exceptionally powerful position which they have continued to defend.

We have seen that the chance of promotion was small for the intending honorary physician or surgeon. In the medical school and in the teaching hospital men were (and still are) cooled-out at various points on the road to consultant status. This has meant that there has been no creation of permanent hospital grades below consultant level — all are in fact training grades however senior the period in them may be. Many has been the blocked career and numerous the ways of over-coming the blockage. Junior physicians and surgeons gradually took over the work done by the apothecary, who was squeezed out of the large teaching hospitals between 1850 and 1890. Thus the juniors came to do the basic medical work of the hospital, at first without any pay at all. Some students were in fact asked to pay for the privilege. Gradually however small salaries were introduced — £50 or £100 *per annum*. In many provincial hospitals even the most senior registrars were forbidden to engage in private practice, thus protecting the monopoly enjoyed by the senior consultants. In the middle years of the nineteenth century some of these hospital doctors whose careers were blocked reacted by starting out-patient clinics for particular diseases, or using new and special techniques. But the full development of a speciality requires equipment and a group of beds in a hospital. Often the aspiring specialist was again blocked by seniors or governors whose consent was necessary and who alone could decide whether or not to allocate resources.

One reaction to this was to become a medical entrepreneur and start a special hospital. In London the middle decades of the nineteenth century saw numerous foundations of this type. Between 1860 and 1870 no less than sixteen were founded. Some, such as lying-in hospitals, had of course existed since the eighteenth century but obstetrics was firmly placed by the President of the Royal College of Physicians, when he said in 1827 'that midwifery was an act foreign to the habits of a gentleman of enlarged academic education'. Nevertheless maternity hospitals founded by specialists in obstetrics were justified by the risk of cross-infection, as were the smallpox hospitals, fever hospitals and the Lock hospitals for venereal disease. (Some of these special hospitals were founded by the state.) A range of hospitals including those for the eye, for children, and for incurables, were founded by enterprising medical men. Whereas the general hospitals had been founded by laymen, this new kind were created by doctors with the energy and ability to raise funds. Inevitably the new specialists began to compete with the existing hospitals and even with the general practitioner.

There was an outcry in the profession against special hospitals when it was realised that self-diagnosis of ear, nose, throat or eye troubles would lead the patient to by-pass his regular medical attendant and go straight to the special hospital. Though some hospitals and treatments turned out to be spurious, many made an important contribution to the welfare of particular classes of patient. Specialisation did not necessarily lead to the creation of new hospitals, but a range of specialities could be exploited by younger men. They were able to convince wealthy patients that though they could not outstrip their seniors in overall knowledge, yet they already had a reputation for treating a particular condition.

The growth of Poor Law infirmaries in the latter part of the nineteenth century was of particular importance in opening up careers in the public service for men whose chances of promotion had been blocked in the voluntary hospital setting. When Dr Rogers founded the Poor Law Medical Officers' Association in 1840 he was perhaps not aware that, by encouraging the more exalted members of the profession to take an interest in the Poor Law hospitals, he would bring about a transformation in their staffing to the detriment of general practitioners in relation to the Poor Law infirmaries. During the previous year Wakley, owner of the *Lancet*, commissioned three doctors to visit the workhouses. The visit was very much at the instigation of the Poor Law medical officers. Two of the visiting members were from the London teaching hospitals and looked at the workhouse wards in the light of their own high standards. They were very critical of the conditions they found, and also of the position of the medical officers whom they reported to be overworked and underpaid. They believed it to be quite wrong for the medical officers to be required to pay out of their own pockets for dispensing and drugs. The report produced by the visit led to the foundation of the Association for the Improvement of the London Workhouse Infirmaries. It said the 'State hospitals are in work-house wards'. It was these that the Association intended to see improved. Powerful members included Sir Thomas Watson, President of the Royal College of Physicians, Charles Dickens and John Stuart Mill (Abel-Smith 1964:72-3).

In 1867 there was a new political initiative relating to the Poor Law which was of great consequence to the medical profession. A Bill was devised which carefully balanced central direction and local autonomy and had some measure of rate equalisation built into it[1](although this was not stressed at the time for fear of the political consequences). The Metropolitan Poor Act enabled both the creation of isolation hospitals in London for fever and smallpox and also quickly led to the foundation of the Metropolitan Asylums Board. The creation of a central fund pooled from the rates of the numerous districts of the metropolis was crucial because in the extreme case of the Metropolitan Asylums Board most of the costs were met by the fund. Also, the particular Guardians who sat on the Board had to pay less immediate heed to the pressures of local electors when authorising expenditure. In addition the fund was used to meet the salaries of medical officers by reimbursing the local Guardians, if and only if, they provided infirmaries of which the Poor Law authorities approved. Provided capital expenditure was not too great initially, there was a built-in incentive to create separate

141

infirmaries. Thus the Poor Law Board was at last given real powers if it chose to use them. Also the Act was an acknowledgement of the responsibility of the state to provide hospitals for the poor. In this sense it represented an important step towards the creation of the National Health Service eighty years later.

For the medical profession the outcome of these changes was a takeover of the senior posts in the improved Poor Law hospitals by men whose careers had been blocked in the voluntary hospitals. These young men, be it noted, were patronised by some of the most exalted consultants in the profession. Doctors trained in the voluntary hospitals brought new knowledge and ideas into the Poor Law system, and implicitly challenged the whole philosophy underlying it. By the mid-1860s two free hospital systems had emerged. The small sector of voluntary hospitals, financed by voluntary contributions and working on a very selected basis to a high standard, and the 'real hospitals of the land' which were to be found under the auspices of the Poor Law and which were still very inadequate. Soon the poor even gained the right to institutional care when they were sick, and were no longer branded as paupers and disenfranchised (Abel-Smith 1964:64-5).

The new doctors took charge of these hospitals, as their forbears had done in the voluntary sector, and assumed control from the lay official. The leading posts of medical superintendent went to former housemen from the voluntary hospitals, who had not achieved a consultancy, and they were often aided by a full-time assistant medical officer. A further mark of the improved position of the public hospitals was their entitlement, after 1889, to admit medical students. Paradoxically it was not long before the problem of frustrated juniors began to emerge in these hospitals as it had done in the voluntary ones, and this was reinforced by the fact that most superintendents were appointed from outside the Poor Law service. Part-timers and general practitioners who had once been the mainstay of these hospitals were finally excluded almost altogether. 'Just as the Royal Colleges dominated medical appointments in the London general hospitals, so a limited group of doctors in each local town controlled the local hospital. The status which had always gone with a hospital appointment in London went with a hospital appointment in the provinces' (1964:102).

We have noted that the apothecary was being excluded from the voluntary hospitals in the 1860s. In the 1870s and 1880s the general practitioner was likewise ousted from the urban Poor Law infirmaries. Only in the rural areas, to which the hospital movement was spreading in the second half of the nineteenth century, did the general practitioner have access. Indeed he had a central role in their creation. In 1865 there were eighteen cottage hospitals and by 1880 the number had increased to 180. Most were started by a legacy or a donation and others by money raised from local subscribers. In some cases a hospital was started with subscriptions from local working people. Typically there was a small committee of management in which a leading role was played by the local parson. Such hospitals were usually open to all local general practitioners and frequently admitted patients on a paying basis. It was in this way that the 'ideal' of the family doctor, a beloved stereotype, came into being. 'Far away from the towns where the "old orders" controlled hospital beds, the rural patient was able to enjoy a continuous relationship with one doctor and had the "privilege of being able to pay something, however small, according to his means, for the treatment he receives" ' (Abel-Smith 1964:103).

In general the hospital movement had been perceived as a threat by the general practitioner and competition became more intense with the foundation of each new hospital out-patient department providing free medical attention. This was one of the reasons why as early as 1836, at its fifth annual meeting, the British Medical Association had concerned itself with the issue of free medical assistance. Doctors who obtained a precarious living by practising among skilled workers and the lower middle class were naturally interested in establishing a stringent definition of those people who should be given medical charity. Their aim, right up to the establishment of the National Health Service, was to ensure that income tests would be applied. They wanted to make sure that persons who could afford to pay, would in fact pay a fee to a doctor and not be allowed to get away with a free consultation. The *British Medical Journal*, in 1853, attacked what it regarded as the abuse of hospitals and dispensaries which it saw as the monster evil of the day. The British Medical Association campaigned against out-patient departments which, it contended, reduced the earnings of all general practitioners working within the catchment area of the hospital. 'Gentlemen's servants, clerks and well-to-do tradespeople with their wives and children absolutely encumber the waiting-rooms of the London hospitals' (*British Medical Journal* 1853:76). Similarly 'yeomen' were said to be depriving local doctors of their fees by travelling to the nearest voluntary hospital. For months the *Journal* was obsessed with this problem. 'We would commence by driving forth, with indignation, from the waiting-rooms, the over-paid and pampered menials of the pseudo-charitable societies' (1853:76). The implication was that the leading men, consultants and specialists, in the voluntary hospitals were stealing patients from the general practitioner, and that some people who could well afford to pay, were wrongfully abusing the system of free medical advice. It was for this reason that cottage hospitals controlled by general practitioners were pay-hospitals. After all, medical men should receive an adequate remuneration. We have already noted that a problem was posed by the free-enterprise special hospitals which charged for a specialist opinion, but at a rate competitive with the general practitioner. From the latter's point of view the system amounted to undercutting.

Public and Private Medical Assistance: their inter-relationship

We have now discussed the opening-up of medical careers in a publicly-funded hospital setting provided under the auspices of the Poor Law. This grew from small beginnings as a development from the system of harsh indoor relief. It is necessary also to note the relationship between the medical practitioner and outdoor relief. The provision of some medical assistance for the poor paid for by parish funds long antedated the 1834 Poor Law. For example, as early as 1717, at Wednesbury, a parish doctor called Richard Hammersley was appointed and paid three guineas a year to attend poor people. By 1763 the parish doctor's annual fee was five pounds. In 1831 Robert Ladbury was appointed parish surgeon at an annual salary of £25 (Ede 1962). Paupers and others, whom church wardens and overseers might see fit to recommend were attended by the surgeon. Such cases included confinements where a mother was not in receipt of parish relief but adjudged to need assistance with doctors fees. In each case the surgeon was paid five shillings. As Marshall points out speaking of the eighteenth century 'just as they contracted for the farming of the poor in workhouses, and for the conveying of vagrants, so parishes contracted for medical attendance of the poor' (Marshall 1969:121).

The introduction of the Poor Law (1834) had involved the parish authorities much more systematically in securing the services of doctors, mostly on a part-time basis, to attend sick paupers. The relationship between doctors and the Poor Law was to be an unhappy one and has coloured the attitude of the profession towards local authority service up to the present time. A number of objectionable features, from the doctors' point of view, soon became apparent. Under the Poor Law doctors found themselves in conflict with the masters of the workhouses, whom they usually regarded as their social inferiors. Workhouse masters were typically recruited from the ranks of non-commissioned officers in the Army or Navy. The medical officer was normally a part-timer with little or no security of tenure and there were but few full-time resident medical officers anywhere in England.

Many guardians were content to hire their doctors at the lowest possible price by advertising vacancies and inviting the local practitioners to undercut each other. In some unions the posts were subject to annual renewal which entailed a yearly round of canvassing by all the local doctors. Older practitioners had to compete for these Poor Law appointments in order to keep potential competitors out of their districts. Young doctors sought these posts in order to supplement their incomes (while they struggled to establish a private practice) and [gained] experience in the lucrative business of midwifery' (Abel-Smith 1964:58). The competition from midwives in this branch of practice could be severe. It is true that some medical officers were reasonably paid, but in many cases the salary was small and the doctor was expected to pay for his own drugs, to defray the costs of any deputising which proved necessary, and in some recorded instances a doctor could make a loss. Presumably in such a case a practitioner thought it necessary to do this work in order to keep rivals out of the district. 'As a result, the *Lancet* commissioners found that "an antagonism is set up and in many cases leads to the most vexatious and mischievous interference by the master with the purely medical orders of the surgeon" ' (Abel-Smith 1964:60).

'When conflict arose, the medical officer could rarely hope for support from either the Guardians or the Central Authority' (1964:61). Unfortunately medical relief proved to be in contradiction to the basic Poor Law principle of 'less-eligibility'. The situation clearly parallels in many instances the relationship between the elementary teacher and the school managers. If the medical officer fell out with the master over any matter, he might find himself refused on some pretext the midwifery fee which he would normally expect. Some relieving officers would vex and harass the doctor in such a situation.

Frequently doctors could not afford to argue, for some of their most valuable patients were members of the Board of Guardians, or were well known to them. A doctor was unlikely to 'quarrel with his bread and butter' (1964:91). Nevertheless, some Poor Law medical officers did send a memorial of protest to the Local Government Board. They wanted higher salaries, the status of civil servants and to be permitted to offer relief to poor people in the home without the intervention of the relieving officer. These points did not impress the Board, which pointed out among other things that servants of the state were prohibited from engaging in private practice. Remarking on the matter of remuneration the Board stated that 'the facility with which, when the office of medical officer becomes vacant, competent medical men are found to fill the vacancies, affords a strong presumption that on the whole the remuneration is not deemed to be insufficient' (Local Government Board 1879:86-8). Such an attitude is strongly remembered in the folklore of the medical profession. Changes in the political direction of the administration of the Poor Law were important to the medical profession and were influenced by it. Eventually the funda- mental principle of Poor Law doctrine namely 'less-eligibility' was breached by the clear instructions of the Central Board which asserted that the cure of illness and the alleviation of suffering should have first priority (Poor Law Board 1867-8:28). 'No longer were the standards of care of the pauper patients to be judged by the standards enjoyed by the lowest paid labourer' (Abel-Smith 1964:96). This entailed a new administrative structure and a transformation, as we have noted, of the work situation of the hospital medical staff. Where the chief officer of the workhouse was a lay official, the leading official in the new infirmaries was a full-time medical superintendent. By 1888 every London infirmary had its own superintendent aided by a full-time assistant medical officer. Often they were recruited from among former housemen from voluntary hospitals who had not achieved a consultancy. In 1905, in London, a superintendent might earn between £350 and £500 as well as such fringe benefits as spacious accommodation, gas, coal and laundry provided free. Some additional fees could be expected for vaccinations and the certification of lunatics.

Assistant medical officers, on the other hand, were mainly young men looking for an introduction to general practice. They were paid much less and did not often serve for more than two or three years. In some cases Guardians only appointed them for a one-year period. Because most superintendents were appointed from the voluntary hospitals the chance of obtaining the highest rank was small for the assistants. Indeed, as previously mentioned, the problem of frustrated juniors quickly manifested itself as it had done in the voluntary hospitals. What was new for the Guardians was the demands made by professional chief officers which it was hard for laymen to refuse. Any layman's opinion was as good as that of a professional when it came to a judgement of less-eligibility, but where the problem was defined as a medical matter the balance of power shifted to the doctors. The standards which they imposed were modelled on those of the voluntary hospitals in which they had worked or trained.

There was a short period in which, due to a change in policy, the amount of outdoor relief granted was considerable. Poor Law dispensaries were set up but they were scarcely operational before another change of official policy reversed its situation and the volume of dispensary orders granted was, by 1873, falling steadily. In their place the authorities were fostering the development of sick clubs and provident dispensaries by pressure on the poor. The growth in membership of these private institutions was immense. It is the opinion of Abel-Smith that 'the Poor Law Board and the Guardians between them managed to direct the organisation of general practice in Britain from the publicly-owned dispensary or "health centre", with its salaried dispenser to the club or "panel" practice and the commercial pharmacy' (Abel-Smith 1964:93). This was to lead to the so-called 'battle of the clubs' in which the British Medical Association played a leading role.

The British Medical Association also did its utmost to bring pressure to bear in the growing local authority medical field with the object of establishing adequate standards of salary and working conditions. For example, it had encouraged the Poor Law medical officers to form their own Association (1846). The British Medical Association continued to maintain the closest relationship with it, acting as its mouthpiece in negotiations with local authorities, and introduced the tactic of 'blacklisting' those authorities that refused to pay adequate salaries. Subsequently, from 1905, a Central Emergency Fund was set up to assist individuals or organisations who suffered as a by-product of the British Medical Association's militant action. Later on in the 1920s and

30s the British Medical Association supported the Society of Medical Officers of Health with whom it agreed a scale of minimum commencing salaries. Many local authorities refused to recognise this but again it was successfully enforced through the tactic of black-listing recalcitrant authorities. The *British Medical Journal*, the *Lancet* and the *Medical Officer* refused to carry advertisements for black-listed posts. As a measure of success it may be noted that in 1926-7 180 vacancies in public health posts were advertised at a figure under the minimum, and in 101 of these cases the scale salary was achieved. The British Medical Association also had a long struggle to get medical doctors accepted as officers rather than non-commissioned officers in the Armed Forces and to obtain adequate salaries and conditions. 'The point was finally won after a report on the alleged unsatisfactory conditions in the Army had been sent to the Dean of every medical school asking that it might be brought to the notice of every man who contemplated entering the service' (Carr-Saunders 1933:97).

If the British Medical Association was important in the struggle to get the Medical Registration Act of 1858 on the statute book, by 1888 it was called 'the greatest power in the profession' (Laffan 1888: 131). It has had a 'persistently skilful leadership', (Carr-Saunders, 1933:91) a succession of unusually able permanent officials, and doctors willing to give much of their time to the affairs of the Association. It has often pressed its policies upon the General Medical Council either directly through its representatives suggesting British Medical Association policies or by gingering up the General Medical Council for example to make greater use of its disciplinary powers, and issue warnings about advertisement. The Association has dealt with the less serious matters of professional misconduct which fall outside the sphere of the General Medical Council.

The nineteenth century witnessed a truly remarkable growth in self-help organisations of which the friendly societies were a formidable example (Gosden 1961). These expanded at a remarkable rate at least up to 1870, but after that time they, if anything, were outpaced by the vigorous expansion of the trade union movement. The growth of friendly societies, trade unions with friendly functions, and provident clubs, and dispensaries run on a charitable basis increasingly involved the employment of the services of doctors under conditions determined by these organisations and their officials, rather than by the doctors themselves. Doctors found themselves under the control of committees made up of working men which 'it is not a pleasant matter for an educated gentleman to serve under' (*British Medical Journal* 1875:484).

The impact of the crusade against outdoor relief (1871) which was rooted in the doctrines of economic liberalism and stressed thrift and the importance of each individual making private provision for sickness led to the growth of provident clubs into which working people were pushed by deliberate government policy. This was done by the stark enforcement of the Poor Law. In this situation commercial insurance interests could exploit the opportunities thus created. For the general practitioners the threat existed that in the long run he could be reduced to the status of an employee of the large Commercial Insurance Company.

From the 1870s onwards the state encouraged, more positively than before, the development of private insurance schemes, and also strengthened the long standing government commitment to fostering the Friendly Society movement. Both of these affected the work situation of the general practitioner because the growth of private aid medical institutions run by lay committees, usually consisting of people ignorant of professional standards, were concerned to hire doctors as cheaply as they could; they advertised and canvassed to augment their clientele and imposed patients upon their medical servants in such numbers and under such conditions as to render honest and efficient service impossible.

The British Medical Association became involved in 'the battle of the clubs'. After a considerable struggle the Association succeeded in persuading the General Medical Council to institute an enquiry into the problem, which eventuated in a ruling (1894) that it was unprofessional for a registered doctor to associate himself with a canvassing institution. The friendly societies had also begun to utilise some of the methods of the medical aid institutions. From 1900 until 1911 the Association struggled to combat the evil in this new location. Eventually the leadership came to accept that nothing less than some form of publicly-funded medical service would give the profession a chance to overcome the abuses attributable to Friendly Society and Provident Association domination of the cheaper end of the medical market. Political developments at the national level were tending in the same direction leading up to the 1911, National Health Insurance Act. Support for a state organised insurance scheme to finance medical attendance began to seem a possibility within the profession, particularly if it could be confined to the poorer end of the market. Doctors who depended precariously for a living upon practice among skilled workers and the lower middle class were naturally interested in establishing a stringent definition of those people who should be given medical charity. Their aim right up to the establishment of the National Health Service was to ensure that income tests would be applied, so that persons who could afford to pay would in fact pay their fee to a doctor and not be allowed to get away with a free consultation.

The national organisations such as the Royal Colleges or the British Medical Association did not in fact lay down national minimum scales of fees. The role of these organisations in national bargaining with the state only emerged in the twentieth century. The same was true for the trade unions (Royal Commission on Trade Unions and Employers' Association 1968). In the nineteenth century small medical associations, or the local branches of the British Medical Association in particular, did in fact set a scale of recommended fees for use by local practitioners. Such a tariff of medical fees, for example, was issued by the Manchester Medico-Ethical Association and published in 1865. Thereafter revised editions were published from time to time and such an edition appeared in 1879. It states that the Association

'disclaims a wish to dictate either to its own members or other medical men [and is] convinced that the subject of medical charges must remain forever a somewhat open one, so long as the profession, unlike all other trades and professions, continues to claim its remuneration not according to the abstract worth of its services alone, but also according to the ability of its clients to pay — a compulsory scale of charges is neither possible nor to be desired. Still this Association has found a recommended tariff highly useful in many ways' (Manchester Medico-Ethical Association 1879).

Specifically it mentions cases of disputed charges: preventing litigation and providing friendly settlements. Also as a guide to the junior practitioner in doubt as to proper remuneration it advises that

'the present scale has been fixed at such a rate that the humblest member of the profession need not hesitate to make it the basis of his charges. Indeed, it may be observed that the rates have been fixed rather according to what is usual than according to what would be necessary to enable the profession to maintain its due status, in the presence of the greatly diminished value of money and the increase of wealth and luxury among other classes in the community. Owing to these causes it will certainly be necessary before many years have lapsed to ensure that a considerably higher tariff should be adopted; the present period of commercial depression, however, does not appear to be the proper time. It is to be hoped that nothing in the present tariff will prevent those members of the profession who by reason of seniority or enhanced reputation, are in a position to do so, from making higher charges when the circumstances warrant.'

Continuing its advice the Association says that

'the necessary division of patients into classes has been a difficult point in the formation of a tariff. This Association was the first to recommend rental of the patient's residence as the basis of classification instead of income as being easier of discovery and less inquisitorial and fallacious. It need hardly be said that many exceptional cases will be met with where the practitioner must use a wide discretion though not so many as if he attempted directly to ascertain the income of his patients' (Manchester Medico-Ethical Association 1879).

The writer goes on to mention the style of life of the patient as relevant in judging his ability to pay. The tariff uses house rentals in the categories between ten and twenty-five pounds, fifty pounds, a hundred pounds and over this figure. But the author observes that people paying less than £10 annual rent can often afford to pay 'somewhat for medical advice and whom it is desirable to preserve from the necessity of consulting druggists and other unqualified persons'.

'Although it has been considered impossible to give a scale of fees suitable to the means of such of the poorer classes, the Association would impress on its members and the profession generally the advisability of attending them, when their other engagements will permit, at a rate of charges reduced even somewhat below the lowest here given. This would not only be a boon to the poor themselves, but in the case of practitioners inhabiting thickly populated districts, would not be unremunerative. Such small charges should be made for ready money, but when this is not possible, monthly accounts are recommended. In all other cases quarterly accounts are advised' (Manchester Medico-Ethical Association 1879).

By this time the general practitioner had distanced himself socially from his predecessor, the apothecary, whose main source of income was the sale of drugs. On the question of payment for medicines the Association says

'this has been deliberately ommitted, and will serve to mark the sense of the Association that medical men *should, in all cases, base their title to remuneration upon the value of their time and skill*. The practice of supplying medicines at all has died out almost everywhere except in England and the day will probably arrive when it will do so here. Balancing in every light the advantages, to patient and practitioner, of supplying medicines or prescribing, the Association concluded that this tariff is equally applicable to both cases, and recommends it whether medicines are supplied or not. Of course no extra charge for them is understood as their cost is amply made up by the greater hold the practitioner has on his patient' (Manchester Medico-Ethical Association 1879).

This quotation nicely illustrates the dilemmas of the general practitioner's market situation: the need to establish a minimum scale of fees, but the realisation that such a scale could never be applicable to the poorest patients without modification; the knowledge that unless they served such patients their territory might be invaded by others; and finally, following the lines of tract we have quoted, a statement that surgical fees laid down by the Poor Law Board should be used as the *minimum* for all kinds of surgical work.

The problem posed for the profession by the existence of patients who could not afford to pay, but who needed care, was seen from another point of view by Reeney. 'Those patients who cannot afford the smallest fee, are certainly entitled to gratuitous medical aid, but not necessarily gratuitous medical aid given by the profession.' Such help should be provided by the state by some method not making the recipient 'but one step removed from the criminal' (Reeney 1905:44). It is evident that, by the 1870s, general practitioners were using scales laid down by the Poor Law Board and even by Act of Parliament, as guide lines for judging remuneration in the private market. This indicates the extent to which publicly stipulated scales had penetrated the medical world by then. For example, in the Factory & Workshops Act of 1878 the surgeons and the occupiers of a factory may agree a fee between them but in case of disagreement, a scale of fees was laid down (Rivington 1879:240).

The 'battle of the clubs' was essentially about contract practice. Complaints about the 'evils of contract medical practice' are older than the British Medical Association itself (Little 1932:199). According to the Webbs,

> 'when kindly philanthropists in the [1830s] started provident dispensaries and sick clubs as an alternative to Poor Law medical relief, it seemed to the medical profession of the time that for doctors to take contract service from the Committees at a capitation fee, or a part-time salary, was to be commended as at any rate a preferable alternative to service under the Board of Guardians. Later on, when the Friendly Societies had developed into a network covering the whole kingdom, and including not only manual-working wage-earners, but also many members of the lower middle-class, and when points of difference between Friendly Society Committees and doctors had multiplied, it was not the abuses of the system, but the system itself, that was denounced as inconsistent with the proper relation of the practitioner to his patients' (Webb 1917:12).

There were two principal types of contract practice. From the point of view of the medical profession 'the least objectionable was that of the private club, in which a practitioner agreed to attend his poorer patients for a small annual sum to be paid weekly, whether the patient were well or ill'. Little takes the view that 'this was a form of charitable relief coming out of the doctor's pocket, for he knew that these club patients could not afford to pay adequate fees' (Little 1932:199). It is important however to notice that no outside body intervened between doctor and patient and that it was for the doctor alone to settle the terms upon which patients would be admitted to the club.

The other and more formidable type of contract practice was carried on through the agency of the Friendly Societies, who were intermediaries between doctor and patient, and were in effect the employers of the doctor. He was expected to treat 'whatever patients the society chose to allot to him' (Little 1932:199). Among the Friendly Society Medical Clubs, there were some which were fostered by Boards of Guardians in an effort to relieve the rates.

151

Doctors felt that the remuneration provided under contract practice was wholly inadequate and that the lack of any restrictive clause as to the election of new members of the clubs who could make a call upon the doctor's services tended to cause him to be overworked. There were some cases of unmerciful 'sweating'. Attention was drawn to this problem in a leading article in the *Provincial Medical & Surgical Journal* on 26 January 1848 by citing the case of the Dorset County Friendly Society. At a meeting of Dorset practitioners it was thought desirable to restrict medical relief to the labouring population and journeymen mechanics and a conference was proposed with a committee of the society.

The societies were in a strong position *vis-à-vis* unorganised medical men, as was the case among Poor Law medical officers in the early days, and as a result every effort was made to find 'one among the local practitioners whose poverty or whose anxiety to get into practice induced him to accept their niggardly terms' (1932:200). One important reason why Friendly Societies obstinately resisted the efforts of doctors to establish a wage limit above which members should be ineligible for medical benefit, was due to the fact that this was only one of their several concerns. Generally speaking, unemployment benefits and benefits paid to members during sickness were much more important than the payment of medical benefit for the purpose of getting the attendance of the doctor. Societies opposed a wage limit for medical benefit because 'they could not exclude a member from one form of benefit and admit him to others' (Little 1932:201).

By the 1890s a new form of association, the medical aid association, was developing rapidly. These provided a new threat to poorer practitioners since they offered only medical and surgical treatment to their members. 'Some practitioners employed by large societies undertook more patients than they could properly attend personally, and therefore employed unqualified assistants, who would accept a lower wage than a qualified man.' This form of contract practice was regarded with great disfavour by the majority of general practitioners who together with the vast majority of the profession 'cordially supported the attempts of the Association [British Medical Association] to get the evil system mended or ended' (1932:201).

In 1892 the General Medical Council summoned a practitioner to answer a charge of 'covering' in connection with a medical aid association and also of employing an unqualified assistant. Although the practitioner in question was able to get off because the case was not proven it was the beginning of positive action against contract practice. A Committee of the General Medical Council was set up to consider medical aid associations and it reported in 1893. It stated that

'a medical practitioner is acting in a reprehensible manner (*a*) if he holds a medical aid appointment the duties of which are so onerous that he cannot do justice to the sick under his care; (*b*) if he consents to give certificates where in his opinion they are not justifiable on medical grounds; (c) if he accepts or retains employment by an association in which canvassing is used to attract members' (1932:202).

The General Medical Council did not adopt the recommendations of its Committee and many in the profession thought that it had shirked its responsibilities. In 1894, the *British Medical Journal* (1894:831) discussed the increase in medical aid associations which it attributed to the impecuniosity of medical men. It suggested that during the previous decade there had been a steady increase in the ratio of medical practitioners per one thousand of the population, and at the same time a continuing rise in the amount of charitable medical relief offered particularly in the large towns. It was thought that 'consequently the struggle for existence generally within the ranks of the profession had become annually more and more keen' (Little 1932:203).

The outcry against contract practice reached its greatest pitch in the first few years of the twentieth century. Attention was particularly focussed on the oppression of the medical aid associations and the British Medical Association was drawn increasingly into this struggle. A fund was opened for practitioners in Cork 'who had resigned their positions as officers of clubs and benefit societies rather than submit to their terms' (1932:203). The annual meeting of the British Medical Association 1903 carried a motion to the effect that the Association's Medico-Political Committee investigate contract practice, and that the Ethical Committee examine the situation with regard to canvassing and the acceptance of posts which other practitioners have conscientiously declined.

As a result of this a publication on contract practice appeared as a supplement to the *British Medical Journal* (1905). This was a particularly important document which covered not merely contract practice as defined above but also provident dispensaries and public medical services. There was a general acknowledgement that there are districts where contract practice is necessary but it insisted that 'the profession is the best judge of the classes and individuals who are entitled to such a concession on their part, and that therefore the ideal system is that contract practice in every area should be arranged by and under the control of the medical profession itself'. It should be especially noted that this report was extremely influential as it subsequently 'formed the basis of many of the negotiations which ended with the passing of the National Health Insurance Act in 1911, and although this Act excluded the creation of such a medical service as was contemplated in the Report, the investigation supplied valuable evidence upon which to negotiate' (Little 1932:204). The whole report rested on the first principle that the medical profession 'should itself prescribe the rules and conditions under which it will enter into agreements to give medical attendance by contract. It was largely over this principle that the unequal battle between the profession and the Government of the day was waged in the discussions of the Insurance Act' (1932:204).

The earlier refusal of the General Medical Council to act on the matter of contract practice was taken up by the British Medical Association and its branches. They argued that

'these commercial undertakings depended to a great extent for their success on advertisement and canvassing. This view of the matter was pressed home by the direct representatives on the Council, (General Medical Council) which at least decided that medical practitioners serving canvassing societies would be acting in an infamous manner in a professional respect' (1932:205).

Together with the decision of the Council that the employment of unqualified assistants amounted to 'covering', the Association (British Medical Association) was given two strong weapons which it used effectively in dealing with contract practice until the Insurance Act abolished these medical companies. The Friendly Societies had a long history but the medical aid associations lasted scarcely more than forty years. The first one was probably opened at Preston in 1869, and by 1911, the Medical Alliance (of Medical Aid Associations) claimed a membership of seventy-five, and upwards of 100 of these organisations were known to exist throughout the country.

Doctors and the State

During the middle years of the nineteenth century medical men, both locally and nationally, were the spearhead of the growing movement for sanitary reform. This inevitably involved calling upon the state to intervene in the health field. Under pressure from public opinion as a result of the repeated cholera epidemics, Parliament established a General Board of Health under the Public Health Act of 1848. Although the General Board of Health was served by energetic and intelligent men, its role was poorly planned and it was perhaps too early, given the climate of opinion, for a central authority to act firmly in the health field. It was certainly true that the Board lacked a direct connection with a Ministry and was in any case, subject to clashes of personality. At all events, the Board was universally unpopular and the press rejoiced when, in 1854, it was abolished. Among its enemies had been the influential Royal College of Physicians. A new, reconstituted Board was set up on an annual basis until, in 1858, its responsibilities for public health were transferred to the Privy Council.

Sanitary reformers still continued to press, in spite of the failure of the General Board of Health, for greater central direction in health matters. One prominent advocate of this view was John Simon, who himself was Medical Officer of the Privy Council from 1858-71. He conceived the state's role as 'superintendent-general for health'. In the 1860s there was still no single national health authority concerned with the administration of the government's expanding role in preventive and curative medicine. On the one hand, the Medical Office of the Privy Council was extending the scope of its work in the surveillance of sanitary problems and the control of infectious disease, and on the other the Poor Law Board was administering the medical relief of the poor under the Act of 1834. Poor Law medical officers were appointed in every parish, some serving full-time, and others part-time. Fixed salaries were payable as well as additional payments for particular types of cases from the parish Boards of Guardians. Remarkably little supervision was exercised by the Poor Law Board over the 'parish doctors' and there was little concern expressed by the medical reformers for improving curative as opposed to preventive medicine. It is true that occasionally complaints were expressed in medical journals about the quality of Poor Law practice in the context of the penny-pinching attitude of Boards of Guardians, but the chief concern was the denunciation of the 'Guardians for underpaying parish doctors' (Brand 1965:5).

By the mid-1860s England was already in advance of other countries in its development of sanitary legislation. The Royal Sanitary Commission (1868-71) 'was directly attributable to medical men, both within and without the government' (1965:8). A number of medical witnesses pressed for a strong central health authority capable of acting decisively at both national and local level. The Royal Commission preceded the Local Government (Board) Act of 1871, which provided for 'a merger of the staff of the Poor Law Board, the staff of the Local Government Act Office, the staff of the Registrar-General's Office and the staff of the Medical Office of the Privy Council, into one, new Local Government Board, which was to exercise the functions of its old components' (1965:14). The government in presenting the Bill to Parliament stated that it was merely a first step in carrying out the Royal Sanitary Commission's recommendations. Sir Lyon Playfair, who was the unofficial parliamentary spokesman of the medical profession, gave the measure hearty support. Mr James Stansfeld was appointed President of the new Local Government Board. In 1872 a new Public Health Act was introduced to the House by Stansfeld which proposed to divide England into new urban and rural sanitary districts. Simon noted 'that the Bill was drafted to favor the appointment of poor law medical officers as the health officers of the newly created administrative districts'. A storm arose in the medical profession on the grounds, as the *Lancet* suggested, that 'a new, unwelcome class of state physicians might develop as a result of the Act' (Brand 1965:16). The Poor Law Medical Officers Association opposed the Bill and it was urged by the *Lancet* that some provision be made for the appointment of health officers at a superior level to supervise the districts if only because no local official, medical or otherwise, could be expected to oppose the interests of 'his vestrymen and other (important) patients' (1965:17).

He could not tell them, for example, that a house of which one of them was landlord was unfit for human habitation. When the Bill became law, in 1872, some at least of the objectionable features were modified.

The Medical Department of the Local Government Board exerted little influence on policy both because of the domination by the personnel of the old Poor Law Board and the eclipse of the role of the former Privy Council group, not least of whom was their chief, John Simon. He eventually resigned in 1876. The medical officers employed by the Local Government Board were confined in an administrative straight-jacket which only served to strengthen the spirit of retrenchment inherent in the old Poor Law administration. In 1895 the Chief Medical Officer of the Local Government Board said that 'concentrated medical officialism is not a desirable thing in this Country . . . A religious adherence to the negative implications of this doctrine constituted one of the reasons for the Medical Department's weakness' (Brand 1965:81). Such a view, however, was also widely advocated for many decades outside government circles and even a liberal medical man like Dr Henry Acland, in an important address to the National Association for the Promotion of Social Science, pressed this line of thinking on his audience. The Webbs noted as late as 1910 that the Chief Medical Officer of the Board still had no regular share in advising the Board's President on health matters (Webb 1910:223-4). There is no question that 'the lack of a strong, forward-looking central medical authority undoubtedly delayed the expansion of government into the personal health services'. Nevertheless, within the narrow scope of its role, the Medical Department of the Board 'maintained and widened the concept of State intervention for the control of disease (Brand 1965:82).

As the General Board of Health is considered to be the forerunner of a Ministry of Health it seems extraordinary that it took sixty-one years from the demise of the one to the creation of the other. The forces underlying the struggle for the Ministry of Health have been thoroughly analysed by Honingsbaum (Honingsbaum 1971). Apart from the fact that, as we have seen, 'with few exceptions, the Local Government Board's Poor Law functions smothered its concern for public health' (1971:9). We note that delay in the creation of a durable department may be laid partly at the door of the doctors. While it is true that from the middle of the nineteenth century public-spirited practitioners were to be found in every campaign directed towards the creation of a Ministry of Health down to its establishment in 1919, yet

'the bulk of the profession showed interest in the subject only when it held out hope of strengthening their economic position. What they wanted most of all was protection against the competition of unqualified practitioners. Here, however, the 1858 Medical Act and the 1911 National Health Insurance Act satisfied much of their needs — the former, by confining Friendly

156

Society (as well as public) posts to registered doctors; the latter, by extending this protection from one-tenth to one-third of the population. After 1911, medical interest in a Ministry weakened and it revived in 1918 only after the profession saw how much protection could be extended further without running the risk of bureaucratic control' (Honingsbaum 1971:10).

As Sir Bertrand Dawson once put it, the Ministry 'was brought about by public opinion and not, unfortunately, by medical opinion' (1971:11).

The Poor Law medical officer, or ' "parish doctor" (was overworked and underpaid, [and] he could rarely satisfy both the medical needs of his patients and the shilling-pinching demands of his tough-minded employers, the local Boards of Guardians' (Brand 1965:85). In the middle years of the nineteenth century, the Poor Law medical officers had formed themselves into a well organised group within the medical profession and were becoming increasingly vocal on the necessity of urgent reform of Poor Law medical care (Hodgkinson 1967). From the 1870s Poor Law medical officers, who prior to the Act of 1858 were often only partially qualified, were increasingly recruited on a more selective basis because the Poor Law Board would now employ only fully qualified and registered practitioners. 'This is not to say, of course, that all parish doctors ranked with Harley Street men. But their status within the profession and in the eyes of the public had increased remarkably' (Brand 1965:88). Despite the variations in salary, Poor Law medical officers were employed on a fairly permanent basis and often in the large cities were full-time medical officers to the workhouses. Moreover, by the end of the century the posts were more hotly competed for because they carried among their several advantages 'a publicly guaranteed introduction to the neighbourhood' (Sprigge 1899:146). This was based upon the fact that the Poor Law Board, from 1868, had discouraged the use of unqualified assistants to Poor Law medical officers and the rate of medical scandals in the service, frequently alluded to in the 1840s, were much reduced by the 1860s.

The division of functions within the Local Government Board, which as we have seen reduced its Medical Office to a very minor position, makes sense of the fact that there was no proper development of a central medical advisory staff to oversee the work of the Poor Law medical officers. Central inspection was in the hands of the Board's lay inspectors, not physicians. These men were imbued with the principles of retrenchment upon which the Poor Law itself had been founded. Such directives as were issued from the centre were sporadic and without the adequate force of authority or inspection which would ensure compliance and the development of national standards of Poor Law medical care. Brand's view is that 'permissive regulation made for not only considerable variation in performance but outright abuse' (1965:92). The struggle over the provision of 'medical extras' was a constant source of friction between Guardians and medical officers. The authorities believed that to give the Poor Law medical officer free reign over medical extras would send the cost of medical relief soaring.

With the passage of time, the impact of the evangelical revival with its new humanitarianism towards the poor, the dramatic effects of the cholera epidemics before which rich and poor were equally vulnerable, helped to temper the harshness of the principle of less-eligibility. In this process the Poor Law Medical Association played an important role as a pressure group. Originally, it had sprung from the Poor Law Committee of the Provincial Medical and Surgical Association and remained closely linked with the British Medical Association. As in the case of the latter Association, it had involved the merger between metropolitan and provincial medical interests. Through the pages of the *Lancet* it had obtained considerable publicity and in alliance with the Association for the Improvement of Workhouse Infirmaries, it had been important in the legislative field, not least, in the passage of the Metropolitan Poor Relief Act 1867. The Association sought reforms through pressure on the Local Government Board. They asked its President, Stansfeld, for reform of the service, the appointment of more medical officers, greater autonomy for Poor Law doctors and payment for drugs from the rates, rather than out of the officers' pockets, and improved pay. At this stage their efforts were not particularly effective. The Association was also concerned with the defence of individual medical officers who were in dispute with their local Guardians, and in the 1890s directed their efforts to obtaining superannuation, payment of medical witnesses and improvements in salary scales. By this time, the climate of opinion within the Poor Law Board and the government was more sympathetic to their case, conceding for example that in future anaesthetics could be provided at public expense in the treatment of the poor, and in 1897 the Poor Law Officers Superannuation Act was passed.

One of the consequences of the sanitary movement was the introduction of local medical officers of health. The first was appointed in Liverpool in 1847. From 1855 onwards the appointment of medical officers of health was compulsory in London. Prior to 1872 some fifty of these new posts had been created outside London, but the Public Health Act of that year made it mandatory throughout the country. Only gradually did medical officers of health come to be specially trained in that branch of medicine, although the Local Government Board required that these officers be registered doctors. A Society of Medical Officers of Health was founded which by 1877 was able to comment on the great improvement in the training available. In spite of the importance of the 1872 Act which established a nation-wide corps of medical officers of health, it contained a grave weakness in that it failed to specify whether such officers should serve part-time or full-time and this opened a loophole through which recalcitrant authorities were able to evade their new responsibilities. The relationship between the medical officers and the Board was tenuous. Lyon Playfair noted in 1874 'the utter confusion' (Brand 1965:113) which he believed resulted from the failure of the Local Government Board to consult its own state officers, including John Simon. The Society of the Medical Officers of Health tended to be in advance of public opinion and, indeed, of the rest of the medical profession in pressing for state intervention in many aspects of preventive medicine. In the sixties and the seventies they were particularly concerned with the issue of 'the extent to which the individual should voluntarily surrender "personal liberty" in order to live, in health, in a healthful community' (1965:115). They pressed for action on matters of infectious disease, including hospital and isolation facilities, and the registration and notification of disease. They also took an active part in influencing public policy on housing standards for the working classes. In addition, they were involved in the sanitary aspects of industrial legislation, including industrial nuisances and the sanitary control of food and drugs. The Association was, in other words, concerned with an expanding conception of public health and a widening scope of co-operation with government departments. It was however never a radical reforming body, but rather adopted a pragmatic, professional approach to public health.

The Involvement of the State in Personal Health Services

In the early twentieth century the state began, in a step by step manner, to develop personal health services to ever-increasing categories of the community. Infectious disease was now treated free of charge in isolation units and quite literally bishops and paupers might be found in the same ward. A similar process of personal service was established in relation to tuberculosis, and the increasing consciousness of maternal and infant mortality led to the development of welfare services in this regard. The health of the school child became a recognised problem and the Education (Administrative Provisions) Act 1907 was a major piece of social legislation, which is usually considered as the legislative beginning of personal health services in England. Under the auspices of this Act, a new Medical Department was created within the Board of Education which authorised the creation of a complete medical inspection service (Honingsbaum 1971:16-17).

In 1905 the appointment of the Royal Commission on the Poor Laws signalled a major review of policy which could deeply affect medical interests. The battle was joined between those who wished to see continued the principle of deterrence and the new social reformers. Beatrice Webb recalled that while listening to the evidence presented by the Charity Organisation Society, which argued in favour of restricting medical relief to the technically destitute, 'it suddenly flashed across my mind that what we had to do was, to adopt the exactly contrary attitude, and make medical inspection and medical treatment compulsory on all sick persons, to treat illness, in fact, as a public nuisance to be suppressed in the interests of the community' (Webb 1948:348). The British Medical Association was reluctantly forced to admit that the profession was split on the subject of the creation of a state medical service, although it recorded its opposition to the municipal funding and control of voluntary charity hospitals.

The Majority Report of the Commission recommended that the Poor Law medical service in England and Wales should be separate from public health services run by local authorities. It opposed rigorously the idea of free medical service on the grounds that it would tend to create a dependence of virtually the whole population on it, and would thus be a crippling burden on the Exchequer and the rates. Also it asserted that voluntary organisations would be ruined, as would the practices of almost all medical practitioners.

The Minority Report was infused with the elegance of Beatrice Webb's style, and was in many respects a radical departure from the *status quo*, especially in society's attitude towards poverty and the extent of government intervention. It proposed the establishment of a county public medical service and rejected the principle of deterrence in medical relief. It did not go so far as to suggest a free medical service to all applicants but, rather, a scale of charges which would allow those who could afford it to pay on a basis related to the size of their income. The essential principle of the Minority Report was the recognition of a duty on the part of the state to provide curative treatment for those in need of it.

Interest on the part of the medical profession, and especially by the British Medical Association was intense. A rumour to the effect that a public medical service might be recommended was enough to provoke the observation 'that the medical profession would not agree to becoming a branch of the Civil Service' (Brand 1965:205). After the Report had been published, the British Medical Association 'stated only that any system of medical assistance which might be adopted must include two principles in order to be satisfactory to the medical profession. First, medical services rendered to the state should be paid for by the state, and second, payment should be adequate and in direct accordance with the professional services rendered' (1965:205). Moreover, in a major editorial on 3 July 1909 the *British Medical Journal*, while recognising the urgent need for reform admitted that 'it is inevitable that what appear to be the selfish interests of the profession will loom largely in our debates' (*British Medical Journal* 1909: 36-7). They believed, however, that the success of any proposal for a public medical service must rest upon the just recognition of the rights of the doctors. In the event the recommendations of the Royal Commission were not immediately implemented but they nevertheless had a profound influence upon the climate of opinion.

Notes

1. Rate equalisation simply refers to the fact that some funds were transferred from rich boroughs to poor boroughs.

8. SEXUAL DIVISIONS AND THE MEDICAL OCCUPATIONS

It is an important contention of our book that sexual divisions in society must be treated as a structural factor which is of equal importance with social class. In a previous paper (Parry and Johnson 1974:2-3) the problem was couched in terms of the division between two ideologies. On the one hand, it was argued there existed in our society a 'familial' ideology which enjoins the idea of co-operation rather than competition and the concept of duty and responsibility between parents, children and relatives. This stands in sharp contrast to the 'market' ideology which is based upon the notion of the supremacy of the individual and his freedom and rationality. It was suggested that in our society both these ideologies to some extent constrain and motivate the behaviour of individuals but that it is still expected that the women will be committed to a greater extent to the familial ideology, and the man, to the market ideology. These ideological perspectives articulate the sexual divisions in our society at the structural level. They are the product of social forces operating historically over a long period.

Writing about the situation of women in the seventeenth century Clark argues that 'capitalism was the means by which the revolution in women's economic position was effected in the industrial world' (Clark 1919:295-6). She suggests that there were three important elements in this revolution. The first was the substitution of an individual wage for a family wage, giving men the opportunity to organise themselves in the labour-market 'without sharing with the women of their families all the benefits derived through their combination'. Secondly, there was 'the withdrawal of wage-earners from home-life to work upon the premises of the masters, which prevented the employment of the wage-earner's wife in her husband's occupation'. Thirdly, it was 'the rapid increase in wealth, which permitted the women of the upper classes to withdraw from all connection with business'. Even in the seventeenth century, it was possible to discern that 'once the strong hand of necessity [was] relaxed there [was] a marked tendency in English life for the withdrawal of married women from all productive activity, and their consequent devotion to the cultivation of idle graces; the parasitic life of its women has been in fact one of the chief characteristics of the parvenu class' (Clark 1919:296).

We have already explained in our discussion of the declining guild system that as the wealth of masters increased under incipient capitalist organisation, the craftsmen and journeymen were reduced to wage-

162

earners. Clark points out that 'the incidental result [was] that women were excluded from [the] ranks [of] the more highly skilled trades' (1919:297). The older system of family industry had united both labour and capital in the family group so that women had been directly involved in the productive enterprise. By contrast the individualism inherent in capitalist organisation caused men and women to vie with each other in the labour market to secure work and wages from the capitalists. Under the old system 'craftsmen had been free to employ their wives and daughters in any way that was convenient allowing the widow to retain her membership in her husband's guild or company, with full trading privileges' (1919:298). The new system closed such opportunities to women, including married daughters and spinsters.

The new theory of the state founded upon individualism and characteristically expressed in the writings of such social philosophers as Hobbes and Locke conceived of the family as a private sphere. Only the male head or other adult males had a function in the wider world. The voluntary associations characteristic of English society which were concerned with the pursuit of trade, education, or science all excluded women from their membership. 'Any association or combination of women outside the limits of their own families was discouraged and the benefits which had been extended to them in this respect by the Catholic Religion were specially deprecated' (Clark 1919:303). It is not that there was a conscious demarcation of the respective spheres of men and women in the occupational world. Rather, because the idea that women's place was in the home 'was regarded as an immutable law of Nature' (1919:299-300) the effects of the changes mentioned above on the social position of women was an unanticipated consequence of these developments. Excluded for the most part from the public world outside the home 'women were forgotten, and so no attempt was made to adjust their training and social status to the necessities of the new economic organisation' (1919:299).

> 'Thus came about the exclusion of women from the skilled trades, for the wives of men who became capitalists withdrew from productive activity, and the wives of journeymen confined themselves to domestic work, or entered the labour market as individuals, being henceforward entirely unprotected in the conflict by their male relations' (1919:289-99).

It is the view of Clark that 'the subjection of women to their husbands was the foundation stone of the structure of the community in which capitalism first made its appearance'. It is for this reason that the subjection of women to men as such cannot be explained by the rise of capitalism. She regards the increasing exclusion of women from the skilled trades and the developing higher professions as very much a result of their exclusion from specialised education and training. Such training required the investment of time and money and the rearing of children has always caused the withdrawal of women from productive work, particularly of a specialised kind, for a significant part of the life-cycle. Even before industrialism within the context of domestic industry the available evidence suggests that many of the more specialised tastes requiring greater training tended to fall within the province of the male and that processes requiring 'general intelligence and commonsense' fell to the female. While both sexes were engaged in domestic industry both reaped the advantages accruing from the trading privileges and social position of the particular family enterprise. Only when industry was reorganised under capitalism was the woman 'driven to fight her economic battles single-handed and women, hampered by the want of specialized training, were beaten down into sweated trades' (Clark 1919:303). Women's lack of specialised training was a disadvantage when industry had been reorganised on the basis of individual bargaining in the labour market. Men were freed to some extent from economic dependence on their wives and as a result were able to engage in the formation of exclusively male economic associations separated in large measure from the family sphere.

In the sphere of the medical occupations the seventeenth and eighteenth centuries witnessed an increasing division of labour and a concomitant exclusion of women from the higher and more lucrative branches of practice which were gradually emerging. By the mid-nineteenth century this process was so complete and so deeply institutionalised in society that it was necessary to rediscover the fact that women had been engaged in the healing arts in earlier times.

Manton points out that 'early Christian missionaries to Britain introduced the order of deaconesses who, among their religious duties, visited the sick in their homes or cared for them in hospital. The boundary between nursing and medical practice was vaguely defined but by the tenth century the ecclesiastical law of Edgar and his adviser, Saint Dunstan, was explicit' (Manton 1965:56). Women were given a legal status to practise medicine.

'The Norman Conquest brought to England an established tradition of medicine practised by women from castle to cottage. Ladies were the ordinary practitioners of domestic medicine and the skilled chatelaine could reduce fractures, probe and dress wounds or burns and prepare herbal remedies. Certain religious orders had, of course, a special vocation to tend the sick, which included diagnosis in the light of existing knowledge as well as treatment and everyday nursing. The most famous hospital in medieval Britain was probably the nunnery at Sion on the Thames. At Wherwell in Hampshire there was a Benedictine House with an infirmary directed by the abbess Euphemia. Male physicians were rare, since time and desire for study were almost confined to monks, Jews and others debarred from the supreme masculine occupation of fighting. Professional women doctors, trained by apprenticeship to men, by reading medical books and by continual practice in the empiric method . . . emerged to meet the need. None in Britain attained the fame of the women professors of Salerno, but they flourished well enough to take in their turn male apprentices' (Manton 1965:56-7).

In the fourteenth century 'Queen Phillipa, wife of Edward III, is said to have appointed as Court Surgeon Cecilia of Oxford, and by the close of the fourteenth century a few women were even recognised as surgeons by the Guild of Surgeons founded in 1389'.

It was 'in 1421 [that] the Surgeon's guild petitioned Parliament that no man should practice without having graduated [at a university] . . . and that no woman should practise under pain of long imprisonment' (Power 1921). By contrast the Royal College of Physicians which received its Charter in 1518, excluded women from the start. Yet though the College denied them full rank women continued to practise medicine during the sixteenth and seventeenth centuries, both as amateurs and even as professionals. Following the lead of Bishop Bonner of London, the bishops issued licences to practise physic and surgery within their jurisdiction, and at least sixty-six such licences, in seven dioceses, have been traced to women. Female apothecaries were also sometimes admitted to membership of the Society of Apothecaries after apprenticeship, usually to a relation. Bishops in the course of visitation to the parishes for which they were responsible, regularly enquired 'whether any man or woman, within the Parish hath professed or practised Physick or Chyrurgery'.

Throughout the seventeenth century St Bartholomew's Hospital employed women as official members of its medical staff, for the treatment of skin diseases (Manton 1965:58). 'The last women to treat skin cases was appointed as late as 1708' (Moore 1918:733). The 'descendants of the medical chatelaines played the part of military surgeon to both armies in the civil war . . . Lady Anne Halkett, who had studied medicine and surgery in order to help the poor, received the thanks of Charles II for her care of gunshot wounds and mangled limbs on the battlefield at Dunbar' (Nichols 1875:59). The care of the sick poor demanded not only charity but study, and domestic medicine was a serious art. Lady Falkland supplied 'antidotes against infections and other several sorts of Physick' on a hospital scale. Mrs Bedell 'was very famous and expert in Chyrurgery which she continually practised upon multitudes', while Mrs Bury studied morbid anatomy until her skill in diagnosis was remarkable. Jane Barker read medical books with her brother at Cambridge and issued prescriptions which were filed 'with those of the regular physicians'. She was said to be 'particularly successful with cases of gout'. In the opinion of Manton 'the lady amateur of medicine, though excluded from official scientific education was probably no more of a menace than the Hogarthian surgeon-apothecary of the early eighteenth century with his bleeding bowl and swingeing doses of calomel and antimony' (Manton 1965:59).

Apparently there were also a number of number of successful female quack and Mrs Map of Epsom who worked as a bone-setter ran her own coach and six (1965:59-60). Some sceptical people in the eighteenth century felt that there was not much to choose between the wise woman and a learned holder of degrees. As Adam Smith put it 'do not all the old women in the country practise physic without exciting a murmur or a complaint?' (Turner 1958:118).

'The credit of the woman medical practitioner declined steeply in the second half of the eighteenth century. A combination of historical circumstances worked against her. The great wars on land and sea produced numbers of men who had served a rough-and-ready training as surgeon-apothecaries in the armed forces of the Crown. It has been said that by the end of the century more than half the medical men in practice in Britain had service qualifications. They had entered the profession with no pre-liminary education, apart from a chance meeting with the recruiting officer or the press gang, and many of them were remarkably tough customers. Competition with them was cut-throat competition and the women could not survive it.'

The growth of middle class aspirations to live in the style of the gentry brought about, as we have already noted, 'the devitalising ideal of lady-like idleness, which was to be such a bane to high-spirited Victorian girls' (Manton 1965:60).

'By the end of the eighteenth century . . . good-class medical practice had closed to women, apparently for ever. The Royal College of Physicians had established a thriving oligarchy in which royal patients, appointments at the great new voluntary hospitals of the century, university Chairs and knighthoods rotated among the Fellows, to the fury of the surgeons and even of their own licentiates. There was still less room for women within that circle of privilege. At the same time social and economic changes were forcing them out of family practice. The same process was at work in France, where women were forbidden by an edict of 1758 to practise medicine or surgery except midwifery' (1965:61).

Of particular interest to us is the relationship between professionalism and the changing structure of sexual divisions in society. Clark shows the extent to which while 'social organisation rested upon the basis of the family, as it chiefly did up to the close of the Middle Ages, many of the services which are now ranked as professional were thought to be specially suited to the genius of women, and were accordingly allotted to them in the . . . division of labour within the family' (Clark 1919:285). By the beginning of the seventeenth century the traditional attitude towards women was undergoing rapid modifications. While a thorough historical analysis of the period characterised as 'traditional' may demonstrate far less stability in the structural relationships obtaining between the sexes than is commonly supposed, yet it is certainly true that new forces were at work 'deciding the scope of women's professional activity within the seventeenth century' (1919:285) and thereafter. The teaching and healing arts were increasingly emerging from the domestic or family sphere and were subject to opportunities for professional organisation. In the context of the family girls were able, to a large extent, to obtain the same training and experience as boys. Women had always acted as teachers of young children within the family and they continued to be employed in the dame schools attended by the common people. With increasing specialisation of labour however, even

> 'governesses employed by gentlefolk, or the schoolmistresses to whom they sent their daughters for the acquisition of accomplishments [considered] appropriate to young ladies were seldom competent to undertake the actual teaching themselves; for this masters were generally engaged, because few women had gone through the training necessary to give them a sound under-standing of the arts in question.'

Clark points out that 'as knowledge became more specialized and technical, the opportunities which home life provided for acquiring [it] proved inadequate; and consequently women were soon excluded from the higher ranks of the teaching profession' (1919:287).

A similar effect is observable in relation to the arts of healing 'when no professional services were available, it was to the women of the family, rather than to the man, that the sick and wounded turned for medicine and healing'. In spite of their traditional 'affinity for the care of suffering humanity, women were excluded from the sources of learning which were being slowly organised outside the family circle, and were thus unable to remain in professions for which they were so eminently suited' (1919:288).

The exclusion of women from the upper ranks of the teaching profession and their total exclusion subsequently from the medical profession was not as was often suggested by contemporary writers due to women's incapacity to practice these arts, but rather resulted from their lack of specialist training. She refers to

> 'the remarkable history of Midwifery; which from being reserved exclusively for women and practised by them on a professional basis from time immemorial, passed in its more lucrative branches into the hands of men, when sources of instruction were open to them which were closed to women. Just as the amateur teacher was less competent than the man who had made art or the learned languages his profession, so did the woman who treated her family and neighbours by rule of thumb, appear less skilful

than the professional doctor, and the uneducated midwives brought their profession into disrepute. The exclusion of women from all the sources of specialized training was bound to re-act unfavourably upon their characters, because as family life depended more and more upon professional services for education and medical assistance, fewer opportunities were offered to women for exerting their faculties within the domestic sphere and the general incompetence of upper class women did in fact become more pronounced' (1919:288-9).

The exertions of male practitioners in excluding women from their traditional practice of midwifery brought about a situation in which the midwife was destined to decline both in numbers and social status. 'By 1827 . . . the number of midwives was so reduced that in many places pauper mothers in workhouses were delivered by boy apprentices under sixteen.' The situation was one in which 'the character of medical practice [(was so changed that it)] promised to exclude women finally and completely from the profession'. In the early nineteenth century 'although the best physicians might be both learned and scrupulous, the profession as a whole could not claim the respect given to the Church or the Law. If a doctor was called to a large country house in early Victorian times, it was customary to offer him refreshment in the housekeeper's room' (Manton 1965:62-3).

The case of midwifery, to which we have already alluded, is uniquely important to the changing structure of sexual divisions within the medical occupations. These divisions in turn reflect the powerful forces, of which we have been speaking and which were operating throughout society. The development of self-governing professionalism as part of the emergence of modern types of occupational association involved the exclusion of women from the higher branches of several occupations, including midwifery. In a recent thesis Donnison has thoroughly explored the problem (Donnison 1974).

From the 1720s onwards there was a marked increase in the number of male practitioners engaging in midwifery. Whereas at first, they were called in for abnormal labours, increasingly they began to encroach on routine cases in direct competition with the midwife. As Donnison puts it, 'what for centuries had been a female occupation and, in particular, the resort of the woman with a family to maintain, was now in danger of being lost to men' (Donnison 1974:43). The use of midwifery forceps, which by custom only male practitioners could use, may have influenced this development, but following the trend in France where the ladies of the court first began to employ male practitioners, the custom spread to England not only among the highest social levels but to the 'middling' classes and eventually to the artisans. In midwifery, as in other occupations, male remuneration tended to be higher than that offered to the female, and it was probably a matter of status to the tradesman aspiring to gentility to show his neighbours that he could afford the higher priced article (1974:44). An important factor, Donnison suggests, which worked directly to reduce the social standing of the midwife was the decline and disappearance of the system of episcopal licensing which, as we have noted, had been intended to establish legal control over the practice of midwifery. This system had at least conferred a recognised status on the occupation. Its disappearance destroyed the independent basis of the midwife's position and made it possible for her to be reduced to the role of assistant to the male doctor.

Midwifery was important to the young surgeon or apothecary seeking to establish himself in practice because having attended a woman in labour, he would hope to become established as the medical adviser of the whole family. It was in this context that the concept of general practitioner began to emerge. The formation of the Obstetrical Society in 1826 crystallised interest in incorporating midwifery as part of the medical curriculum. Although the Society of Apothecaries was sympathetic, the Colleges of the Physicians and Surgeons took a negative view. Among the medical fraternity there were those who wished to see the traditional midwife pass into oblivion. They envisaged that her work would be taken over by the emerging male general practitioner. No case of parturition, they argued, was ever without danger. Only a man could combine the necessary scientific and anatomical knowledge with physical strength and precision in the use of obstetric instruments which would allow him safely to practice midwifery. Donnison notes ironically that an illiterate Irish woman, Mary Dunally, had performed the first successful Caesarian operation recorded in the British Isles after which both mother and child survived (Donnison 1974:93). The march of male encroachment on midwifery practice nevertheless gained strength as the nineteenth century advanced.

The decline of employment opportunities for women was the object of attention by the Clapham Evangelicals as early as 1804 when they set up a 'Ladies' Committee for Promoting the Education and Employment of the Female Poor'. They were concerned about the relationship between the magnitude of prostitution as a social problem and the lack of suitable work for women. In many occupations they observed that women were being ousted by men and from some they were entirely excluded (1974:96-7). In particular the situation of the middle class woman, and especially of the middle class girl, became the object of attention of a number of early advocates of women's rights. Young single women began for the first time to find a place in midwifery and in nursing. The surplus of women over men in the population during this period led to pressure for the opening up of new occupational opportunities for the single female. No longer could the institution of marriage absorb all of them. The suggestion was put forward that young ladies who had received some education and who for economic reasons found it necessary to compete for work in a depressed market for unskilled female labour might be afforded the opportunity to train as midwives. It was even hinted that such a programme might be financed at public expense. Donnison reports that a correspondent of the *Examiner* went further by suggesting that female pupils should go beyond midwifery and encompass in their studies all the diseases specific to women. It was proposed that a 'female college' should undertake to train women for this work. Its object should be to produce well-trained midwives who would serve the poor under charitable auspices and who equally would be available for private practice among the ring. After the establishment of the British Ladies' Lying-in Institution the supervision and instruction were given by a woman 'Consulting Midwife', however, after 1858, following the general trend, she was replaced by a male 'Surgeon-Accoucheur'. The introduction of training for midwives undoubtedly arrested the decline of the female midwife but it failed to return the control of midwifery practice into female hands; rather it subordinated the midwife to the doctor.

As the modern medical profession became established hostility to the training of midwives declined, and its utility from the point of view of the medical practitioner was more clearly discerned. 'For some years medical men had complained of the lack of competent women to watch labours for them and call them when necessary. A good nurse was essential to the doctor, saving him hours of waiting at the bedside without loss of his fee' (1974:99). The British Lying-in Hospital began to train monthly nurses who would attend the households of the middle classes or the wealthy thus opening up a new source of employment for women. The 1858 Medical Act did not recognise the subject of midwifery as an integral part of medicine, but within the recently unified medical profession the former man-midwife had established a new status. As a subject midwifery was already required for qualification by several of the medical examining bodies. The Royal College of Physicians admitted a number of distinguished obstetricians (the term was a new one) to the dignity of the Fellowship and in 1852 the College of Surgeons declared that medical practitioners of midwifery were eligible for election to its Council and also offered a new licence in midwifery. Obstetricians in London formed the Obstetrical Society – the earlier body of the same name having been rather short-lived. Membership was open only to registered medical practitioners. The problem of midwives was discussed at the outset and the dominant view among the membership was that obstetrics could never become a major medical speciality until women had been ousted from the practice of midwifery altogether. This was an assertion warmly supported by most general practitioners.

Whereas several other occupational groups who shared a common field with the medical profession were progressing towards some form of independent occupational control, midwives were not. Even before the Medical Registration Act of 1858 the Pharmaceutical Society was successful in obtaining state registration for qualified chemists (1852). Soon after the passing of the Bill, the Royal College of Surgeons instituted a licence in dental surgery. The midwives however contained among their numbers few who were sufficiently well educated or respectable to organise for professionalism. Midwives as a group were weak and scattered with little opportunity to form their own associations. It seemed probable that without some outside impetus midwifery in the hands of women would continue to decline and be taken over by the all-male medical profession.

As part of the feminist movement which was concerned to extend the range of remunerative employment for ladies, an organisation called the Female Medical Society was founded in 1862. Shortly afterwards it instituted a Ladies' Medical College for the purpose of instructing women in midwifery and medicine. The hope was that by this means midwifery could be reopened as an occupation for gentlewomen who, through their training and respectability, would be suitable to attend such ladies as might request their services. Dr James Edmunds held unusual views for a medical man of his time. He was a leading light in the foundation of the College and proposed the separation of ordinary midwifery from medical practice on the ground that this would spare the sensibilities of modest women and more significantly would also save the doctor much of the time-consuming business of waiting during labour. He pointed out that although midwifery was a useful entrée into general practice those practitioners who had become well established very quickly took the opportunity either to engage a deputy to relieve them of this arduous work or alternatively they were inclined to raise midwifery fees to a level designed to discourage all but the better off. Dr Edmunds stated his belief that ladies were quite as fitted as men to undertake midwifery and appealed to his fellow doctors to remember their sisters as well as their brothers (Donnison 1974:132). After all, 'many womenfolk of medical families were put to desperate shifts on the death and disablement of the breadwinner. Midwifery could provide such women with the means to maintain themselves in independence' (*Lancet* 1866:614).

The question of training for midwives led inevitably to a discussion of the possibility of midwives' registration. The Obstetrical Society confronted the issue when considering the problem of the high infant mortality rate and the measures by which it might be reduced. Public opinion was also aroused because the problem of baby farming and abortion was raised by several scandalous cases in the 1860s and early 1870s. The lack of any response to these matters from either the Royal College of Surgeons or the Society of Apothecaries led the Obstetrical Society to set up its own examination for midwives with a view to ensuring that they remained under medical control. The Society set out to make certain that any legislation creating a register would confirm medical authority over the midwives. The Female Medical Society took the opportunity to propose a solution in which qualified women would be admitted to the Medical Register as licentiates in midwifery. A Bill was mooted to promote this object but it was bound to meet with opposition from the medical profession because it would have given a group of women equal status with medical men. Miss Maria Firth was a leading member of a new organisation 'The Obstetrical Association of Midwives' but the Royal College of Surgeons successfully resisted pressure from this quarter to establish a licence in midwifery for women. An appeal was made by the women to the General Medical Council's Committee which was set up to consider the issue. Naturally, it received opposing suggestions from the male-dominated Obstetrical Society. There was deadlock and the *status quo* was reaffirmed by inaction. The problem was soon shifted to the Local Government Board which, because of its responsibility for the Poor Law, became involved in the midwife registration question. Stansfeld, then President of the Board, was bound to disappoint the British Medical Association and the Obstetrical Society because he was a strong supporter of the women's movement. He tended to favour a mode of registration involving two classes of midwife, one highly educated and the other subordinate and less well qualified. Maria Firth was opposed to the all-male Obstetrical Society's alternative proposals which involved annual licensing on the model of 'stall-holders and publicans'. She regarded the proposal as humiliating to women.

At this stage the supporters of midwives' registration failed to achieve their objective and attention shifted to the possibility of founding a medical college for women. In 1874 the London School of Medicine for Women was founded by Sophia Jex-Blake thus eclipsing the activities of the Female Medical Society. The Society had been important in paving the way for the entry of women into the medical profession and this is demonstrated by the fact that several of the students of its associated College went on to become successful doctors. The College itself faded away.

An important impetus to the cause of medical women came from those who wished to see an improvement in the moral character of society. Josephine Butler, for example, devoted herself to the rehabilitation of prostitutes. She asserted that the attendance of male medical practitioners on women in purely female matters was repugnant to female modesty as well as permanently injurious to a woman's moral nature. It was her belief that the 'wicked custom' by which women were excluded from the practice of medicine was a hindrance to the 'moral renovation' of society. The excessive prudery which was encouraged by the mores of the middle class in Victorian society were regarded by Mrs Butler as sanctified by God. The paradox was that girls sheltered by the strict upbringing of the middle class family were required, if they were to practice midwifery, or to become

medical practitioners, to undertake work regarded as fitting only for
lower-class women or men. In practical terms the introduction of well
trained midwives or 'lady doctors' would, it was hoped, not merely
allow an easier relationship between the patient and the professional
attendant in which symptoms could be more uninhibitedly described
and discussed, but also lead to a greater interest and concern by women
doctors in the diseases of women and children.

Two years before the Medical Registration Act a woman had
formally applied both to the University of London and to the Royal
Colleges of Physicians and Surgeons to seek their ruling on whether a
woman might be admitted to their examinations. She was Jessie
Meriton White, the daugher of a Liverpool ship-owner. As Manton says

'in May 1856 she wrote to the Registrar of the University of
London, asking whether a woman could become a candidate for a
diploma in medicine if, on presenting herself for examination, she
produced all the requisite certificates of character, capacity and
study from one of the institutions recognised by London
University. Two months later, after taking Counsel's opinion, the
Senate of London University passed a resolution that "Miss J.M.
White be informed that the Senate, acting upon the opinion of
the legal adviser, does not consider itself empowered to admit
females as candidates for degrees" ' (Manton 1965:65).

The attitude of the medical profession may be gauged by the derisive
amusement with which the matter was dismissed in the pages of the
British Medical Journal (1856:653). Elsewhere though, the decision was
pointedly criticised by linking it with the charge that the medical
profession was motivated by a 'sordid spirit of monopoly' of the type
which Florence Nightingale had been forced to contend with in the
Crimea. Donnison describes the reaction of the medical profession to
the efforts of women to enter it as, 'hostile'. For example, the Lancet
dismissed the movement as merely a 'perverse' and morbid agitation on
the part of 'ambitious ladies to open up to women the one occupation
for which they were least suited' (Lancet 1858:44; 1861:117).
There were however also those who argued for the introduction of
female physicians. Among them was S. Gregory who wrote a letter to
Ladies in Favour of Female Physicians (1850). Browne also asserted
that women were 'all but born doctors', and that the 'mothers of
England' should take up the fight (Browne 1859).

The first woman to practice medicine in England in modern times
was Elizabeth Blackwell, unless Dr James Barrie be so considered.
'Barrie, a remarkably fresh-faced subaltern who entered the army
medical service in 1813, rose to the rank of Inspector-General of the
Army Medical Department, and was found after death to have been a
woman' (Manton 1965:65). Dr Elizabeth Blackwell had graduated in
medicine from the small university of Geneva, New York State, in 1849
and opened her own dispensary among the immigrant women and

children of the New York slums. She had been born in Britain and returned to her native shores to practice medicine prior to the Medical Registration Act 1858. Under the terms of the Act the newly created General Medical Council was obliged to add her name to the register as one of those who had been in practice before 1 October 1858. This was a once for all procedure which other women would be unable to follow.

A committee was set up with the task of campaigning for the admission of women to the medical profession. It obtained substantial support both in the middle and upper classes. One argument used to justify the exclusion of women from the medical profession was that delicacy would forbid the entry of girls into the harrowing experiences of medical training. One commentator (Dale 1875:preface *iv*) said 'women cannot study medicine in mixed classes, we judge, without unsexing herself – it shocks one's sense of propriety – it destroys that seemly modesty which is her chief adornment'. From the other point of view, it was argued that the delicate sensibility of the lady would require at the very least that she should have the opportunity to consult either a male or female practitioner. Throughout the eighteenth and nineteenth centuries a continuing controversy raged over the propriety of involving men in midwifery or gynaecology at all. There were those who attributed a decline in sexual morality to this cause, and indeed claimed that the very fabric of society was being undermined by the lascivious activities of the 'touching gentry'. If ladies were to have the opportunity of consulting a woman it was first necessary to have women qualified as doctors. Evidence was said to exist that some women refused to consult a male doctor even if in dire need of medical attention.

Support for the entry of women into the medical profession was growing. Immediately after her admission to the register, Elizabeth Blackwell was to be found proselytising on the theme of medical education for women. Among those whom she inspired with a determination to become a doctor was Elizabeth Garrett, the daughter of a successful Norfolk merchant. Arrangements were made for Miss Garrett to work for a time under the guise of a nurse at the Middlesex hospital where she could obtain some practical experience with a view to making a final decision. She determined to dedicate herself to the daunting task of becoming a doctor and was allowed informally to become a student in the same hospital. She obtained honours in every subject but this only caused a caucus of male students to engineer her removal. The Society of Apothecaries had at first refused to admit her to their examinations but after seeking legal opinion it was established that, because the 1815 Act spoke of 'persons', women could not technically be excluded. Miss Garrett was able to claim that her private tuition constituted an apprenticeship which was at that time legally acceptable for qualification at Apothecaries' Hall. To prevent such a thing occurring again the Apothecaries' Society changed the rules.

Henceforth education in a recognised medical school was also made a pre-requisite for qualification 'with the deliberate purpose of excluding women' (Newman 1957:301). Eventually Miss Garrett sat the examinations, passed and became a qualified practitioner. Her success in practice was considerable both among the well-to-do and the poor. Subsequently she also obtained an MD in Paris, the first woman to do so (1870), though she was refused in Scotland at St Andrews where she had also made an attempt to break down the barriers against women. In the latter case she lost on a legal technicality relating to the university charter (Manton 1965:137). Her services at the Marylebone Dispensary for Women and Children which she herself founded were in great demand (1965:173). She also founded the first hospital for women, staffed exclusively by women.

If other women were to follow suit and qualify as doctors it would be necessary for them to obtain access to medical schools. The first four women who became medical students at Edinburgh University were forced to do their practical chemistry in a room separate from the men and the examiners claimed that consequently their work was invalidated. By this strategem they were prevented from sitting the examination. There were other difficulties. For instance, Sophia Jex-Blake was not merely prosecuted for libel as a result of controversies with male students but also given a nominal fine which meant that she had to bear the heavy costs of the case. Even when women managed to gain access to the examinations they had to meet the obduracy of the examiners who could simply refuse to pass them. This happened to Sophia Jex-Blake in Edinburgh and she only qualified eventually by going to Dublin where she persuaded the examiners to pass her.

In most cases women could not legally be excluded from qualifying in medicine because none of the laws or by-laws of the qualifying bodies had been framed with them in mind. But the informal barriers faced by women who wished to break 'into a highly self-respected profession of a singularly pompous kind' were formidable (Newman 1957:301-2). As Newman puts it, 'it was thought natural, in a way, for women to nurse: they had always done so in the home; but for the theoretically subordinate sex to assume the function of making decisions in a Victorian world was quite another matter' (1957:302). Certainly the doctors saw the advantage of maintaining a male monopoly and feared that the entry of women into the practice of medicine would be likely to reduce the status of the profession and probably damage existing levels of remuneration. For many Victorians, both men and women, the concept of the equality of women was beyond their comprehension. Much medical teaching was conducted in a somewhat obscene and indecent atmosphere and indeed the teachers of anatomy relied greatly on imparting a mass of unmemorable details through the use of indecent mnemonics. Opposition to the entry of women to the profession was extraordinarily strong and the right for men to be obscene among themselves was stoutly defended in Victorian society.

The battle was by no means over even for women already established in the profession. In 1874 Elizabeth Garrett Anderson having by then a considerable medical reputation, applied for membership of the Obstetrical Society, but was blackballed. The following year Sophia Jex-Blake and two other women who had qualified in Edinburgh decided to confront the Royal College of Surgeons by applying to take the separate midwifery diploma which had been introduced in 1852. Unintentionally the diploma became recognised as sufficient for registration under the 1858 Medical Act because it had not been specifically laid down that this diploma should be conferred only on those who were already practising members of the College. In 1876 three women with the requisite experience applied to the College to be examined and 'the College was advised that legally they had no right to refuse the application. To prevent any repetition of such a dangerous occurrence the examiners in midwifery resigned, no new appointments were made and the examination fell into abeyance until 1881' (Franklin 1950:144). It is no surprise to discover that the examiners in midwifery were all leading figures in the Obstetrical Society the members of which believed that they had most to fear from female competition.

The exclusion of women from the medical profession was in large part defeated through the training given at the London School of Medicine for Women. The success in gaining access to clinical instruction at the Royal Free Hospital was the key, for without it the School would have been doomed to failure. The Governors drove a hard bargain. They wanted monetary guarantees against loss of income should subscribers withdraw their support and also demanded higher fees from women students compared to those asked of men in other medical schools (Manton 1965:252). It was established that women could qualify through the Irish College of Physicians and the University of London, whose degree conferred a qualification in all three branches of medicine. Slowly, the other qualifying bodies relented but there remained many hindrances to full equality of opportunity for women in medicine.

Ladies had gained a foothold in the medical profession but the general practitioner was becoming more afraid of another threat, as he saw it, this time from midwives. Dr Rentoul was an active campaigner against midwives' registration and he was a staunch advocate of the general practitioners' cause. It was his belief that the Midwives' Institute, which was pressing for the registration of midwives, would not rest content with the achievement of that objective. He feared that registration would tend to create an inferior order of practitioners which would not only rob the general practitioner of midwifery, but which — subsidised by the state after the continental pattern — might one day supersede the public vaccinator and the Poor Law Medical Officer. The Institute's real object, Rentoul contended, was to gain for women, access to medical practice through a back door, thus increasing the competition already suffered by the 'overstocked' profession from the prescribing chemist, the unqualified practitioner and the quack (Donnison 1974:202). Having lost the battle over the entry of women into the medical profession, general practitioners like Rentoul, were quick to reverse their former arguments by insisting that if women wished to practise midwifery they should take the full medical curriculum. The old apothecary had gone; now the lady doctor should replace the ancient midwife (1974:202).

Rentoul's campaign against midwife registration included a tactical move to get the General Medical Council to act against any registered doctors who involved themselves in the process of examining and awarding certificates of qualification to midwives. A short-lived success was obtained in 1894 in the case of the Obstetrical Society's examination. Surprisingly, the General Medical Council declared that the Society's qualification was a 'colourable imitation' of a medical diploma. The society successfully evaded the force of this judgement by the simple expedient of substituting the word 'diploma' for the term 'certificate'. In spite of the efforts of Rentoul and Dr Bedford Fenwick, who at this time was opposing registration especially from the editorial pages of the *Medical Times*,[1] a considerable body of medical opinion was coming round to support midwife registration provided only that it was under complete medical control. Mrs Bedford Fenwick, at this stage, sided with her husband and was assiduously courted by the opponents of midwife registration. She became convinced that the midwives were an anachronism doomed to disappear and that the very word 'midwife' would soon be no more than an historical curiosity. The midwife would be replaced by what Mrs Fenwick called the 'obstetric nurse' whose duty would be to work solely under medical supervision. The struggle between those who wished to see the complete subordination of midwives to the medical profession and those, representing the interests of midwives themselves, who wished to obtain some degree of control over their own situation, was a fiercely contended issue in the 1890s (Donnison 1974: chapter 8).

Maria Firth's movement which was intended to achieve the registration of the midwife on 'equal terms with the medical practitioners' had failed. It was evident that a successful campaign would require the co-operation or at least the acquiescence of the medical profession in general and the obstetricians in particular. The problem was that while the medical profession insisted that midwives be clearly defined as a lower level group than doctors and subject to the oversight of medical men, the feminist movement resisted such a compromise. It should be remembered that in the 1890s women were not merely excluded from the management of general hospitals but even from that of lying-in-hospitals. Their participation in government was negligible and amounted to membership of a few school Boards and Boards of

Guardians. Membership of women on the Board governing the examination and registration of midwives would have been stoutly opposed even by many medical men who were supporters of midwives' registration. Indeed, as Donnison points out (1974:197), one doctor writing in the *Nursing Record* in June 1895, about his experience as an active member of the British Nurses' Association referred to his experience on a 'mixed Board' as one he would not care to repeat. In his view, the thought of women members on the Midwives' Board would strike terror into the hearts of their male colleagues.

In 1890 a Bill for the Registration of Midwives was brought before the House of Commons. It was promoted by the Midwives' Institute which had taken the precaution of having prior discussions with the Obstetrical Society. It was based on a draft Bill which had been prepared by the British Medical Association in 1882. The proposal was that registration was to be under medical control not, as some supporters of registration had suggested, under the local authorities. There were to be new Local Boards with general practitioners included on them. The Board's powers were to include examination and registration of midwives as well as responsibility for suspension or erasure from the Register. There was to be a right of appeal to the Central Board and to the Privy Council. The Central Board was to be wholly composed of senior obstetricians.

The Bill was brought forward under the private members' procedure and had the appearance of backing from powerful sources, not least the British Medical Association. It was opposed by Dr Tanner, who was member of Parliament for Mid-Cork, on the ground that many general practitioners feared that the registered midwife would compete with them for patients to the detriment of the doctors' livelihood. The free-thinking member of Parliament, Charles Bradlaugh, opposed the Bill not only on the general ground that it was another example of government interference in the lives of individuals (by the creation of innumerable regulations) but that it discriminated unfairly against women. Under the Bill women wishing to register as midwives would be required to produce a certificate of good character in addition to demonstrating their competence to practise: no such requirement was made in the case of men registering under the Medical Act. The Bill was talked out by Bradlaugh.

After the failure of the Bill the government itself became interested in promoting legislation for the registration of midwives. The Bill underwent some redrafting by the Privy Council and a Select Committee. The proposal which emerged was that the oversight of registration should be in the hands of the County Councils since these had the necessary staff and could raise funds. This proposal was objected to by the British Medical Association and the Obstetrical Society which insisted that the registration of midwives should be in the hands of the medical profession. A compromise was reached whereby the administration would be undertaken by the local authorities but control of examinations and discipline would be vested in the General Medical Council.

It soon became clear that the rank and file general practitioners were still not at all convinced that the registration of midwives was in their interest, no matter what the leaders of the medical profession might say. Indeed it was only after the failure of the 1899 Bill that the controversy reached a crescendo. Extreme anti-registration candidates were elected by the medical profession to the British Medical Association and the General Medical Council. The Medical Practitioners' Association in particular supported militant candidates. At the grass roots level, some general practitioners took direct action by refusing to 'follow' midwives, and others continued to claim (wrongly) that they were forbidden to do so by the rules of the General Medical Council. They contended that they were at risk of being struck off from the medical register for 'covering an unqualified practitioner'. Direct action of this kind had its dangers and rebounded to the detriment of the doctors' case. Massive publicity was given to the refusal of three doctors at Swanscombe in Kent to attend a woman in labour where a difficult birth was well beyond the competence of the midwife who was present. The doctors had agreed among themselves to refuse to 'follow' a midwife and in the event the woman died. The fact that a substantial body of practitioners clamoured in support of the Swanscombe doctors' stand could only cause damage to the public image of the profession. Dr McCook Weir a practitioner who had himself some years earlier similarly refused to answer a call wrote to the *British Medical Journal* saying that he was glad that 'the mere male was still master of the situation. Medical men', he urged, 'should drop their sham philanthropy and unite for the common good of the profession' (*British Medical Journal* 1901:1379).

Those promoting legislation for the registration of midwives were hindered by their dependence upon the Private Members' Bill procedure for a chance to introduce a Bill into the Commons. But the opportunity came in 1902 and from this moment things moved speedily. Seeing that midwives' registration had become a distinct possibility Mrs Bedford Fenwick suddenly dropped her disapproval of it. After moving through a stage in which she tried to link the registration of nurses to that of midwives so that both could obtain registration together, she finally decided (on tactical grounds) to support midwives' registration because she regarded it as a useful precedent for nurses' registration. Moreover after

> 'her break with the medical leadership of the Royal British Nurses' Association, Mrs Fenwick, in spite of her husband, did not remain as keen as she had been on medical control over nurses and midwives. She now proposed that medical men should serve only as consultants on the regulating bodies of these

occupations and, like other campaigners for women's rights, she regretted that midwives themselves were not to constitute the majority of members of the Midwives' Board' (Donnison 1974:274).

The medical profession had lost in her an important ally inside the women's movement, and the public were offered the spectacle of Dr Bedford Fenwick opposing in one medical journal the views propagated by his wife in another (*Nursing Record* 1974:273).

The Bill was taken up by the government and was supported by both the Home Office and the Local Government Board. The Privy Council rather than the General Medical Council was to exercise control. All this was against the interests of the medical profession which firmly opposed the Bill. The interest of the relevant Departments of State in the matter of midwifery registration and midwifery services was also an important asset to the success of the Bill's promoters. An attempt was made during the passage of the Bill to get a Royal British Nurses' Association representatives on the proposed Central Midwives' Board. This was obviously a tactic of the medical profession to increase medical influence at the very moment when it became apparent that the Bill might well succeed. The Royal British Nurses' Association remained under the control of medical men and its representative would be likely to support their interests. The only substantial amendment achieved by the British Medical Association was a clause banning unqualified practice. Its attempt to impose the humiliating condition of annual licence was rejected but under the terms of the Act annual notification was required.

Many in the medical profession felt that the failure to obtain medical control and supervision of midwives by the General Medical Council constituted a defeat for the medical profession at the hands of both parliament and public opinion. They tended to blame for this state of affairs the activities of the more militant and extremist groups in the profession. Yet in some respects, as Donnison points out, midwives were put 'in a uniquely disadvantaged position among the professions' (Donnison 1974:287). They were not only unique in being subject to the licensing procedures of local government but could be struck off from the midwives' register for a wide range of ill-defined and petty ethical misdemeanours which even included minute regulations governing their dress. Moreover, although the medical profession was not to have complete control, through the General Medical Council, of the administration of midwives, nevertheless this 'rival profession was to have a dominant voice in their government' (1974:288). This was an outcome entirely consistent with the interests of the medical profession although some medical commentators felt that the victory had not been as complete as they would have wished. One such commentator argued that the control of midwives by the Local Authorities was detrimental to the medical profession which ought to have been vested with the necessary administrative powers. He also suggested that the midwives had been given an opportunity legally to prescribe drugs. The fact that many were not required to keep a register of any drugs they used in the course of their duties 'assumes that the prescribing of drugs by a midwife is correct and right. Such an assumption raises the position of the midwife to that of a qualified doctor' (Reeney 1905:113). Such protestations continued for a time but it soon became apparent that the Midwives' Act had drawn a sufficiently firm boundary to sustain the dominance of the medical profession.

The medical field was a battleground over which the campaign to secure male dominance was fought. Nursing especially was reformed on a basis which accepted the doctrine of male superiority, particularly as embodied in the stereotype of the male doctor. As an occupation for women, nursing lent itself well to the purpose of early feminism precisely because the conventional definitions of woman's 'natural' attributes could most easily be applied to it. As Hill points out, in the 1860s the call for religious sisterhoods to become engaged in nursing, especially in the lunatic asylums, was not only based on an argument for the emancipation of women and the assertion of their rights, but on a claim that women had an *'hereditary right* to care for the afflicted' (Hill 1973:275). In many ways nursing duties were not far removed from the domestic tasks thought appropriate to women and in some cases even the nurses' uniforms closely resembled those of the Victorian domestic servant. Florence Nightingale saw nurse training as essentially practical 'within the capacity of the country girl. The probationer was disciplined to handle competently and effectively all the situations she encountered in the hospital ward. And from this discipline came the strength and confidence needed to meet the heavy emotional and physical demands of nursing work' (Dock, Stewart 1938:254). There was no intention on the part of Florence Nightingale to create a category of 'Lady Nurses', but her own class background, and the aura of her success in organising nursing services for the British Army in the Crimea, caught the imagination of middle and upper class girls who came forward to offer themselves for a vocation in nursing. The scene was set for the entry of the divisive element of class into nursing. The paradox was that the search for professionalism among nurses was more an expression of the antipathy felt by the status conscious lady-nurses towards those recruited from the working class than it was an effort to establish a self-governing profession of nursing. The leaders of the Nurses' Registration Movement continued to have more in common with doctors who came from a similar class background to themselves than they had with the mass of ordinary nurses.

It is instructive, in this regard, to examine the case of the British Nurses' Association which was founded by a group of 'Lady-Nurses' with the intention of seeking registration. The leading personality was Miss Ethel Gordon Manson who was the daughter of a medical doctor

181

and eventually also married one. On marriage, she took the name of her husband, Dr Bedford Fenwick. He was already an established figure in medical politics. Mrs Bedford Fenwick entered nursing politics and pressed her views uncompromisingly throughout her long career. In the late nineteenth century

> 'an extremely varied group of people were engaged in the practice
> of nursing. Ladies with excellent instruction and servant girls with
> a minimum of training belonged to the same occupation, and
> there was little by which the general public could judge their
> professional competence. To remedy this situation, a group of
> ex-lady-pupils, urged on by feelings of insecurity about their own
> status, banded together to introduce a firm distinction between
> the trained and the untrained by establishing a register of nurses'
> (Abel-Smith 1960:61).

Mrs Bedford Fenwick believed that if 'the highest possible standard of nursing' was to be maintained 'this could be secured by confining entry to the profession to the daughters of the higher social classes' (1960:63). She thought that nurses should be recruited 'from a class of women who had been trusted for so many years that the failures would be the exceptions' (Select Committee 1905:33). Clearly defined educational and financial barriers should be established in training schools to exclude unsuitable recruits. Rather than be paid a salary they should themselves pay a training fee. Mrs Bedford Fenwick thought that the longer the training, the tougher the rituals of initiation, the greater the intellectual requirements the higher the status of the profession would be. 'The very fact that every woman thought she could nurse made it the more necessary to emphasise and exaggerate training requirements' (1960:62). Such a restriction of recruitment would have made the shortage of nurses acute. The lady nurses thought that many respectable and well-educated women were discouraged from entering the profession by the reputation of some of the 'lower' elements in nursing which were associated with scandal or even crime.

The views of Miss Nightingale alluded to above and those of Mrs Bedford Fenwick were bound to conflict. Among senior medical men at several of the London hospitals there was at first opposition to Mrs Fenwick's views. 'They were firmly opposed to any measure which would narrow the field of recruitment to the nursing profession' (Abel-Smith 1960:66). As Sydney Holland of the London Hospital put it (Select Committee 1905:39), 'the numbers of women in the upper classes are comparatively small who wish to nurse'. He believed that registration rather than adding to the supply of nurses would actually reduce it and that the proposed registration fee would exclude many excellent women from taking up nursing. He thought that the educational standard should not be raised too high and that girls who came from a background of domestic service, some of whom became excellent nurses, should not be excluded. Openings into the nursing profession should be as wide as possible. Holland summed up his position in these words: 'we want to stop nurses thinking themselves anything more than they are, namely the faithful carriers out of the doctor's orders. The other side are always talking about nursing being a profession and "graduates" in nursing, just as they do in America' (1905:37). He thought that 'superior' nurses are unsuitable in the households of gentlefolk (it should be remembered that much nursing was done at this time on a domiciliary basis). In this context the best nurses come from the servant class.

Most of the nursing associations followed the conception of an 'open' nursing profession favoured by Miss Nightingale rather than the elitist and restrictive idea proposed by Mrs Fenwick, but the conflict about the status of nurses at the turn of the century was made complex by the cross-cutting divisions of interest. For example, matrons in certain provincial hospitals were in some cases supporters of registration because they hoped that the certificates they awarded would place them on a parity with the fashionable teaching hospitals. They believed that in this way they would be able to attract the 'better type of girl' and improve their own status. The smaller hospitals in the provinces took a stand against registration because they feared that if it were introduced they would not receive recognition as schools approved for the purpose of training nurses. In a few instances hospital matrons were opposed to registration because they believed that it would affect their total autonomy in the hospital by introducing an element of outside interference.

A counter proposal for registration was put forward by H.C. Burdett who was a pioneer of hospital administration and who was serving as vice-president of the Seaman's Hospital, London. The type of register he proposed was totally different from that envisaged by Mrs Bedford Fenwick. It was simply an administrative device by which matrons or medical men could assure themselves (by consulting the register) of the character and capability of any woman who presented herself for employment as a nurse. This idea was objectionable to Mrs Fenwick who dismissed it on the grounds that it was just a 'central registry office similar to that in vogue for domestic servants' (*Nursing Record* 1893:110). The views of Burdett and Mrs Fenwick were irreconcilable and their relationship became embittered. After a meeting in 1887 which resulted in an open breach, the hospitals' association led by Mrs Burdett started its own register of trained nurses. It was however very little used. The 'Lady-Nurses' under the militant leadership of Mrs Bedford Fenwick founded the British Nurses' Association. It sought to achieve professional status for nurses. Effective power in the association was placed by the Constitution 'in the hands of the doctors and the London hospital matrons. The Infirmary matrons, the provincial matrons, and the ordinary working nurses were "kept out in the cold" ' (Abel-Smith 1960:70). The Association campaigned for an official register of nurses and Dr Fenwick persuaded the British Medical Association to pass a resolution to the effect that a Bill should be prepared providing for the registration of nurses. Mrs Fenwick and the British Nurses' Association obtained the support of Princess Christian, a daughter of Queen Victoria, who graciously consented to become Patron of the Association. This was a shrewd move because it inhibited the expression of overt opposition by the opponents of registration. Florence Nightingale was afraid that the nursing profession would be split on the registration question. Although she objected to it, her opposition was covert but no less effective for that. She used her influence to prevent an Act of Parliament thus forcing the British Nurses' Association to turn to the alternative method, (which they regarded as less satisfactory) of applying for a Royal Charter by which the Association itself would be granted the power to register nurses. The Privy Council considered the matter in 1893 and conferred on the British Nurses' Association various powers, but not the one it chiefly wanted. The Charter did however divide power equally between doctors and nurses within the Association. Florence Nightingale managed to have the last word, the term 'register' was struck out and the word 'list' was the carefully chosen substitute. In a letter to *The Times*, Nightingale and her allies came out into the open and pointed out that 'the list will have nothing in common with legal registers of the medical or other professions, but will simply be a list of nurses published by the Association' (*The Times* 1893:7). The proudly named Royal British Nurses' Association as thus deprived of any real powers over nurse training schools or qualifications. The opportunity for nurses to have their names on the 'list' was taken up by very few. Although Florence Nightingale was attacked for her attitude, she had, for the time being, prevented registration. It was not long before the Royal British Nurses' Association reverted to its former campaign for powers of registration through an Act of Parliament. But the affairs of the Royal British Nurses' Association were in fact soon disrupted by internal controversy. The Fenwicks clashed with the other leading personalities and Dr Fenwick resigned the Treasurership in 1894. Before the end of that year Mrs Fenwick herself was forced to resign from the General Council of the Association although she was supposedly a permanent member. From being founders and friends of the Association, the Fenwicks became its enemies, and Dr Fenwick in particular probably had a deep influence on the attitudes in the medical profession. In any event, when the Association reversed its policy in 1896 and passed a resolution against state registration for nurses the doctors on the Council were blamed. In fact it was very probably Florence Nightingale herself, acting behind the scenes, who had worked effectively to ensure that such a resolution was passed.

The medical profession was in disagreement on the question of the desirability of the registration of nurses. The London consultants tended to support the idea 'in the belief that registration would lead to more good nurses and this would serve the interests of their patients both in hospital and at home'. It is important to realise that the relationship 'between doctor and trained nurse was already clearly established in London teaching hospitals. The supremacy of the medical profession on medical matters had been conceded; its position was unassailable. The consultant depended very heavily upon good nursing in his domiciliary practice' (Abel-Smith 1960:75). As one doctor put it as tactfully as he could, 'the consulting man is not able to watch the case quite so thoroughly as the general practitioner would do, I mean to say, as thoroughly but not so closely' (Select Committee 1905:79).

By contrast the general practitioner tended to view with nearly as much suspicion the possibility of the registered nurse as of the registered midwife. In the early twentieth century many general practitioners felt that the British Medical Association, whose ambition it was to be the only voice of the medical profession, was in fact no longer wholly representative of their interests. Although it had 20,000 members in 1905, yet it was 'very largely officered by the West End consultants in London and the consultants in the big towns' (1905:78). The Incorporated Medical Practitioners' Association claimed to represent the general practitioner. General practice in the provinces neither commanded the same status nor anything like the same income as the London consultants. It was reported that country doctors feared the competition of the new district nursing service because they thought that 'people are very apt to send for the nurses when they might otherwise send for the doctors' (1905:82). A nurse with a certificate was believed to be a serious rival who would undoubtedly undercut the doctor by charging smaller fees. The doctors' attitude was openly expressed to the Select Committee of 1905. The British Medical Association supported registration for nurses and had in mind the Midwive's Act 1902. They even wished to make it a criminal offence for unqualified women to practise as nurses but by what methods this could be done was not specified. The Select Committee came out in favour of registration but proposed that the register should be set up and supervised by a state-appointed organisation created for the purpose. This central body would admit trained persons to the register and approve the schools in which they trained. It would be an offence for persons other than those listed on the register to call themselves 'Registered Nurse', although it envisaged the institution of a separate category of persons whose training would be of a lower standard and who would be entitled to nurse. As Abel-Smith points out, it was almost forty years before a register of assistant nurses on the lines suggested in 1905 was actually established but registration for the trained nurse came more quickly. After the presentation of numerous bills by rival associations the government finally brought in an Act of its own which received the Royal Assent in December, 1919.

Notes

1. This was the journal of the Medical Practitioners' Association or The General Practitioners' Union as it was formerly called.

9. THE DOCTORS AND THE STATE: FROM NATIONAL INSURANCE TO NATIONAL HEALTH SERVICE, 1911-48

Lloyd George had several objectives which he wished to achieve through the National Health Insurance Act of 1911. He particularly wanted 'to break up club practice, not the Poor Law. His interest in social reform . . . embraced the working class as a whole and could not be satisfied through a programme confined to those below the poverty line' (Honingsbaum 1971:18-19). The Webbs, on the other hand, were interested in the unification of health services which were administratively fragmented. Rather than breaking up club practice they wanted to 'raise up the casual labourer into a position in which he could become a possible recruit for the great Friendly Societies'. As Honingsbaum put it 'this was the last thing that Lloyd George – or the doctors – wanted but the Webbs never understood that' (1971:18).

We have already remarked that, during the decades prior to the 1911 National Health Insurance Act, the development of privately-run charitable and provident schemes controlled by lay-men posed a serious threat to the doctors' hold on a large part of the market for medical care (see Chapter 7). In fact the British Medical Association suggested a state scheme to meet this problem and indeed had prepared a draft. It did not approve of the government's particular proposals for a system of national health insurance. What it really wanted was a 'public medical service organized and administered by itself for the benefit of the lower levels of the working class. In this way private practice would be preserved for all except those least able to pay' (Lindsey 1962:9). The British Medical Association was determined to transform the original draft of the government Bill in which control of medical benefit was to be left in the hands of Friendly Societies, thus perpetuating what the doctors regarded as the most objectionable feature of the existing form of organisation in the new state scheme.

The Act of 1911 was in many respects modelled upon Bismark's legislation in Germany (1883). The major political aim was to deliver a considerable part of the working population out of the hands of the Poor Law without placing a heavy burden upon the Exchequer. The scheme was to be largely self-financing; it would thus be paid for and used by the working class. Lloyd George's intention was to provide a state organised scheme which levied compulsory contributions on manual workers, or indeed others, who had an income less than £160 a year. Workers made contributions of 4d a week to a society approved under the Act. Their employers and the state contributed 3d and 2d respectively. An insured person was entitled to a limited cash benefit in

187

time of sickness, and to the services of a general practitioner together with the free prescription of drugs. Hospital and specialist services and appliances, such as artificial limbs, were excluded. This meant that the general practitioner was involved in a state administered scheme, while the voluntary hospitals and consultants were not. The tuberculosis scheme, which was introduced at the same time, was seen by some as the beginning of a full state hospital service. In fact, such a service was not to materialise until 1948. What the 1911 Act did for general practitioners was to provide them with 'a regular and reliable source of income at a not ungenerous rate' (Abel-Smith 1964:238).

Lloyd George wished to introduce his national health insurance scheme as quickly as possible and he appointed that formidable administrator, Robert Morant, to the Chairmanship of the new National Insurance Commission. Morant at once had a fight with the Treasury over the issue of appropriate accommodation, staffing and resources for he feared that unless a larger allocation of resources was put at his disposal he would be unable to see the Act implemented by the specified date – 15 July 1912. In a surprisingly tough manner for a civil servant he wrote to Lloyd George and suggested that unless more staff and resources were forthcoming there would be 'a public scandal of the greatest magnitude – a scandal which will not only destroy irretrievably all chances of making the Act work well and be acceptable to the people, but will involve the Government in criticisms so serious and damaging that it will be impossible to withstand it' (Allen 1934:273-4). Morant was saying to Lloyd George in effect: either give me the resources I require or postpone the date on which the Act is to be implemented. Lloyd George refused to postpone the date, but he immediately gave instructions to the Treasury officials which resulted in Morant getting all the staff and resources he required. Within seven months, using many brilliant young men whom he chose from various departments of the Civil Service, he was able to build up an effective organisation and launch the great system of national health insurance on schedule.

The public were but dimly aware of the problems of administration which Morant confronted. But more in the public mind was the well-known opposition of the medical profession to the scheme. From the outset the doctors took an active interest in the scheme 'and had exerted themselves to obtain such modifications of the Bill as would make it acceptable to the profession' (1934:275). The doctors had agreed among themselves upon six cardinal points which they wished to see achieved in the new legislation. The points at issue were as follows:

1. An income limit of £2 a week to be applied to those receiving medical benefit.
2. A free choice of doctor by the patient, subject to the consent of the doctor to act.
3. Medical and maternity benefits to be administered by the

proposed insurance committees instead of by the Friendly Societies.[1]

4. The method of remuneration of medical practitioners adopted by each insurance committee to be fixed according to the preference of the majority of the medical profession of the committee's district.
5. Medical remuneration to be fixed at an amount which the profession considered adequate.
6. The medical profession should be adequately represented on the central and local administrative bodies which might be set up to administer the scheme (Little 1932:326-7).

'During the passage of the Bill through the House they were able to secure the adoption of amendments under which most of these points were met. On one point, however, the remuneration to be paid to doctors for medical treatment, the position was left unsettled. The actuarial calculations on which the finance of the Bill rested were based on a calculation of an average payment of six shillings per head for every person on a doctor's panel. This amount was regarded by the British Medical Association as entirely inadequate, and after the Bill had become law on 16 December, an important representative meeting was held in London to consider whether the doctors should at once refuse to have anything to do with the Act' (Allen 1934:276).

One tough-minded view was expressed by Sir James Barr who argued in a letter to the *British Medical Journal* that the doctors should strongly resist. Drawing on the analogy with the Merchant Shipping Act of 1883, a piece of legislation fostered by Joseph Chamberlain, he recalled that the seamen of Liverpool had adamantly refused to carry out one of its sections which, as a result, Chamberlain quietly allowed to remain inoperative. Barr suggested that resistance by the doctors could have a similar effect in defeating 'the Act of the "little Welshman" '. It was suggested that Mr Lloyd George (then) retire with his Act into that obscurity from which he should never have emerged (1934:276). Among the doctors' representatives the majority took a less extreme line. They suggested that

'as no figure for doctor's remuneration was mentioned in the Act, it would still be open for them to obtain an increase in the amount by negotiating with the Chancellor for an increased Treasury grant; and it was accordingly decided that the profession should only refuse to work the Act if they were unable to secure complete satisfaction on their six cardinal demands. All members of the Association were asked to sign an undertaking to this effect, and by the middle of that month [January 1912] over 26,000 doctors [out of a membership of 32,000] had agreed to sign.'

In February the British Medical Association formed a State Sickness Insurance Committee, to which it entrusted the task of drawing up detailed proposals for submission to the insurance commissioners. These proposals, which were approved by a special representative meeting of the profession, contained the first definite statement of what the doctors' demands for remuneration were. Their request was that, instead of the capitation fee of six shillings (inclusive of drugs) which had formed the basis of the actuarial calculations for the Act, the doctors should receive a fee of 8/6d (exclusive of drugs). The demand was sent in to the insurance commissioners on 29 February 1912 (1934:277). This was not the best time for Morant who was in the midst of his great administrative task of creating the complex machinery of the new insurance system. After his victory over the Treasury, however, he turned his mind to the problem of medical remuneration. He conceived the idea of undertaking an impartial enquiry into existing levels of remuneration. Sir William Plender, later Lord Plender, was asked to carry out a detailed investigation of the terms on which medical treatment was given in six representative towns (Plender 1912; Cd 6305). At the same time the medical profession was asked to appoint representatives to a joint advisory committee which would undertake to discuss medical remuneration with the insurance commissioners. Lloyd George, fully aware of the power of the doctors, made a conciliatory speech in the House of Commons in which he underlined the government's anxiety to work in co-operation with the British Medical Association. The Act was implemented on 15 July 1912, although the question of doctors' remuneration remained unsettled.

Time was short for a settlement with the doctors with only six months remaining before 15 January 1913, when medical benefit was to be paid out. The annual representative meeting of the British Medical Association was held at Liverpool only a few days after the launching of the Act. Barr, the extreme opponent of the Act, was elected President and an overwhelming majority of the meeting called upon members of the profession not to give medical treatment under the Act until the demands of the Association had been met in full. In the interim doctors were urged to withdraw their services from the advisory insurance committees. The attitude of the doctors was summed up in a comment in the *British Medical Journal* 'the country could perhaps do without Mr Lloyd George, but it could not do without the doctors. That is the strength of our position' (Allen 1934:278). Nevertheless Morant and his staff issued provisional regulations for the guidance of doctors and insured persons and they were issued to the profession for consideration. Lloyd George decided to act, and on 23 October he called together the doctors' advisory committee and told them of his final decision on the question of remuneration. He was able to point out that Sir William Plender's enquiry showed that

'the average capitation fee paid to doctors under contract practice was 4/2*d*, together with 3*d* for extras and 5*d* for drugs – total 4/10*d*. The government's original proposal had been 4/6*d* together with 1/6*d* for drugs – total 6/0*d*. He had now, however, succeeded in getting additional funds from the Treasury and he was prepared to increase this allowance by at least 50%, the amount proposed being 7/0*d*, together with 1/6*d* for drugs and a "floating amount" of 6*d* (for either drugs or remuneration) – total 9/0*d*. Special provision was also to be made for epidemics' (1934:279).

The British Medical Association on hearing of the offer appointed a delegation of five doctors to carry on negotiations with the commissioners. Resulting from this, the government issued a final statement in which they said that 'while many of the points put forward by the doctors' representatives had been met, some either could not be accepted without amendment of the Act or were matters for settlement by local insurance committees' (1934:279). The matter was referred for consideration to the British Medical Association's local divisions who were required to vote upon the question of acceptance or rejection and then to send delegates to a plenary representative meeting to be held on 21 December. Despite the concessions made by the government there was almost a universal rejection and a resolution was carried at the representative meeting which stated 'that it is prejudicial to the interests of the profession for practitioners to apply for service under the Insurance Committees and the Regulations now issued. The Association therefore calls upon all practitioners to refrain from placing their names on any panel under Government control or to accept any whole-time office' (1934:280).

By this time, however, invitations had already been issued by each local insurance committee to the doctors in each district to submit their names for inclusion on the panel. The matter now rested with individual doctors. Would they abide by their undertaking to the British Medical Association or would they be attracted by the more generous rates of pay already being offered by the local insurance committees? For Morant and his colleagues it was an anxious moment because 27,000 doctors had signed a British Medical Association undertaking not to serve upon the panels until the appropriate terms had been accepted by the government. On the other hand, millions of insured people would begin to claim benefit on 15 January for which they had already been paying contributions. Moreover, in certain popular newspapers there was significant support for the British Medical Association if only because the press was anxious to embarrass the government. The government did, however, have some powerful cards up its sleeve. To start with, it was known that the views of the British Medical Association did not represent the views of the whole profession. Not all doctors belonged to the Association and, the moderates who did, were unable to make their voices heard in favour of more conciliatory

191

measures. 'Morant and his staff proceeded to build up "a skeleton army" of men who were prepared to step into the breach on 15 January and prevent British citizens from being robbed of the medical treatment to which they were entitled' (1934:281). The government put it about, especially through the Liberal press, that it intended to set up a state medical service of salaried doctors which would be financed by a heavy increase in income tax. In addition, rumours were circulated that after a given date the panels would be closed and doctors who had not already signed would no longer have an opportunity to join the state insurance scheme. 'Those doctors who were already working on contract practice in the large towns and were receiving a payment per head of little more than 4/0d could not be expected to throw away the chance that the Government scheme gave them of doubling their incomes, and at the beginning of the New Year there were signs of a change in the medical ranks' (1934:281). Numerous doctors wrote to the Association asking to be relieved of their undertakings, but the Association always replied that this could only be done by the decision of the representative body. Many doctors, in spite of this undertaking, agreed to support the government and on the appointed day the panels, established by the government, were found to have their appropriate quota of doctors ready to carry out the provisions of the Act. Within three days the representative meeting had released the 27,000 doctors from their pledges. In all this Morant had been highly important. He had enabled 'a British Cabinet Minister to defeat a revolt against an Act of Parliament' (1934:282). The doctors had yielded; and yet they were really victorious. This Gilbertian situation was well described by a writer in the *Westminster Gazette* when he said: 'we all admire a man who does not know when he is beaten. The trouble about the British Medical Association is that it does not know when it has won.' Shortly afterwards, when one of the commissioners was asked about his task he said, 'we are engaged in ramming down the doctors' throats the rare and refreshing fruits of their own victory' (1934:282).

The medical profession had gained a very adequate rate of remuneration. The agreements arising from these negotiations were the basis not merely for higher incomes for general practitioners after the Act, but more regular and reliable incomes. The general practitioners gained concessions from the government by vehement action. They achieved emancipation from the direct lay control of Friendly Societies, something which they had long sought. State intervention would simply have meant the continuation of existing institutions and practices in the market for medical care, had it not been for the exercise by the British Medical Association of its power, negotiating skill and its single-minded pursuit of the strategic goal of overall medical control of the market for general practitioner services. Where the original Bill had left control of medical benefit with the Friendly Societies, in its final form they were to be administered by local health committees with strong medical representation. In addition, there was a statutory recognition of a new animal, the medical committee. This operated at the local level representing the profession within the domain of each health committee. Describing the position of the medical profession under the National Insurance Act Beatrice Webb wrote,

> 'the statutory constitution of the Medical Profession down to the passing of the National Insurance Act of 1911 consisted of the General Medical Council and its constituent elements — namely, the ancient medical corporations, the old and new universities and the whole body of registered medical practitioners of the United Kingdom. The Insurance Act of 1911, for the purpose of the medical benefit under that Act, set up a supplementary constitution for the profession' (Webb 1917:8).

Not only were all medical practitioners entitled to be 'on the panel' for their district and to receive a capitation fee for each person on the list but each doctor had to provide 'adequate' treatment as defined by the Act. He was required also to fill up certain forms, issue certificates, make returns to the local insurance committee and also provide certificates of incapacity for work, noting the causes thereof. The approved societies were empowered to send their own medical man to judge the correctness of the diagnosis. The costs of prescriptions were liable to be scrutinised and if judged extravagant, the doctor could be surcharged. This was a new situation in which all doctors accepting service under the Act came 'automatically under the control of lay authorities, namely, the Insurance Commissioners of England, Wales, and Scotland respectively' (1917:9). In the case of the domiciliary treatment of tuberculosis they even came under the Local Government Board.

On the other hand, under this new constitution medical men secured a strengthening of self-government. In order to protect the panel practitioner from any unfair treatment by the local insurance committee, medical doctors were given considerable scope to participate in the administration of the Act. The whole body of medical practitioners within the area of each local insurance committee had the right to elect, not only two representatives on the insurance committee itself but also half the members of a sub-committee of the insurance committee (the medical service committee) to which certain questions relating to medical benefit must be referred. In other words, the National Insurance Act provided for a local medical committee elected by medical men and representative of the whole profession within each area, and also a panel practitioners' committee representative of just those members of the profession who accepted service under the Act. To these committees were referred, for investigation and report, all complaints made by one practitioner against another, all questions as to whether a given service was, or was not, of a kind properly undertaken by a practitioner of ordinary competence and skill and complaints of extravagant prescribing and other malpractices by panel practitioners. The insurance committee was, in effect, obliged to accept the decision of these representative bodies unless it chose to appeal to the insurance commissioners. Also, the insurance commissioners in each of the three countries of the United Kingdom included one medical man appointed by the government, more or less on account of his representative standing (Webb 1917:9). Medical representation was further strengthened when the administration of the scheme was put into the hands of the Ministry of Health which was created in 1919.[2] Such representation was then located in the Central Advisory Committee.

It has been argued by some writers that the tactics of the British Medical Association failed. Admittedly the British Medical Association at one stage in the negotiations over-reached itself, by deciding, after holding a referendum which resulted in an overwhelming vote against participation, not to accept service under the Act on the terms offered by the government. But as we have observed this position was soon undermined when individual general practitioners quickly accepted service on the panels. At a hastily called meeting the British Medical Association's earlier decision, not to participate, was revoked. In fact their policy enabled them to emerge 'from the negotiations on health insurance as a formidable power' (Stevens 1966:37). For the first time general practitioners, through the Insurance Acts Committee, achieved national recognition by the state because that committee negotiated directly with the government. On the other hand, the general practitioner had the advantage that he was not in any sense directly an employee of the state. Like certain other occupations, especially those with organised trade unions to represent their interests, the general practitioners were now engaged in a system of collective bargaining. Nevertheless, the state was only indirectly established in the medical market place, but the doctors for their part had obtained more than a footing in the apparatus of administration and decision-taking. They were thus afforded many opportunities for advantage which accrued from that position. The fact that the general practitioners were well organised, prior to the direct entry of the state into the medical market place and on a national scale, was an important basis for this achievement.

The 1911 Act as we have seen, left the whole matter of remuneration unsettled. It was to be a subject of negotiation by collective bargaining. One test of the success of the Act and of the new administrative machinery was, from the British Medical Association's point of view, the crucial question of doctors' remuneration. They obtained the right to choose the method by which they would be remunerated (they chose the capitation fee) and also the amount paid was 'to be what the profession considered adequate for the work performed' (1966:36). An important result of the National Health

Insurance Act, in spite of its limitations in respect of the people covered by it (only the wage-earner but not his family was insured), was to expand the effective demand for medical care. It ushered in a period in which the general practitioners collectively consolidated their control in the medical market place and improved their status position in society. By 1938 forty per cent of the population of England and Wales were covered by the scheme and all but ten per cent of all general practitioners were involved in it. It has been estimated that between 1936-8 over a third of the income of doctors (on the panel) was derived from health insurance work (1966:53). There seems little doubt that most general practitioners favoured the system if only because it provided an assured income. Through the effectiveness of medical representation and bargaining during these years the general practitioner's income, improved as it was by panel practice work, brought him closer both in income and status to the consultant than he had been before (1911). There is evidence that the net average income of the general practitioner in 1936-8 was about £1,000 a year (Hill, Roy 1951:26).

To a great extent the income and social position of the general practitioner after 1911 depended upon the success of the approved societies, which were the lynchpin of the national health insurance scheme. It had been assumed that the outbreak of war in 1914 would result in an economic depression with a consequent fall in income from contributions, and a rise in claims. In fact the boom conditions of war-time allowed the stronger approved societies to accumulate large surpluses, while the actual number of societies fell by a half. The problems they faced during the war included shortage of staff, and there was a shortage of doctors as more and more men were drawn into the armed forces. For the doctors this provided a good bargaining position because of their scarcity value. The pre-war strain between the profession and the approved societies was replaced by noticeably better relations. But boom meant inflation, and quickly the upper income limit for eligibility of the national health insurance scheme (£160) was passed by many workers. This was not important for manual workers who were covered at any wage, but more and more non-manual workers either lost their eligibility or were threatened with its loss. Often employers were generous enough to pay their 3d contribution as a gift, so that the worker might retain his eligibility. This anomaly needed to be ironed out for it was technically illegal, and in 1919 the maximum income for eligibility to the scheme was raised to £250. It continued at this rate until the beginning of the Second World War, when it was raised to £420. The British Medical Association was unwilling to see it raised too far for fear of damaging doctors' income from private practice.

The wartime inflation also affected doctors' incomes. The capitation fee paid to general practitioners working for the national health insurance medical service, was agreed in 1912 at between 8/6d and 9/0d per head, depending upon whether the doctor provided medicines or not. 'This rate had substantially increased medical incomes and nearly doubled the price of medical practices offered for sale' (Gilbert 1970:267-8). However, the effects of inflation during and immediately after the war created dissatisfaction among doctors with their income and conditions under the scheme. This resulted during 1919 in

> 'complaints from Insurance Committees about the low standards of attendance and casual treatment by doctors in their employ. If doctors were genuinely dissatisfied with their conditions, and the government failed to give them a substantial increase in income [so the Cabinet was warned] . . . the likely result would be a strike which would do nothing for national health insurance medical service, nor for the reputation of the Coalition Government' (Gilbert 1970:268).

The mood of the day in government circles was towards economy and it became increasingly difficult to find the money to give doctors a pay rise. The state already contributed £1,700,000 annually as part of its agreement with the profession to support the level of capitation fee which had been necessary to break the deadlock with the British Medical Association and buy off the threatened boycott by the doctors. It became clear that the doctors were already receiving higher remuneration than the approved societies could afford to pay from their reserves, and thus, any new award would have to be a charge on the government. In 1920 the matter reached Cabinet level, the only time it was to do so between the wars. Evidence was put that '75% of medical practitioners working for national health insurance received less than £500 a year from the scheme' (1970:269). Over the protests of the Chancellor of the Exchequer and others, the Cabinet finally agreed to increase the capitation fee from 8/6d to 11/0d.

By 1921 growing unemployment and the search for government economies began to affect national health insurance as it did almost every area of government financed activity.

> 'Most immediately hit was the medical profession. The settlement in the spring of the previous year of 11/0d as the capitation fee had satisfied no one. The doctors had asked for 13/6d while the approved societies had believed that 7/3d was ample. Like a man with two masters, the Government was able to serve neither well and found that only by contributing from its own funds was it able to force an agreement' (1970:271).

A new financial crisis caused the Ministry of Health to decide that after 1 January 1922 doctors would be paid only 9/6d per patient. The action was taken at the insistence of the Treasury and was not caused by the infamous axe of the Geddes Committee. In the spirit of national sacrifice, the doctors accepted 'the reduction in their fees grudgingly' (1970:271).

196

The Ministry promised that the new rate would be guaranteed for two years and that during this period a general enquiry would be held into doctors' pay.

> 'Approved societies, on the other hand, had always felt that the doctors were overpayed. This prejudice on the part of the societies gained unusual force in the spring of 1922 when, as a result of the Geddes Committee recommendations, the Government announced that it intended to end the grant of £1,700,000 toward the cost of the medical benefit that David Lloyd George had procured in 1913 as a means of breaking the doctors' strike at the inception of the health insurance programme.'

Confusion resulted from the decision and the approved societies were angry because '£1,700,000 represented approximately the difference in cost between the 9/6d per head that the doctors actually received and 7/3d which was the amount that the increase in insurance contributions would in fact permit toward the payment of the capitation fee' (1970:271). If the government withdrew its subsidy then the approved societies would have to meet the cost and, as we have seen, they happened to be in surplus. They reluctantly agreed to carry the extra cost for two years, but told the government that they would reduce the amount paid to doctors at the end of 1923 if the government did not stump up some money. It was clear that additional revenue could not be raised from the contributions of the working class beneficiaries during a time of economic depression.

The Bill reducing the capitation fee caused the doctors much unhappiness and the Cabinet had been warned that

> 'to remove all State assistance . . . would be to surrender the weapon which the State can use in dealing with the doctors and to hand them over to the approved societies. To do this would raise a storm of opposition in the medical profession and gravely endanger the structure of the medical benefit now embodied in the National Health Insurance Act' (PRO Cab 1922).

The medical profession feared the societies, who were pressing for a reduction in the capitation fee, and were aware that they were using their political influence to obtain pledges from Members of Parliament not to use society funds for payment of doctors above 7/3d.

In the event, the government offered (1923) a capitation fee of 8/6d for three years or 8/0d guaranteed for five years. In the letter to the Insurance Acts Committee in which the government's offer was made, it was pointed out that despite the reduction in the fee made in January 1922, there had been a sharp drop in the cost of living and that even under these conditions 552 doctors had been recruited into the scheme. It was contended that the average salary of a full-time doctor was about £1,200. The British Medical Association was not to be persuaded and the offer was rejected. Preparations were made by the doctors to strike. The British Medical Association claimed that 97 per cent of panel practitioners had put their resignations at the disposal of the Insurance Acts Committee. At the same time the profession was demanding an independent Court of Enquiry to look into medical remuneration. Such a move, the doctors confidently expected, would be of benefit to them just as it had been in the case of the arbitration panel of 1920. This had offered a capitation fee of 11/0d. The government (particularly the Treasury) and the approved societies were reluctant to submit themselves to an agent over whom they had no control. Nevertheless under the threat of a strike, the Ministry of Health capitulated and an offer was made of a capitation fee of 8/6d for five years, and the appointment of a Court of Enquiry — whose findings would bind both sides. Indeed they went further and promised a Royal Commission to examine the whole question of the national health insurance scheme.

The award of the Court of Enquiry raised the fee to 9/0d and recommended that it remain at this level until the end of 1927. This was a happy day for the doctors, but the approved societies repeatedly asked where the money was to come from, and kept pointing at the government. The money was found, after some statistical mystification, and the capitation fee, except for a short period in 1931, remained at this level until 1946. The ensuing Royal Commission, supported by the evidence it took from the British Medical Association expressed itself well satisfied with the situation of doctors under the scheme.

The greater security and improved incomes deriving from the national health insurance scheme was the basis for the contemporary feeling that 'a better class of man' was being attracted into general practice. The *British Medical Journal* was suggesting in 1937 that 'medicine gives to those who follow it an honourable position' and naturally addressed its remarks to prospective medical students attending public schools (*British Medical Journal* 1937:445). The profession 'was staunchly middle class' (Stevens 1966:57).

Undoubtedly such an average figure betrayed differences between geographical areas in the income of general practitioners especially in relation to the amount of private practice which could be added to the bread and butter income arising from the health insurance scheme. But perhaps the most significant consequence of the Act was the disappearance of large numbers of very poor practitioners due to the firm financial underpinning provided by the state scheme in the medical market. A lower boundary to the income of general practice had been established below which it was not difficult for a full-time practising doctor to fall. The feeling of belonging to a successful profession, which many general practitioners experienced in the inter-war years, was articulated by the British Medical Association. In 1935 it was exhorting the American Medical Association to take courage in the fact that 'the much greater experience of the British Medical Association in collective negotiation and bargaining indicates that the power of the organized medical profession, reasonably exercised, is very effective' (*British Medical Journal* 1935:365). Since the published evidence it had given to the Royal Commission on National Health Insurance (1926), it had come out as a strong supporter of the scheme. It had provided a degree of financial security and an increase in levels of remuneration far beyond those in existence prior to 1911, and the legislation changed the relationship between general practitioners themselves as well as between the latter and specialists. It should be remembered that the hospitals and specialists were excluded. There was a considerable growth in the number of partnerships and a consequent decline in single-handed practice because partnership facilitated the sharing of duty periods and expenses. By 1938 it was thought some forty five per cent of general practitioners were in a form of partnership. On the other hand, the division of general practitioners into panel and non-panel practice tended to militate against specialisation among them on the pattern which grew up in America. The gulf between the general practitioner and the specialist was if anything widened, and the system of referral which was by now traditional did not encourage general practitioners and consultants to form common partnerships. Under a by-law (157) of the Royal College of Physicians of London, fellows were debarred from entering such partnerships without obtaining the express permission of the Censor's Board of the College. General practitioners customarily sold the goodwill of a practice like any other business, but fellows of the Royal College of Physicians were forbidden to do so.

From the standpoint of the general practitioner, the national health insurance scheme was most advantageous in ending the fierce competition with out-patient departments of the hospitals. The general practitioner received his capitation fee whether or not he referred a case to hospital, which naturally encouraged him to send any difficult cases. The danger lay in his becoming a mere signpost. The trend towards the exclusion of general practitioners from the hospital was reinforced, thus confirming the separation between the respective work situations of the hospital doctor and the general practitioner. The number of specialists who practised without the seal of respectability conferred by a hospital appointment declined into insignificance. Nevertheless, the general practitioners still had access to the cottage hospitals and to the consultants via the referral system. The British Medical Association was the representative organ of the profession to the state. The general practitioners, through the British Medical Association, had shown that they were able to use the private power generated by their well organised and entrenched position to force the state to concede the professions' claims on almost all the key issues. Paradoxically, they were able to use state intervention as a means of restoring and enhancing their power, which had been threatened by the growth of lay control and private medical organisation during the last part of the nineteenth century. There is little likelihood that doctors would easily have been able to redress the balance without harnessing the state to their cause.

In the years between the two World Wars there was considerable convergence of views among non-socialist organisations on the fundamental problems of health organisation and on measures for its improvement. After the First World War, the problems of the hospital were perceived as paramount. Charity was no longer an adequate source of funds for voluntary hospitals and a public Voluntary Hospital Commission was set up, with a large sum of money from the Exchequer to aid the private hospitals. At first it was envisaged that this would be necessary only on a temporary basis but after its demise, a new body was created adopting the same name, but this time it was under the auspices of the British Hospitals Association (1935). It recommended that all hospitals should be co-ordinated by strong regional committees and that specialists should be paid in order to secure a more equitable distribution of their services.

In the 1930s there was a shift in the focus of policy on health matters within the Labour Party. Hitherto the Fabians, and particularly the Webbs, had been opposed to the concept of free medical services to all. Socialists were enormously suspicious of the medical profession and it remained true that curative medicine was still fairly primitive. On the other hand, it was recognised that preventive medicine generally, especially the sanitary movement, had made a vast contribution to public health. There was an awareness of the need to strengthen and develop curative medical services and during the 1930s no outspoken anti-medical group existed on the Left. Within the medical profession, the Socialist Medical Association was small but became influential within the Labour Party after its affiliation to the Party in 1931. Two years later it published a definitive programme which was adopted by the Party's Annual Conference in 1934. The Labour Party asserted that medical services should be free to the public and that doctors should be public employees on a full-time salaried basis. It was agreed that health centres should be the principal organisational feature of medical services. These points are of interest because of the subsequent Labour victory in the General Election in 1945.

Perhaps more important than Labour policy, as articulated at this time in the formation of the future National Health Service, was the experience of the doctors, the consultants in particular, during the Second World War. The approach of the war with its threat of aerial bombardment of the cities caused the government to introduce an Emergency Medical Service (EMS) to cope with the vast numbers of civilian and military casualties which were expected. The military planners turned out to be wildly over pessimistic — which was fortunate for the country. But it was in this context, under the threat of

200

impending devastation, that negotiations to set up the Emergency Medical Service took place. Feelings of patriotism, loyalty and national urgency caused the Royal Colleges to urge doctors to accept the scheme and make it work. For its part the government's usual peace-time caution in regard to expenditure and control was greatly relaxed. There was to be no interference in the internal affairs of hospitals whether voluntary or municipal. Initially there was a corps of Emergency Medical Service doctors including not merely house-officers but also consultants who were paid a salary (£800 to £950 *per annum*). Compared to their pre-war situation this must have been hardship for even reasonably successful consultants. When the specialists who had moved out of London found themselves still shouldering the burdens of maintaining town houses and consulting rooms, not to speak of massive life insurance premiums, they were beset by considerable anxieties. They feared that their private practices would melt away in their absence. The fact that in the early days of the war, the so-called 'phoney war', the anticipated massive aerial bombing was conspicuous by its absence meant that they soon ceased to believe that the Emergency Medical Service arrangements were necessary.

Under these circumstances, the British Medical Association and the Royal Colleges moved quickly to persuade the Ministry to revise Emergency Medical Service terms of service. The President of the Royal College of Physicians became chairman of an advisory committee whose recommendations were accepted with alacrity by the Ministry. The success of these negotiations was achieved within three months of the outbreak of war. Consultants were enabled to return to private practice, but their services were retained on a standby basis at a salary of £500 *per annum*. Later, a House of Commons Select Committee was to remark that it did not regard the terms as in the best interests of the country. They did, however, 'shed light on the strength of the medical profession in influencing national policy, and they introduced the Royal Colleges, together with the British Medical Association, to negotiations with the government over conditions of service' (Stevens 1966:69). The experience of the Emergency Medical Service was soon to have a remarkable and favourable effect on the attitude of the profession towards the idea of the National Health Service. This was particularly true of the consultants and, indeed, the hospital doctors generally. They, after all, had no previous experience of state service. Certain positive changes in the organisation of medical care were established under the Emergency Medical Service. These included not merely the organisation of a national hospital service, but a national blood transfusion service. At the same time national pathological and public health laboratory services were created. These were advances brought about under conditions of war which it would afterwards be difficult to dismantle.

During the early years of the war there was considerable agreement between the doctors and the Coalition Government on the main principles which should underlie the post-War re-organisation of health services. A professional planning committee was set up in 1940 comprised of representatives of the British Medical Association, the Royal Colleges and the Scottish Medical Corporations and it reported in 1942 (Medical Planning Commission 1942). The report underlined the split which existed between the general practitioner services and the hospitals, and drew attention to the isolation in which the general practitioner worked. It stressed the need for a comprehensive health service to unify the public health, hospital and general practitioner branches of medicine and also recommended the creation of health centres to encourage the growth of general practice on a 'corporate' basis (Eckstein 1958:118-9).

Within the broad agreement about the aims of a new service there were still questions to be resolved about the means through which these should be realised. The British Medical Association, representing the general practitioners, was all in favour of extending the national health insurance principle. This it had already proposed to the Royal Commission of 1926. The question was what proportion of the population should be covered? The British Medical Association had in mind that the new service should be extended to all but the wealthiest ten per cent. In this way private practice would be preserved. There were those who suggested that the new scheme should give coverage to all citizens regardless of income, but, if this proposal was adopted what then would happen to private practice?

The Government White Paper of 1944 took into account most of the issues and attempted to solve them (Ministry of Health 1944). It recommended that the three areas of practice, (hospital, general practice and public health) should be united under the Ministry of Health. A scheme of area planning of service was proposed. In deference to the views and interests of the British Medical Association a compromise was suggested on the organisation of general practice. This would partly be based on new health centres (where doctors might possibly be salaried) and partly on the continuation of individual private practice. A special central medical board would concern itself with the longstanding problem of the distribution of general practitioners and would have the power to refuse permission to doctors to enter public practice in overmanned areas. The right to set up in private practice was to remain inviolate.

From the consultant's point of view the proposal for joint health authorities with local authority participation was totally unacceptable. The fear of coming under the local authorities, comprising a set of attitudes inherited from the conditions of service obtaining with the Poor Law, conjured up in the mind of the voluntary hospital consultant 'the vision of himself reduced to the level of the lowest municipal doctor' (Stevens 1966:71). Nevertheless, reform of medical services became an increasingly urgent problem not least because nearly a quarter of the country's general practitioners were serving in the Armed Forces. They wanted to know what their future was to be.

At the end of the Second World War the Coalition Government which had served the country during the war years under the leadership of Winston Churchill was replaced, after the General Election of 1945, by a Labour Government in which Attlee was Prime Minister. Aneurin Bevan was appointed by him to the Ministry of Health. Bevan's plan was to introduce a free health service available to all without limit of income, and he was determined to nationalise the hospitals. Bevan believed that the Willink proposals were unsatisfactory.

> 'Fearing perhaps the dangers of excessive centralization, Willink had sought to shift responsibility from the centre to the periphery. When the profession protested that this would mean the municipalization of medicine, which they hated more than any alternative, Willink had devised a compromise which restored some of the apparent power to the centre, while blunting the instruments to wield it. Both voluntary and local authority hospitals would be left in their existing ownership and the planning bodies to be set up at area and regional level would become solely advisory. All the various "interests" were thereby mollified, since nothing could be too rapidly or drastically changed' (Foot 1973:131).

Bevan regarded this question of the hospitals as the gravest weakness of the scheme and he decided to confront the powerful vested interests of local authorities, which controlled the municipal hospital system, as well as the voluntary hospitals by his decision to expropriate them, leaving only the

> 'teaching hospitals [with] a separate status, [allowing them both] a special control over their endowments and a special method of nomination of their Boards of Governors. Here indeed was one of Bevan's crucial decisions, for only by attracting the best and the most prestigious medical brains into the service could he hope to make it *universal*, covering the whole or nearly the whole population. This was the key to so much else he had to keep in mind – outflanking the British Medical Association, enlisting public support, averting left-wing attack, winning over the Cabinet' (1973:131-2).

This solution had never been proposed by any of the earlier reformers, not even the Socialist Medical Association, which had not included this demand in its proposals which were agreed in a resolution at the 1945 Labour Party Conference. The views of Herbert Morrison, a powerful advocate of local authority interest (especially of the London County Council), had to be overcome in Cabinet. Foot sums up the situation when he says 'it is difficult today to recall the widespread sense of shock which the plan aroused . . . by the same stroke Bevan was challenging two of the most powerful and respected vested interests in the country' (Foot 1973:133).

Foot tells us that 'no-one in the previous Parliament had protested more vigorously than Bevan that precise negotiations with outside bodies about major legislative measures subverted the authority of the House of Commons; it meant that a Minister came before Members of Parliament with his hands tied, unable to accept amendments' (1973:118). On the other hand, he was perfectly prepared to consult and negotiate with the bodies representing the medical profession about terms of service or specific regulations at a later stage. Already the Ministry had amassed evidence about the doctors' views and Bevan himself, at a series of early meetings, sought not only 'to allay the doctors' fears, he explored and exploited the political ramifications of the profession with mischievous zeal and delight' (1973:120). In many crucial respects he had anticipated the attitudes which would be taken up and when he finally unveiled his plans to the British Medical Association and other bodies in January 1946, it suddenly dawned upon them that these were the 'consultations' which he had promised. In point of fact the doctors found that 'they had been mobilizing on a battlefield where no battle would be fought' (1973:140). Eckstein in summing up Bevan's concept of negotiations says 'from the beginning, Bevan appeared to act on three principles: that the views of the profession were already well-known; that, while these views should be taken into account, there certainly should be no prior professional approval of the Government's scheme; and that he would negotiate over terms of service but never over the organization of the Service itself' (Eckstein 1959:158).

The National Health Service Bill (1946) introduced a tripartite administrative apparatus organised around the traditional structures of medical care, (public health, hospital and general practice). The only locus of co-ordination was at the level of the Ministry of Health. Even at the time it seemed to many people more sensible to proceed on a basis such as that which was proposed in the Dawson Report (1920), namely to create a more unified and integrated service. But such a scheme flew in the face of the organised interests of the profession. The Minister may have been tough and a socialist but he was also a realist. He was ready to compromise in order to get the National Health Service started quickly. In an imperfect world ideal solutions were not politically feasible.

The government was aware that the method and amount of remuneration would be a crucial issue and sought advice from a committee set up for the purpose. Even the *Lancet* had recognised that 'the truth is that the doctor-patient relationship in modern form needs improvement rather than preservation; it can never be wholly satisfactory while the doctor (as someone has put it) is not only a friend in need, but also a friend in need of his patient's money; nor while there is competition rather than co-operation between him and his colleagues' (*Lancet* 1946:503). The Spens Report was cautious on the form of payment, but was at least marginally favourable to the continuation of the capitation fee (Ministry of Health 1946). This was highly satisfactory to the general practitioners and their reaction was not disturbed even by the thought that it might introduce a greater division between them and the consultants who were likely to be paid by salary. The doctors thought that Bevan favoured a salaried service. It was no surprise to them when the Minister announced only a qualified approval of the Spens recommendations. This was the reason why Bevan's statement, that he wanted to introduce an element of salary (£300) into the general practitioners' remuneration, was rejected by the British Medical Association even though it was intended to help young doctors who were just starting out in practice. The doctors believed that this move on the part of the Minister was the thin end of a wedge which was intended to reduce them to the status of salaried civil servants. Many consultants, on the other hand, were already salaried university teachers, or in salaried posts in the municipal hospitals. They did not fear salaried service as the general practitioners did, since many consultants were already combining fees from private practice with a salary. 'The part-time consultant continued as he had before as an "honorary", but with the added prize of a monthly cheque; emotionally, this was felt to be a fee for consultant duties rather than a part-time salary' (Stevens 1966:77).

It was in this setting that the profession as a whole had to decide how to represent its interests to the government. Feelings ran high between the general practitioners and the consultants, re-opening old wounds. The Royal Colleges brought a new-found political interest and sophistication to bear. They also had more room for manoeuvre. The British Medical Association on the other hand, regarded itself as the organisation which should negotiate exclusively for the profession. It was becoming obvious that the consultants would want to be separately represented by the Royal Colleges in the coming negotiations. The British Medical Association feared that Bevan was hoping to exploit these differences on the well-tried principle of divide and rule. Whether this was true or not, the antagonism between the interests of the two sides of the profession was to be carried forward into the structure of National Health Service. After the National Health Service Act became law there was still plenty of room for negotiation. The British Medical Association had decided to conduct a plebiscite among its members to discover their views. The Royal Colleges were already committed, by their Presidents, to a policy of co-operation but there was some suspicion among both the physicians and surgeons that their leaders were moving ahead of the opinion of the majority. The view was expressed for example, that everything should be done to assure the general practitioners 'that the surgeons were with them and not against them' (Stevens 1966:80). Nevertheless, the Royal Colleges informed the Minister, in January 1947, that they would enter the negotiations on a separate basis. For his part, the Minister assured the Colleges that their decision to negotiate would not prejudice their right at the end of the day to refuse, if they so decided, to enter the National Health Service. In addition, the Minister pledged that there would be no interference with the clinical freedom of any doctor and that individuals would be free to join the service or not on either a full-time or part-time basis. He reaffirmed that consultants could continue to treat private patients in nationalised hospital beds, subject only to availability. Summing up the position in a debate in the House, the Parliamentary Secretary to the Minister of Health said 'no body of public or private employees has ever had the same freedom as the medical profession will have under this Bill' (Lindsey 1962:44-5).

In the event, the profession entrusted the negotiations to a committee of thirty-three. The appointments were made jointly by the British Medical Association and the English and Scottish Royal Colleges. The British Medical Association participated only on the understanding that any agreed terms would be subject to a plebiscite of the profession and that the option of fresh legislation should remain open. Mr Bevan indicated his willingness to accept these conditions. The negotiations themselves were shrouded in secrecy and were protracted. On matters where agreement was reached early on, the new machinery was quickly set up. For example, by the summer of 1947 members of regional hospital boards were being appointed. In November 1947 the state of the negotiations emerged, at least in part, from under the wraps of secrecy in which they had long been shrouded. It became clear that no final agreement had been reached on the organisation of general practice. The question of the sale of the goodwill of medical practices and the matter of the powers of the medical practices committee, in regard to the control of the distribution of doctors, were still in dispute. Even powers of negative direction seemed to the British Medical Association representatives to threaten the freedom of the general practitioner. On the matter of the proposed disciplinary machinery, the general practitioners wanted the right of appeal to the High Court. None of these issues were of direct concern to the specialist branch because nothing like them was envisaged by the government for the consultants. The profession was unanimous on one point – that the patient should *not* have the right to consult a specialist of his choice. The traditional referral system was sustained. The Minister made it clear publicly, in December 1947, that the right to sell a medical practice would remain inviolate, but not its goodwill. Partnerships, though, would still be marketable. He also stated that the right of appeal to the High Court was not a possibility as it would conflict with the doctrine of Ministerial responsibility. It soon became apparent that the specialists were reasonably content with the arrangements being made on their behalf, but that the general practitioners were far from happy.

The results of a British Medical Association plebiscite expressed dissatisfaction with the terms being offered, though the British Medical Association stressed that the profession was in no way rejecting the Health Service in principle. The general practitioners began to display considerable militancy of mood and more heat than light was being generated.

The move for compromise was initiated by the Royal Colleges who suggested some easement on the matter of general practitioners' remuneration. The consultants, represented by the Royal Colleges, probably took this accommodating attitude because of the concessions which Bevan had already agreed in regard to them. It should not be forgotten – shades of 1911 – that the National Insurance Scheme was to expire on the day appointed for the implementation of the National Health Service Act and many general practitioners faced the loss of their incomes (Eckstein 1959:162-3). In April 1947, only three months before the date on which the new service was to commence, Bevan showed himself to be in a conciliatory frame of mind. He agreed to make it clear, in an amendment to the Act, that a whole-time salaried service was not his intention. The capitation fee was preserved; though an optional basic salary was available. A salary element would be paid only to new doctors in their first three years of general practice. Unlike civil servants, doctors would have absolute freedom to publish their views on the working of the National Health Service. The general practitioners wanted also to retain the right to buy and sell practices, including goodwill, but the government were against it. On this point the general practitioners compromised and accepted generous compensation for the loss. Members of the public began to register after 5 July 1948.

The geographical maldistribution of doctors soon became apparent. Some had lists which were growing embarrassingly large; while others were disappointingly small. After 5 July 1948, when the National Health Service became operational, doctors with small lists were soon starting to invoke the protection of the Medical Practices Committee. They sought declarations that their areas were overdoctored so that new practitioners would be prohibited from setting up in practice. As Stevens put it ' "negative direction" had begun' (Stevens 1966:88). In these circumstances further negotiations on the issue were otiose. The British Medical Association was successful in preventing the introduction of a salaried service and protecting the right to engage in private practice. In addition, the new local health executive councils (which were to administer the family practitioner services) were simply expanded versions of the old insurance committees but with increased professional representation. The executive councils were also granted the right to elect their own chairman, thus preventing him being a nominee of the Ministry of Health. In fact, the organisation of the general practitioner services was a rather conservative extension of the former panel practice system to virtually the whole population.

Relative to the consultant and to the hospitals, the situation of the general practitioner changed only gradually. The fact that the general practitioner had more secure and higher remuneration in the years 1911-48 meant that the social gap between the consultant and the general practitioner had narrowed. Moreover the consultant had been dependent on the goodwill of general practitioners for the referral of private patients and it was to his advantage to cultivate good relations. Now that the consultant was on a salary, as a result of the incorporation of the hospitals in the National Health Service, this relationship was somewhat attenuated.

In any case, the consultants had also become politically organised and the Royal Colleges, through their cultivation of the government achieved notable successes in the negotiations. The British Medical Association always regarded itself as the organisation which should negotiate *exclusively* for the profession. In the event, the structural division of interests between the two sides of the profession were carried over into the National Health Service and even accentuated. This division is not always manifest but has been a latent force in all negotiations with the state.

What is very evident, looking back on the inception of the National Health Service is that 'the medical profession as a whole emerged as a strong force from the negotiations surrounding the Act'. As one medical man said at the time, the profession is 'in a more powerful position than ever before' (Stevens 1966:93). From the Central Health Services Council right down the administrative ladder there was substantial medical representation. The right of part-time service and private practice were retained and, with the introduction of a distinction award scheme, large sums of public money were allocated by consultants to consultants. On the matter of appointment of specialists, appointing committees consisted of at least five doctors (out of a total of seven persons). Review committees to assess and grade hospital staffs were entirely made up of specialists. As Stevens said, summing up the position, 'so far the National Health Service had not inhibited professional freedom; on the contrary, the leaders of the profession had more control over the future of doctors than ever before' (1966:94). The nationalisation of the hospitals and the re-organisation of general practice eventuated in a profession-dominated National Health Service which achieved for the medical profession a constitutional position in the realm matched only by the Church and the Law.

The hospitals had been a crucial factor in Bevan's plans. They were scarcely affected by the legislation of 1911, but the impact of the First World War and the increasing cost of medical care in the hospital context, as well as the greater saliency of the hospital as a place of medical care for all segments of society, were the basis for the

208

incorporation of the hospitals under the National Health Service Act in 1946. The Emergency Hospital Service, which had been created as war became imminent, had already brought the consultants into the organisation of a national hospital service for the duration of the war. The consultants were simply charged by the government with this responsibility and given the resources to get on with it. There is no doubt that the mixture which the government had inadvertently prescribed, which was autonomy plus resources, suited the hospital consultants very nicely; they flourished on it. The outcome was that the consultants came very willingly into the National Health Service, especially as the voluntary hospital movement was running out of funds from charitable sources. The Royal Colleges soon proved themselves to be consummate negotiators. Hitherto the British Medical Association had represented the medical profession to the government, now, in the new situation the consultants declined to be represented by the British Medical Association. Once again the ancient rift between consultants and general practitioners was re-opened.

Representing the general practitioners the Association held bitter protest meetings against certain provisions in the Bill.

'Its mood of calm reasonableness evaporated, and it seemed to have forgotten its earlier dicta on the influence of the profession in the National Health Insurance scheme. Meanwhile the Royal Colleges gave impressive and cordial dinners for members of the government. Their aristocratic lineage held firm; at times their links with the royal family appeared stronger than those with their brothers in general practice. The Princess Royal visited the Royal College of Surgeons, of which she was an honorary fellow, to look at their plans for rebuilding, in the month in which the Bill was placed before Parliament' (Stevens 1966:77-8).

At this crucial time the Queen accepted office as Patron of the Royal College of Obstetricians and Gynaecologists, and in the same month the Prime Minister attended a dinner at the Royal College of Surgeons. As it turned out the incorporation of the hospitals, especially the voluntary hospitals, and the consultants into the National Health Service was done on terms which largely conserved the existing arrangements while bringing certain additional benefits to the hospitals and the consultants themselves.

A structure of Regional Hospital Boards and Hospital Management Committees in each local hospital were set up, but the great teaching hospitals associated with university medical schools were not included. Instead they were treated as 'regions' in their own right with direct links to the Ministry of Health. Though teaching hospitals, when nationalised, formed the basis of a region they were nevertheless independent of it, and were in fact separately administered by a special board of governors including representatives not merely of the university, the regional board and the local authorities, but significantly the senior staff of the hospital itself. Moreover the boards continued to have control of the endowments of the voluntary teaching hospitals, some of which were extremely wealthy. The consultant or specialist was employed on a full-time or part-time basis and could continue in private practice outside the service. Private pay beds were provided in the hospitals (for those who could pay the whole cost) where consultants could continue to treat these private patients at fees they themselves determined.

The Ministry of Health hoped to encourage specialists to feel they were all ' "members of one team" in whichever hospital their duties lay' (1966:88). The object was to overcome the old distinctions between voluntary and municipal hospitals. In fact the reaffirmation of the split between teaching and non-teaching hospitals, with the corollary that each should be empowered to appoint their own specialists, went against the principle of a unified specialist service. The long standing jealousies between the former voluntary teaching hospitals and the rest remained, because it 'continued to be more prestigious and lucrative to be attached to a teaching hospital' (1966:89). The teaching hospitals had more private beds than the others and were empowered to select their own cases rather than act as district-general hospitals with responsibility for accepting such cases as were referred to them.

On the question of consultants' and specialists' salaries the Spens Report (1948), published just prior to the implementation of the National Health Service Act, stressed the need for proper negotiating machinery, but the matter of who should represent the specialists was a tricky one. In fact the pay scales met with general approval, so that Lord Moran, President of the Royal College of Physicians, who was himself a member of the committee was later to call the terms 'so generous that they have been attacked in most quarters outside the medical profession' (1966:91).

Nevertheless the differences between the British Medical Association and the Royal Colleges became more marked, for the two branches of the profession entered the service on a very different basis; the one by salary, the other by capitation fee. Once they were together in the new service the vital question, which had not previously arisen, came into prominence; namely, the differential payment between the general practitioner and the specialist. In fact Spens did not directly address the problem, though he gave a clear advantage to the specialist. The British Medical Association itself created a dual structure to represent the two interests, but in the end a compromise was reached to which the colleges and the British Medical Association agreed to the formation of a Joint Consultants' Committee, and the British Medical Association 'lost its right to speak with equal authority for all categories of doctor' (Stevens 1966:93). As Paul Ferris put it

'the Central Consultants and Specialists Committee (of the

British Medical Association) nominates half the members to a more exalted committee further up the line, the Joint Consultants; the Royal Colleges and Scottish medical corporations nominate the other half, and so ensure that the British Medical Association, with its trade-union, general-practice atmosphere, is kept at a decent distance when consultants meet the Ministry' (Ferris 1965:143).

Notes

1. Some writers refer to insurance committee, some to health committee and some to health insurance committee. We use these terms interchangably.
2. For the politics of this development see F. Honingsbaum 1971.

10. THE DOCTORS IN THE NATIONAL HEALTH SERVICE 1948-75

The implementation of the National Health Service Act after 1948 was a high watermark of security and status for the medical profession. Rather than a Service run on socialist lines, which the doctors had feared with the appointment of Bevan to the Ministry of Health, there was in fact a strengthening of the controls exercised by the doctors collectively over the institutions and organisations of medical care. As Eckstein put it 'the collectivization of medicine, in short, has led to the growing corporatization of the medical profession and given the medical corporations, especially the BMA, great powers *vis-à-vis* the government' (Eckstein 1960:48). Although it has been commonly believed that the British Medical Association, in particular, is in constant warfare with the Ministry, it is in fact — as Eckstein among others have demonstrated — engaged for the most part in continual co-operation with it 'a highly useful adjunct to the Ministry's machinery of administration which, had it not already existed, the Ministry would have had to invent' (1960:48). It can be asserted that, through the statutory redefinition of its role and function in society, the medical profession now held a place, in terms of power and prestige, not altogether dissimilar from the legal profession. It now had an established constitutional position in the realm. The medical profession was willing to accept the state as a partner in the provision of medical care (the general practitioners in 1911, the hospital doctors in 1948). The reason for this was that at both of these historical moments it seemed that only the state could provide the necessary quantity of financial resources essential to maintain and improve both the standards of medical care and the degree of security and levels of remuneration which the doctors regarded as appropriate to the profession. The problem of funding the National Health Service and of determining levels of medical remuneration has therefore not been defined as simply a matter for trade-union bargaining in the accepted manner, between parties who see themselves integrally bound together as employers and employees in an industrial system. At every stage the doctors have judged their 'partner', the state, by the extent to which it is willing to fund the Service adequately — on their definition of adequacy — and maintain appropriate levels of remuneration — on their definition of appropriate. The general practitioner has maintained his position as notionally an independent contractor who can withdraw from the service either individually or collectively if he regards the terms of the contract as no longer adequate. This view is also held by the consultants and the other hospital doctors, although it is much less realistic in the context of a salaried service. This is a crucial point in so far as an obsession with finance among medical men seems if anything to be greater because of it than in the case of other professions.

Rudolf Klein, referring to Beveridge, points out that the National Health Service was launched on a tide of idealism and miscalculation (Beveridge 1942).

> 'The miscalculation was general. It was assumed — not for the first or last time — that it would be possible to make a massive policy innovation without making a massive financial commitment. This assumption reflected the optimism of the Beveridge report, which had calculated that the cost of a health service, put at £170 million a year, would be the same in 1965 as in 1945, because expenditure on curing people was clearly self-liquidating' (Klein 1973:739).

Because of this assumption the ever-rising expenditure on the National Health Service attracted accusations of extravagance. The Guillebaud Committee was appointed to look into the question of costs and demonstrated that much of the rise was due to inflation (Guillebaud 1956). Nevertheless the damage had been done and 'the NHS was on the defensive. The main anxiety of its administrators seems to have been to protect themselves against accusations of wasting public money, rather than explore the best ways of spending it' (Klein 1973:739). In this climate of opinion, the 1950s 'was an essentially negative sterile era' (1973:741).

The National Health Service was a negotiated compromise between competing interests which resulted in an administrative division between the hospital service on the one hand (over which the hospital doctors had much greater control with the nationalisation of both the voluntary and the local authority hospitals) and the general practitioner service on the other. Only the rump of local authority health functions, particularly the medical officer of health and the school medical service, remained under local authority control. Essentially there existed a *unified* medical profession operating within the context of a *divided* administrative structure. Clearly, such an administrative division could exacerbate tensions within the medical profession but, provided professional unity was maintained, there were advantages to the doctors in facing a divided administration. Moreover, as Eckstein points out, the Ministry of Health which after Bevan's day was separated from housing and local government, was a weak department usually without a Minister in the Cabinet. This enabled a well organised medical profession to achieve many of the objectives it desired in the detailed day-to-day running of the Service. The major problem remained the overall financing of the Service for which a strong Cabinet Minister would have been a useful ally in obtaining more resources. Without a strong Minister of Health the views of the Treasury, which is above all concerned with the control of expenditure, tended to prevail and consequently expenditure on health grew less quickly than in some other areas of public expenditure, such as education.

Prior to the National Health Service, particularly in the period between the two World Wars, the general practitioner had achieved certain advantages relative to the consultant. The income and social status of the general practitioner rose during these years and was assured, in large measure, through the government sponsored national health insurance scheme. The relationship to the consultant was sustained on a favourable basis by the fact that the latter needed the general practitioner in order to get paying patients and thus make his livelihood. He was inclined to treat the general practitioner nicely. As Stevens puts it 'the financial as well as the social gulf between the two branches had shrunk' (Stevens 1966:95). General practitioners were also well organised politically through the British Medical Association whereas the consultants were not.

We have previously discussed the effects of the Emergency Medical Service in drawing the hospitals and the consultants into the ambit of government policy. This was an important reason why the Royal Colleges came to be politically involved in the process of negotiation with the state. During the negotiations to set up the Health Service it became apparent that in many ways the interests of the consultants differed from those of the general practitioners. This was based on the fact that 'the National Health Service set its seal to a policy of a small number of highly trained and experienced consultants, fed by a relatively large number of general practitioners . . . In 1949 the proportion of consultants to GPs was less than one to three' (Stevens 1966:99). It was under these conditions that an increasing division between general practitioners and hospital doctors was generated.

General practice remained rooted in the practitioner's home or surgery while specialist practice became even more firmly entrenched in the hospital. Added to this was the fact that the general practitioner was rapidly excluded from access to beds in most general hospitals. 'There was a danger . . . of recreating two professions, or at least two demarcated branches of a single profession. Viewed historically, the wheel had come full circle. The inheritors of the teaching hospitals and of the Royal Colleges were once more in control of key hospitals; the general practitioners were once more on the outside.' This had come about not in a situation 'of private enterprise but of government service' (1966: 99-100). The disproportionately fast expansion of the hospital service and the greater prestige associated with specialist practice, together with its financial advantages would, it was feared, cause most young doctors to seek a career as a specialist. The view began to be heard in the profession that the general practitioner was a 'failed consultant' — an intellectually inferior grade of practitioner.

The proponents of this view used in support of their argument, the fact that the introduction of government-financed student grants was enabling bright, but financially hard-pressed students, to complete advanced studies where once they would have had to make do with a career in general practice. Thus, the argument ran, the brightest medical students were being creamed off into consultancy; the rest turned to general practice. By 1956 two-thirds of medical students were in receipt of some form of government grant or scholarship. Not merely was the general practitioner excluded from the larger hospitals and regarded as of lesser intellectual ability than the specialist, but in an era in which specialism was greatly admired he was a generalist. Moreover, unlike the consultants, he had no Royal College of his own. In addition, the promises which had been made to build health centres for the general practitioner service failed to materialise.

The concept of the health centre was originally suggested by the Dawson Committee after the First World War (Dawson 1920). Although the idea as first suggested was frankly woolly, the main purpose was to provide a place where the different elements in the health service were integrated. During the next twenty-five years every effort appears to have been made to make sure that this did not happen. The health services were increasingly fragmented and specialised — infant welfare centres, ante-natal clinics, tuberculosis dispensaries, and venereal disease clinics were only some of the services which were provided on this basis and which had earlier been undertaken by the general practitioner, or the hospital out-patient department, or not at all. In spite of this trend some experimental health centres were brought into being.

Whilst it is true that Bevan, who was also Minister of Housing, realised that the scarcity of building resources after the war made it essential to concentrate on housing rather than on health centres, yet it is also true that family doctors were generally highly suspicious of the concept. They feared that such centres would inevitably be under local authority control and hence that doctors serving in them would be subject to interference from supposed bureaucrats and petty bourgeois councillors (Ryan 1968:41). The suspicion of health centres remained, and the policy of the general medical services committee of the British Medical Association was, that family doctors should own their own premises. In 1966 the government's willingness to create, with the doctors, the General Practice Finance Corporation was the mark of the accommodation of the state to the doctors' point of view. It was recognised that, for the future, the renting of premises (which would be built and owned by the local authority) might become increasingly commonplace. Suspicion remained and early in 1975, to take one example, three out of four group practices in the Hertfordshire town of Harpenden, reneged on their earlier commitment to use the premises of a health centre to be built in the town.

Although the health centre idea failed to take off, with the introduction of the Health Service the organisation of general practice began to change. Already, by 1955, it was reported that the scheme which had been introduced in 1953 to encourage group practice 'had been so successful that, for the moment, the amount of money asked for was considerably in excess of that available' (Ministry of Health 1955: 51-8). The evidence already demonstrated, and has continued to demonstrate, that single-handed practice is in decline. Partnerships have increased and group practice has increasingly become the norm rather than the exception. As older doctors in single-handed practice retired the decline of competition among general practitioners in the health service became apparent.

The reform of the medical pay structure in 1966 included a clause removing the availability of interest-free loans for building group practice premises. This was also a time at which there was a sharp rise of prices in the property market. This made it very expensive for young doctors to buy premises from retiring incumbent practitioners, for although the purchase of the goodwill of medical practices had been abolished in 1948, the premises were still for sale. 'Health centres provided doctors with a haven in an inflationary storm' (Weightman 1975:727). At the same time there was a change of heart at the Ministry where a desire to pare down the burgeoning costs of the hospital service predominated. The concept of community medicine seemed to be one way of providing medical services more cheaply. George Godber, the chief medical officer, supported health centres as did an increasing number of politicians, but the effect of this change of policy varied as between local authority areas. By the 1970s health centres were being opened at a very rapid rate and by 1975 there were approaching six hundred in operation in England and Wales. Most health centres however are still based on a 'group practice' concept not that of a 'health team'. Weightman suggests that in the main health authorities have bowed 'to the demands and prejudices of doctors' (1975:727) rather than taking into account the views and requirements of other health workers such as health visitors.

Health centres or no, it became clear during the 1950s that there was a widespread feeling of dissatisfaction among general practitioners with the British Medical Association. Though the British Medical Association had fought against a salaried service and won, the several advantages of salaried service to the hospital doctors became increasingly visible to general practitioners. For example, consultants benefited from payment during time of illness, they received paid holidays, distinction awards, sabbatical leave, not to speak of a favourable scheme for retirement pensions as well as the support of numerous ancillary services in the hospital, including free secretarial assistance. General practice, on the other hand, was often both poorly organised and inefficient. This at least was the view widely held in the profession.

In 1950 these fears were underlined by the publication of a report on the state of general practice by an Australian, Dr Collings (*Lancet* 1950:555-85). He was particularly critical of the quality of general practice in urban-industrial areas, slightly less critical of standards in urban-residential areas, but he noted that the finest quality of general practice to be found in Britain was in the rural areas. Though Collings did not make the point in so many words, he tacitly suggested that the close proximity of a general practitioner to a teaching hospital or large clinical centre was likely to have a negative effect on the quality of his work. Additional studies, stimulated in part by Dr Collings' report, namely the studies by Dr S.J. Hadfield and Lord Taylor, attempted to refute these allegations, and generally speaking took a more optimistic view. The Ministry of Health and the British Medical Association also began enquiries at this time into the condition of general practice. Whatever the truth or falsity of the various findings, the fact remained that general practitioners themselves increasingly felt that their relative status position had been threatened by the changes occurring under the National Health Service. This view was shared by the rest of the profession and by informed lay opinion.

This feeling was one of the main reasons behind the foundation of the College of General Practitioners. The speed with which the idea caught on among large numbers of ordinary doctors at this particular time is probably a measure of their dissatisfaction with their situation both in the profession and in the National Health Service. The idea was mooted in 1949 by Dr P.K. Murphy, who crystallised the feelings of general practitioners when he wrote that the interests of general practitioners had never been so 'mismanaged and neglected' as in the last few years and that the 'influence, status [and] material prosperity [of general practitioners] are waning' *(British Medical Journal* 1949:124). Doctors in general practice felt that neither the Royal Colleges nor the British Medical Association were able for different reasons to help them in their struggle to maintain their status and improve their position.

The hope was that the new College would 'endow the general practitioner with the kind of status given to consultants by the Royal Colleges' (*Lancet* 1948: 189). With these pressures behind its foundation the College of General Practitioners became a reality (1952) and after a decade had acquired 6,200 members, and associates. The reason for its foundation was retrospectively expressed in these terms;

> 'without headquarters, without academic leadership of their own, without much influence over undergraduate or postgraduate teaching, and without the status of their specialist colleagues . . . General practitioners had muddled along, and time and time again they had found themselves left behind, left out, edged out and even pushed out — as from certain cottage hospitals . . . They had never organised themselves, and they had no one of the standing of the executive of the Royal Colleges to put forward their

claims when big decisions had to be made' (Report of the College of General Practitioners 1953).

The consultants felt that they had been well served by the Royal Colleges under the Emergency Medical Service and in the successful negotiations with the government over their terms of service and remuneration in the National Health scheme. Whereas, between the wars, the British Medical Association had congratulated itself on its successes and had been popular with the bulk of its general practitioner members, now in the National Health Service the consultants were experiencing success through the skilful political manoeuvres of the Royal Colleges. The general practitioners felt that they were playing second fiddle to the consultants and that the British Medical Association had lost the initiative in intra-professional politics. Just as some general practitioners, as we have seen, supported the idea of a college of medicine in the nineteenth century so now the idea was revived. The British Medical Association was not a qualifying Association, but a College of General Practitioners could be, and would establish general practice as itself a specialism in a world increasingly dominated by prestigious specialists.

'GPs were generally recognized only at the lowest and least influential level of the Royal College hierarchy, through the basic LRCP and MRCS diplomas. The BMA represented the general practitioners in negotiations and in matters of general interest, but it did not impose educational requirements. Moreover, after its great efforts to modify the National Health Service Bill, the British Medical Association seemed to have lost its grip. It had not come out of the conflict unsullied. There was doubt as to whether all the noise had really been necessary' (Stevens 1966:103).

In the years after the war the British Medical Association focussed its efforts on general policy reports and there was a feeling among general practitioners that it was doing too little to raise their status.

There was too a growing realisation among general practitioners that whereas in the past the examinations of the Royal Colleges (MRCP, FRCS) had been closely geared to the needs of general practice, now they tended more and more to be applicable to practice in the hospital. Other interests, particularly among specialists were served by the foundation of new colleges, such as that of the obstetricians, which not only improved educational standards but brought rewards of remuneration and status. The hope was that a College of General Practitioners, utilising the fact that medicine was turning back to the community and environmental influences on health and disease, could enable a specialism to be made out of the practice of medicine in the community itself (1966:155).

The question of the relationship between general practitioners and hospital doctors was expressed also in the structure of remuneration.

218

The Spens Committees (1946 and 1948) made recommendations about the scale of remuneration for the two branches of the profession and it should be stressed that the relevant committees considered the pay structure of hospital staffs in complete isolation from that of general practitioners. The level of remuneration was based on the pre-war earnings of each branch and no attempt was made to assess appropriate differentials between general practitioners and consultants. In the event an individual consultant might expect to earn about twice as much as a general practitioner. For the latter, in the age group of forty to fifty years, an income of £1,300 (after expenses) might be expected. On the other hand, a specialist devoting himself full-time to the National Health Service might expect a salary of about £2,500 at the age of forty years. In spite of these indicative figures it was very difficult before the establishment of the National Health Service to make reliable national comparisons of income between the two branches of the medical profession. In general it is clear that income differentials, existing prior to the National Health Service, were carried over into the new structure but the general practitioners and the consultants continued to be organised on a different basis for the purpose of negotiations over remuneration.

At the very inception of the National Health Service the government had agreed that terms of service and remuneration would always be subject to negotiation with the profession, and indeed with the other professions and occupations falling within the domain of the National Health Service. The Whitley Council procedure was to be used. It was already established in some parts of the public health field. Nine councils were set up, each concerning itself with one of the occupations, or groups of occupations, inside the National Health Service. The council for the medical profession was itself sub-divided into three committees. Committee A was intended to deal with the general practitioner service but, because of the pre-existing relationship of the British Medical Association to government under the former National Health Insurance scheme, the committee was never utilised. Committee B was concerned with hospital medical staffs. The Joint Consultants' Committee, set up for the purpose, soon became the most powerful force on the staff side. The employers, for their part, were represented by persons from the Regional Hospital Boards and the Ministry of Health. Committee C was concerned with medical men in the public health sector particularly those employed in the area health authorities (local authorities).

The machinery of negotiation soon proved a disappointment to doctors and others who were working for the National Health Service. Several claims for additional pay by various groups of employees were offered and rejected in the first two years. This was due not only to the national economic crisis but also to the fact that the estimated costs of the service were soon exceeded. In 1951 it was apparent to the

219

profession that 'being tied to a politically dependent service . . . the Ministry of Health as the employer and source of income could not by itself commit government funds in addition to those already granted for the National Health Service by the Treasury' (Stevens 1966:130). It was in this context that general practitioners submitted claims for increases in remuneration and for changes in the mode of its calculation. There was no desire to change from a system of payment by capitation fee as such. But two ways of calculating remuneration from this base were open. Estimates could be prepared (in so far as this was realistically possible) to estimate what doctors would earn on the open market, i.e. a hypothetical situation in which they would be wholly dependent on private practice. Alternatively an agreed fee *per annum* for each patient on a doctor's list, could be used as a basis for calculating each practitioner's income. A development of this second mode of calculation would be to establish an income agreed to be appropriate for the average general practitioner and work backwards to a capitation fee which would meet this level. As Stevens points out the first method suits the profession when the population is rising faster than the growth in the number of doctors. (More patients are being registered per doctor and income thus increases.) The second method benefits the profession when the number of doctors in practice is rising faster than the growth in population. At the start of the National Health Service this first method was adopted but quickly ran into criticism from practising doctors. 'Despite their desire for independence, they were not in favor of the all-out competition implied in this method' (1966:131). Fears were expressed that the medical schools were producing an oversupply of new doctors and that the incomes of established practitioners were threatened. The Ministry naturally favoured the *status quo* which was obviously most likely to hold down the cost of the service.

Negotiations on this issue reached an impasse and the matter was put to arbitration (1951). The arbitrator chosen was Mr Justice Danckwerts. The doctors found the Danckwerts' proposals very favourable, especially as they were promptly conceded by the government. There was to be a nationally agreed income for the average doctor and thus the size of the 'pool' for doctors' remuneration would rise as the number of doctors practising increased. Previously general practitioners had obtained a net average income in 1948, which was sixty per cent above the level recommended by Spens. This 'betterment' factor was now raised to one hundred per cent. The average general practitioner's salary (1951) rose to £2,222 (net) though this figure included all the factors contributing to this from whatever source. The 'central pool' had to be increased to cover the cost of these factors. Another feature favourable to general practitioners was also introduced, namely, special 'loadings' to encourage smaller sizes of doctors' lists.

By this process the capitation fee became a mere artefact. Was it now the case that doctors had become 'salaried' *de facto?* If so might it not have been simpler to acknowledge this by introducing a salaried service? General practitioners remained adamant that the capitation fee suited them and they have continued so to do. This 'indirect method of payment . . . was hallowed by GPs as a symbol of their freedom from bureaucracy' (Stevens 1966:133). It has certainly been no disadvantage to either branch of the medical profession to retain different mechanisms for negotiation. They have been able to play leapfrog for all it is worth. After the general practitioners' success in the Danckwerts award the consultants were soon ready with a new pay claim. They based themselves on the Spens criteria, these reflected income levels obtaining prior to 1939. Used in the 1950s they gave the medical profession an advantage over the other professions because professional incomes had been rising more slowly than the average. Differentials between the professions generally and other occupations were now less than before the war. In the event the gap between consultants and general practitioners was also narrowed.

With the Danckwerts award the general practitioners had scored a notable success. Parliament was forced to cover the award through the mechanism of supplementary estimates. The profession and the Ministry of Health seemed satisfied with the use of an 'impartial' outsider to arbitrate. Nevertheless the government was soon disappointed that the settlement with the profession did not last longer. By 1956 a further conflict on the subject of remuneration once again produced deadlock. On this occasion the committees representing general practitioners and consultants (General Medical Services Committee) and (Joint Consultants Committee) elected a combined team to meet the Ministry. The Whitley machinery was circumvented. Indeed its committees were never again to play more than a minor role. They were henceforth concerned only with the detailed application of income scales after any major settlement. The claim submitted was for twenty-four per cent due, it was argued, because of increases in the cost of living since the last award. The dentists too were solidly ranged alongside the medical profession. This was a difficult situation for the government as arbitration had proved such a temporary solution. This time a Royal Commission was appointed (1957). In an interim settlement both branches of the medical profession received an increase of five per cent, as did the dentists.

There was a suspicion in the profession that the government was using the device of a Royal Commission in order to delay a settlement. The government announcement of the Royal Commission thus did nothing to allay the widespread resentment felt by the doctors. The British Medical Association plan was to ask general practitioners to write letters of resignation. These would then be held centrally by the Association as a means of threatening mass withdrawal by doctors from the National Health Service, unless a favourable settlement was speedily reached. There was also to be no co-operation with the Commission. This policy was undermined by the activities of the consultants in the person of Sir Russell Brain who was chairman of the Joint Negotiating Committee. Moving, as he did, in elite circles, he was able to obtain certain assurances from Sir Harry Pilkington who was chairman of the Royal Commission and from the Prime Minister. The move forced the British Medical Association to reverse its policy of non-co-operation and it was made to look somewhat foolish by the action of the consultants.

The report of the Royal Commission (Pilkington 1960) established that doctors were already doing well financially. After making a series of comparisons with other professions including lawyers, architects, accountants, university teachers and graduates in industry, it demonstrated that in the years 1955-6 the career earnings of consultants were higher than those for any other profession. Taking the median income of professional people in the thirty to sixty-five years age group it was clear that general medical and dental practitioners were second only to consultants in rank order of remuneration among professional occupations. Despite this evidence it was still the opinion of the Commission that medical incomes should be increased. The report was accepted in full by the government and an increase of twenty-one per cent was paid. As part of the package various other factors were included in the agreement concerning a variety of issues, for example, group practice loans. A difficulty which sprang from these detailed changes was that the calculation of general practitioners' incomes became, if anything, even more complex and thus less intelligible to the average general practitioner. Also, comparisons between present and past levels of income became increasingly inaccurate. In order to deal with the periodic review of medical incomes in the long term a small 'Standing Review Body' was set up which, in a formal sense, was outside the National Health Service. The British Medical Association had some reservations about this device because it smacked of the machinery used to determine the incomes of higher civil servants. Nevertheless 'the creation of review machinery could be seen as a successful attempt by the medical profession to overcome some of the penalties of being state servants . . . the Review Body removed from the Ministry's jurisdiction the vital but unpleasant decisions regarding the level of professional remuneration for the most powerful and important group in the health service' (Stevens 1966:137). In the light of the differences between general practitioners and consultants which had emerged in the negotiations it was significant that the Royal Commission had shrunk from the task of determining the appropriate relativities between the two branches. It was reported that in 1955-6 the median income of consultants was £3,130 and for general practitioners £2,160 *per annum.* In other words, general practitioners' earnings were about two-thirds those of consultants.

The success of the doctors in achieving higher levels of income relative to other professions and occupations during this period must to a great extent be attributed to the collective power of the British Medical Association and the Royal Colleges. While it is true that they were dealing with a comparatively weak Health Ministry they ultimately succeeded in the face of opposition from the Cabinet and the Treasury. Eckstein, who made a special study of the negotiations between the British Medical Association and the Ministry of Health concerning Spens and doctors' remuneration (between 1948 and 1951), called his chapter on the subject 'An Unsuccessful Negotiation' (Eckstein 1960:126-50). What he meant by this was *not* that the negotiations had been unsuccessful in producing what the doctors had desired by way of increased income, but rather that the negotiations were unsuccessful because they had deadlocked and an independent arbitrator, Justice Danckwerts, had had to be called in. In fact the British Medical Association had not only obtained a generous settlement from Danckwerts which 'completely vindicated the British Medical Association's interpretation of the Spens proposals' but in fact forced the government, when it agreed to arbitration, to accept that Spens and not the government's own 'economic policy should determine the remuneration of general practitioners in the Service' (1960:148). The real problem which Eckstein discerned was that negotiations were excessively long and produced a fair amount of bad feeling between the doctors and the Ministry. He points to the fact that the main stumbling block on the Ministry's side was the Treasury. Its role was imperceptible at first but increasingly Treasury arguments were stated by the Ministry of Health. The impasse was finalised by the Treasury's decision to put an absolute limit on National Health Service expenditure. On the other hand, the British Medical Association was under great pressure to achieve substantial increases in pay but in spite of its tough gestures could not, in all probability, have produced an effective strike against the service. 'Its rank and file was far too apathetic, too hostile to trade union tactics, and too much afflicted by internal divisions' to act cohesively (1960:150). Eckstein suggests that these factors would generate similar tensions in future negotiations concerning general practitioner remuneration – indeed they have done so with a vengeance. Although Eckstein does not say so, it is a corollary to his analysis that the same problem could face hospital doctors and, as we shall see, the breakdown in negotiations in 1974 and the consultants work-to-rule in 1975 demonstrate the truth of this point.

Writing in 1966 Forsyth said 'although family doctors represent a small minority of those engaged in the provision of health services – about 23,000 out of nearly half a million National Health Service staff – the question of their pay has dominated the National Health Service from its inception' (Forsyth 1966:10). He pointed out that no mere adjustment of pay, 'however substantial, can cure the deep malaise affecting general practice'. He suggested that the struggle between the specialist and the general practitioner, which predated the National Health Service, produced 'as severe a crisis for the British Medical Association as for the government'. For example, the negotiations in 1965 which led to an offer of fourteen per cent by the independent Review Body was the subject of dissatisfaction in 'one of the best paid occupations'. The general practitioners made the provision of clerical help a cardinal point in their negotiations.

> 'The Review Body awarded an interim £5½ million, geared to hiring ancillary staff. Not good enough. The GPs did not, after all, want the money tied in the way they had implied. The Review Body untied the strings, but the doctors' fury seemed to mount with each concession. Now, it appeared, that the grievance was not just the amount of pay but the method of deriving it, although it was the method insisted on by the doctors themselves at the start of the NHS' (1966:10).

The general practitioners had obtained under the National Health Service all the advantages of a salaried health service and none of its drawbacks.

It appeared that one of the chief reasons for the anger of the general practitioners was that whereas under the old national health insurance scheme they had an exclusive relationship with the state, and the British Medical Association was able single-mindedly to represent their interests, under the National Health Service they were constrained to share this relationship with the hospital doctors and the specialists. They felt, probably rightly, that this had worked to their disadvantage and moreover that the British Medical Association, in trying to represent specialists' interests, was failing to serve the general practitioners in negotiations *vis-à-vis* the state with the single-mindedness characteristic of its endeavours before the inception of the National Health Service. It also follows that in so far as the British Medical Association was representing the interest of general practitioners it was failing adequately to represent the specialists. This view increasingly led the latter to seek representation through machinery outside the British Medical Association and was eventually to lead to a dramatic decline in the number of specialists remaining in membership of the Association. In regard to the family doctors' discontent, Forsyth suggests that no reform of the National Health Service is likely to assuage it, and the same could subsequently be said of the specialists. Forsyth is probably correct when he says that only a change in the structure of the medical profession itself is likely to overcome this endemic problem which has been inherited from the past.

One sensitive area for the profession, whether for general practitioners or hospital doctors, has been the question of the supply of medical man-power. We have presented evidence in earlier Chapters to the effect that the forerunners of a united medical profession, the apothecaries, surgeons and physicians were all concerned about the size

224

of the profession and about competition. If there was an issue which consistently evoked general agreement it was the question of unqualified practice. In the twentieth century, when the threat from the unqualified had been brought under control, there was a tendency to consider other aspects of the supply and demand for medical services. We have already noted that the function of professional ethics has been to moderate competition between practitioners. Schedules of fees, or other devices for payment, were introduced which prohibited undercutting. The ban on advertising was a device to enforce this objective. Under National Health Insurance and the National Health Service the general practitioners continued to use their collective power to raise their levels of income through improvements in capitation fees and they endeavoured to achieve for each doctor a predictable income. The hospital doctors were concerned to raise salaries through negotiation with the state. A vital basis for these tactics was the effort to control the supply of new doctors coming into the profession. Under the National Health Service the government 'may be willing to spend a certain amount of money for medical services; but the profession, by influencing the output of doctors, may be able to determine the number of doctors among whom the money shall be shared' (Stevens 1966:243). The *Lancet* was quite frank about this. It asked, to what number of doctors is the nation 'willing to offer the kind of livelihood and conditions of work which professional people consider necessary' (*Lancet* 1957:1043).

Thus, questions of professional status, expectations and style of life have been as important as are sheer economic considerations. The profession has always been conscious of the need to control the numbers of doctors coming into the profession, though there have been variations at different times in the extent to which this issue was the primary focus of professional concern and debate. As Stevens says 'it follows that the profession itself has some responsibility, however informally exerted, for the total number of doctors at a given point in time' (Stevens 1966:243).

It is true that in 1948 the government assumed responsibility for a comprehensive health service, and thus for the supply of a sufficient number of doctors. Unfortunately there were no available criteria for assessing how many doctors of what kinds would constitute a sufficient number. Or rather, such standards as there were had emerged from the past history of the profession. Sizes of doctors' lists gave an indication of requirements. These were measured both by the maximum size permitted and by the average. The other measure arose from the classification of underdoctored and overdoctored areas by the Medical Practices Committee. There were changes from time to time in informed opinion as to the adequacy or otherwise of medical manpower, but in the main it was opinion arising in the profession which counted. The Ministry shrank from planning manpower needs.

An early attempt to suggest ideal ratios in regard to consultants was put forward in a circular (1948) but in the event, the money was not forthcoming 'to pay this number at the agreed salary scales and the circular was quietly forgotten; the choice seemed to be between a limited number of well-paid doctors and a large number of doctors with smaller incomes' (1966:243). In 1957 the *Lancet* asserted that 'from the public as well as from the professional standpoint an excess of doctors would be a bad thing' (*Lancet* 1957:1043). The Ministry was ready to leave the question of medical manpower to the profession. One senior administrator from the Ministry articulated this attitude when he said that it would be 'presumptuous' if a 'lay civil servant was too dogmatic'.

The views of the profession seemed at first sight to be contradictory. For example, in the mid-1950s it was argued both that too many doctors were being trained and that there were insufficient doctors to fulfil the requirements of a comprehensive National Health Service. In fact the contradiction was about whether there should be more doctors who in the actual circumstances of the day — as opposed to some ideal world — would be likely to be less well paid; or whether a tight rein should be put on recruitment to the profession in order to secure the maintenance of remuneration or its improvement for those already in practice. Thus the medical manpower situation depended on the willingness of the country to provide more money for the National Health Service, and also on the outcome of doctors demands for increased remuneration.

In 1955 a Committee was appointed by the Ministry of Health to estimate, on a long-term basis, and with due regard to all relevant considerations, the number of medical practitioners likely to be engaged in all branches of the profession in the future and the consequential intake of medical students required (Ministry of Health 1957). The Committee was made up of seven members of the medical profession to four lay men (who included its chairman, Sir Henry Willink, a former Conservative Minister of Health). It seems to have been receptive to the doctors' view that too many doctors were being produced. There was some appreciable evidence that demand was falling due to Britain's withdrawal from the Empire and the planned run-down in the size of the Armed Forces. The birth rate appeared to have levelled off and the age structure of the profession was now weighted at the younger end. On balance the Committee recommended a cut of ten per cent in the intake of medical students.

In the event the report was quickly rendered obsolete. The fast growing hospital sector was soon suffering from a shortage of junior doctors. 'If both income and numbers could rise together, the professional demands for additional staff would grow in concert.' By 1961 the Platt report was drawing attention to a shortage of consultants whereas only a few years before there was said to be a surplus of senior registrars (Ministry of Health 1961).

In the light of this new information the Minister, now Mr Enoch Powell, agreed that the intake of medical students should be increased by ten per cent *above* the Willink level. After consultation with the University Grants Committee it was decided that the increase could be accommodated in existing university medical schools. It was obvious, though, that this increase could not materialise immediately. The shortage of doctors became apparent as the two branches of the profession began competing for recruits. The Robbins Report was concerned mainly with general student demand for places in higher education and virtually ignored medical education as such. It certainly did not look at the problem from the point of view of the requirements of the National Health Service (Report of the Committee on Higher Education 1963).

The problem of the supply of doctors was again raised in the Todd report which recommended the foundation of some new medical schools and an increase in the intake of students to medical education. Projections of the likely number of doctors required in future years were also made and it was stated that the country faced a serious shortage of doctors both now and in the years to come (Royal Commission on Medical Education 1968). Among the members of the Commission was Professor R.M. Titmuss who had long been a distinguished student of the policies and practices of the health service and a critic of administrative weaknesses. He was well aware of the impediments to the implementation of Bevan's original conception of a socially just health service, including those which arose from the structure and organisation of the medical profession itself. Undoubtedly it was he who encouraged the Commission to exceed its specific terms of reference and to investigate and report on such matters as the provision of medical manpower and the related problem of medical migration.

In the early 1960s a controversy arose over the question of the emigration of doctors, particularly to the USA and Canada. In part this issue came into focus because of the blocked career opportunities for registrars in the hospital service, but it was also put by those, (sometimes the same people), who argued that doctors were seeking to escape from a state-funded and administered National Health Service in Britain and taking the opportunity to seek their fortunes in the private sector arrangements still obtaining in North America. Abel-Smith, then a colleague of Titmuss, had challenged the statistical evidence of those who claimed that emigration of British doctors was high and increasing. The Royal Commission concluded that 'past movements have been erratic and have had many causes [but] the evidence does not suggest that over a long period Britain will experience a heavy net loss of doctors' (1968:146).

The Commission also noted the increase in the numbers of immigrant

227

doctors, particularly those coming from the developing countries, and acknowledged that more of them were settling here than had previously been recorded. While it was conceded that a duty existed to continue offering training facilities in our hospitals for overseas doctors, the report stated that 'the current excessive reliance on the services provided by young doctors from overseas was bad for them and for their countries, and was tending to distort the staffing pattern of British hospitals' (1968:129). The dearth of British-born doctors and the entry into practice of immigrant doctors has become cumulatively more marked since 1968. In his annual report (1974) Dr. Yellowlees, the chief medical officer at the Department of Health and Social Security, stated that the country's reliance on doctors born overseas was proportionately and numerically greater than ever. On the 1 October 1973, some 16.5 per cent of unrestricted principals in general practice were born overseas. In the hospital service, 9,745 of the 28,074 doctors, other than clinical assistants, came from overseas, 725 more than in the previous year. Thus about thirty-five per cent of hospital doctors (other than clinical assistants) came from overseas (Yellowlees 1974).

The shortage of British-born doctors entering the National Health Service might be assumed by the public to derive from a reluctance of suitably qualified young people to enter medicine as a career. Certainly the medical negotiators concerned with raising the level of medical remuneration in the 1950s were inclined to use the argument that increased income for doctors is a vital incentive to attract sufficient suitable candidates into the profession. In fact, however, well qualified young people apply in large numbers for admission to medical schools and are also rejected in large numbers. In recent years medicine has been the most popular subject to study at university, if the ratio of applicants to places is taken to be the appropriate measure.

The medical profession is now complaining, with increasing bitterness, about the number of immigrant doctors currently in practice in Britain. There is a tendency to blame this situation on the National Health Service. In one sense this is justifiable if we recognise that the state, in 1948, accepted a responsibility to provide an adequate health service and hence by implication, an adequate supply of doctors. Some have argued that the state has been too weak and too respectful of the established autonomy of the institutions and organisations of the profession. Because the state has granted a high degree of autonomy to the medical profession, then the profession itself has a responsibility to discharge its duty to society and not to restrict unduly the supply of trained doctors. In 1957 the Willink Committee, composed largely of medical men, recommended as we have seen a cut in the number of doctors in training by ten per cent, yet the government established the Committee because of a widespread feeling that the supply of doctors was insufficient. The outcome of the Todd Report in increasing the number of practising doctors will take some years to become effective.

The supply of home-trained doctors will begin to make a considerable impact from about 1980. This delay is due to the time-lag resulting from the long training at present required of doctors and the length of time it takes to build new medical schools.

The question remains, to what extent was there some deliberate restriction by the medical authorities of the numbers of medical students in training and how far was this due to the traditional fear among doctors of 'over supply'. Was there also a fear of the damage 'over supply' might do to levels of medical income, especially the competitive private market? Was there a fear that a rapid increase in the supply of indigenous doctors would affect adversely the negotiating position of the profession in the National Health Service? On the other hand, is this an overdramatic interpretation? Should we therefore accept the plausible arguments for a reduced supply of home-trained doctors advanced by the Willink Committee and concede that they were reasonable in the circumstances? Was the Committee therefore uninfluenced by considerations of 'over supply'? Whatever the answer to these questions, and it is difficult at the present time to gauge precisely what these might be, the effect has been that, by any of the agreed criteria currently in use, there has been a shortage of home-trained doctors and that the shortfall has had to be made up by immigration of doctors from developing countries. It is evident that compared, for example, with school teaching, where the responsibility for making projections of future teacher-supply (and planning for it) lies with the Department of Education and Science, medical manpower has remained very much in the control of the medical profession. If the profession complains, as it does, about a shortage of doctors and about excessive hours of work, then this arises to a considerable extent from the policies in regard to recruitment and organisation which the profession itself has pursued over the years. It must also be seen in the light of changes in the relationship between the volume and type of work undertaken in general practice compared with the hospital.

It was feared by some doctors that the introduction of free access to the general practitioner under the National Health Service, the cost being borne by the service, would tend to increase the number of 'unnecessary' or 'trivial' consultations by members of the public. The general practitioner has accommodated to this threat by making himself less directly accessible. John Rowan Wilson commenting in 1973 wrote, 'wherever one goes one hears the same complaint, reflected in a spate of articles in the newspapers, that the so-called family doctor is becoming inaccessible. He is walling himself in behind a fortified screen of wives, secretaries, receptionists, unlisted numbers and answering services' (Rowan Wilson 1973:121). The commercially organised deputising service has become increasingly important to the general practitioners since the early 1960s. Such organisations will send another doctor in place of the general practitioner to a patient about whom the deputy

229

knows nothing, in an area which is also likely to be unknown to him. Liberated from the more intense competition of the old-style medical market-place and adopting the changing attitudes of society concerning the 'right' to defined periods of uninterrupted and predictable freedom from work, he will no longer tolerate the possiblity of being badgered at any time of the day or night by his patients. The doctor was at the beck and call of his private patients in the pre-National Health Service era and few of his panel patients would have had a telephone at home. The walk to a telephone box was a kind of deterrent.

The doctors who man the deputising services are often those who are engaged in the statutory one-year post qualification experience in hospital. Many will themselves enter general practice, but others are junior hospital doctors. These have been regarded in recent years as the most put-upon members of the profession though, as we have seen, the problem of the junior hospital doctor, hoping eventually to become a consultant, is as old and intractable as the modern hospital system itself and is integral to the existing structure of the profession. The juniors have long been poorly paid and have been willing also to be exploited by their seniors for the sake of a chance to achieve a consultancy themselves and eventually to become one of a small elite who have access to the most lucrative parts of the private medical market. Just how lucrative this private practice is for doctors who participate in it remains difficult to quantify because evidence is scanty (Department of Health and Social Security 1973).

Private practice was accommodated by the health service from its inception in 1948. Private beds in National Health Service hospitals were available for consultants' private patients and were integral to the continuance of private medicine for twenty-six years during a time when the hospital was becoming more central to medicine than it had ever been before. The prevalent view in 1948 was that the introduction of the Health Service would be likely to strangle the private market for medical care which would wither and die. Even those who regarded themselves as optimists thought that private medicine would exist only as a small residue used exclusively by the rich. The big growth in subscriptions to British United Provident Association during the 1960s was not anticipated. By 1973 it had eighty per cent of the private medical insurance market comprising some 833,000 subscribers paying £28 million in premiums (*Sunday Times,* 12 January 1975:53).

The general practitioner has relatively little access to the private medical market which in the main is concerned with the expensive hospital and specialist services. Most general practitioners have next to no private practice at all and only a small proportion engage in nothing else, some two to three per cent or about 600 in all, have nothing but private patients 'most of them are in London, and to the naked eye many of them look like consultants — these are the consultoids who cluster around Harley Street' (Ferris 1965:135). One of the often remarked changes between general practice and the hospital is the extent to which the general practitioner has been increasingly inclined to send his patients on to the hospital for further tests or for a specialist opinion. The general practitioner still deals with the bulk of everyday cases of illness but increasingly he has been regarded as the signpost to the hospital. His tendency to utilise hospital services more fully has added to the pressure on specialist hospital doctors and technical services. This is due partly to the greater potency of scientific medicine and medical specialisation but also to the fact that the modern general practitioner is no longer in such intense competition with the hospital as he used to be in the past, when the out-patient department provided a free service with open access whereas payment of a fee or subscription was required for a consultation with a general practitioner.

The effect on the hospitals of the increased demand, due to referrals from general practitioners, has been to produce greater pressure of work. Consultants must often see very large numbers of patients in a given time and complain that they are not able to offer the personal touch and the humane approach which they would wish. Pressure of work is even greater on the junior hospital doctors and during the 1960s there was an increasing restiveness amongst them which was manifested in the formation of new ginger groups. In particular, some junior hospital doctors felt that existing doctors' associations, such as the British Medical Association, were doing too little to represent their specific interests and were more concerned either with general practitioners and/or with established consultants. The creation of the Junior Hospital Doctors' Association marked an important step in the political self-consciousness and independence of the junior hospital doctors. There was a new determination to be recognised as a separate and permanent interest within the profession. Dr Francis Pigott, chairman of the Junior Hospital Doctors' Association, made it clear that junior hospital doctors were working excessive hours — eighty-five hours a week was mentioned. He noted that there was an element of blackmail in the relationship between the consultant and the junior hospital doctors because the latter was hoping to achieve a consultant's rank. Junior hospital doctors were too few for public need and expectations. Doctors in these training posts carried consultant responsibilities. In the existing situation, he asserted, the doctors' efficiency was impaired by fatigue. He was either working or on call, without adequate rest, and his private life was disrupted.

We should be careful to distinguish between the causes of the present predicament facing the junior hospital doctor which arise from the organisation of the National Health Service and those which derive from the structure of the medical profession itself, although the two are in practice closely related. We have seen that the problem of the exploited or disaffected junior was already very present in the nineteenth century and therefore cannot be blamed in origin on the National Health

Service. In so far as the health service administration was adapted to the existing structure and interests of the medical profession, it too may be blamed for the inadequacies and lack of proper career structure for the junior hospital doctor. Ferris tells us that 'among the 13,000 or 14,000 junior hospital staff is to be found the most underprivileged, underpaid, pushed-about and generally sat-upon section of the profession' (Ferris 1965:54). Traditionally junior staff have been very apathetic, and for good reason. In London, as elsewhere, 'a few hundred consultants hold the strings: they do much of the examining, they control or influence hospital appointments, and their advocacy, either as official referees or as private backers is eagerly sought by the ambitious student and young doctor' (1965:53). To achieve a consultancy 'doctors commonly wait five, ten, or even twenty years, during which time they must watch their tongue, do their work, pass exams and generally convince their elders that they are suitable candidates for glory' (Ferris 1965:44). In the context of the health service the consultant may look after 'as many as forty in-patients, using them (and the out-patients he sees at hospital clinics) to instruct students and junior doctors'. 'The saving of lives can be mixed up with the advancing of reputations; behind the white clothes and clean hands are all the postures of ambition' (1965:44-5).

The number of junior doctors has increased rapidly under the National Health Service, but as Ferris points out 'it has done this without paying fair salaries. It cheats registrars, and to a lesser extent housemen, on a massive scale, exploiting the fact that they are young, zealous and sometimes more dedicated than their seniors' (1964:54). It is important to notice that within the National Health Service good pay has gone to the well organised consultants and general practitioners. Those who are poorly organised or apathetic have not been spontaneously rewarded by a grateful Ministry of Health on behalf of the state. It has been possible for the medical profession to blame the National Health Service itself, and by implication state medicine, for the situation in which junior hospitals doctors find themselves, but the latter have often been willing to blame *only* the organisation of the health service rather than also identifying the role of the inherited structure and organisation of the profession of which they are members.

It has been argued by a number of writers, including Stevens, that the impact of science and technology in medicine is having a fragmenting effect upon the once homogeneous consultants through the growth of an increasing number of medical specialities. Ferris too, is aware of the impact of the new technologies on medical practice and potentially on the solidarity and unity of the profession. Nevertheless, he provides evidence that

'the London teaching hospitals . . . are still the seats of power. The London system is still rooted in [the] archaic individualism of the part-time gentleman. A registrar may try to be a scientist, but even when he succeeds in doing research and experimental work in wards and laboratories, his appointment as consultant, when he gets it, is unlikely to provide for anything beyond the routine of seeing patients. As a junior he is expected to improve his chances with an impressive list of publications, but to want to go on doing research, once he becomes a consultant is regarded as eccentric' (Ferris 1965:65).

The part-time consultancy is still regarded as the top of the profession combining National Health Service work and private practice. Full-time academic medical research paradoxically is less secure than part-time consultancy and also lacks prestige. Contracts among senior researchers may be for five years and among younger research doctors, the temporary job lasting one, two, or three years is normal (1965:80-81). Having taken a research job or a full-time clinical post the doctor may find that his bridges back to a niche in private practice have been burnt.

It was reported in 1975 that 'nearly half of all consultant doctors are full-timers contracting to work eleven 3½-hour sessions weekly. The great majority of part-timers contract to do nine sessions and are allowed private practice' (*The Times*, 16 January 1975). There is some controversy over the extent to which the health service is exploited by half-time doctors who do not take a joint share of the work. For example, Pappworth, author of the article in *The Times*, argues that although many consultants work additional hours in order to meet the heavy demands arising in the National Health Service and have a strong case for some form of overtime payments, he also claims that 'in spite of vehement denials, there is no doubt that some — possibly a substantial number, especially in the London area — do far less work than they are paid for. Some of the worst offenders are those who have developed large private consultant practices in addition to their National Health Service duties'. Following the publication of this article in *The Times* strong denials appeared in the letter columns stating that while every profession had its black sheep, the vast majority of consultants were not only conscientiously carrying out their duties, in terms of the contract, but were voluntarily doing overtime on a massive scale without being paid for it. On the other hand, a survey carried out by the Junior Hospital Doctors' Association showed, according to Pappworth, 'that over an eighteen-month period in one typical hospital region some forty per cent of all surgical emergencies and eighty per cent of the anaesthetics for them were dealt with by juniors'. While it is true that in this context the word 'junior' includes very experienced registrars, the system does allow the opportunity for consultants to delegate work in ways which would enable them to devote more time to private practice and to minimise the inconvenient demands which must inevitably arise from medical emergencies. Not only clinical work but teaching to medical students may also be delegated in this way. It is difficult to estimate the extent to which the present system is abused by part-time consultants. Indeed the extent of consultant dominance in the National Health Service has precluded the possibility of either independent researchers or the administrators of the health service making an unbiased inquiry. As Pappworth says 'the profession has done nothing to expose and prevent this abuse, [assuming it exists] and would object strongly to any official inspection such as schoolteachers have' (*The Times,* 16 January 1975).

From the point of view of the medical profession the National Health Service represents a partnership between the profession and the state and in 1948 a Labour government, in order to get the service started, agreed to acquiesce in many of the doctors' demands. In a number of important respects, some of which have already been noted, the administrative structure and organisation of the health service was built around the interests of the medical profession and its formation was guaranteed to produce a minimum disturbance to the existing structure and organisation of the profession itself

> 'The result was that the three branches of the service came under separate administration. This was not merely offensive to the bureaucratic mind: it was contrary to the best interests of the patient. For most of the time he would be under the care of his GP, but when he went to hospital for treatment or diagnosis there would be less continuity of care than there should be or generally had been' (*The Times,* 25 April 1974:1).

It seemed that relationships between the hospital doctor and the general practitioner were more distant and that contact was insufficiently close with community health and welfare services under the local authority. Concern with this question was expressed in a minority report from the Guillebaud Committee (1956) which recommended a unified service under the control of the local authorities. The Medical Services Review Committee, under the chairmanship of Sir Arthur Porritt proposed that administrative unification should be achieved under area health boards. 'By 1968 this had become the conventional wisdom, and the Labour Government produced the first of its two Green Papers as to how it should be done.' With the return of a Conservative government a Consultative Document and a White Paper were produced which finally led to the introduction of a Bill which became law on 1 April 1974.

Perhaps the most surprising thing about the reform of the National Health Service in 1974 was the lack of public discussion and debate. Many of those working in the National Health Service, apart from people directly concerned with the reorganisation, appear to be unaware that it was happening and were uncertain of its consequences. There was nothing like the violent public controversy which preceded the introduction of the National Health Service itself. One reason for this has been that the detailed discussions about reorganisation did not appear to challenge the established doctrine of successive governments that 'no service could be run satisfactorily if the professional staff [the doctors] were antagonized too deeply' (*The Times*, 25 April 1974:1). Thus the question under whose control the reorganised health service should be, boiled down to a matter of administrative reorganisation; this was after all the era of managerialism. Improvements in management would, it was hoped, create a better and more coherent service, but the medical associations were determined that such administrative reforms should once again be adapted to the structure and interests of the profession.

> 'What has now been adopted is a three-tier structure, with regional health authorities that will have largely a strategic planning role, with responsibility for appointing most members of the area health authorities below them and monitoring their performance. Each area will be split into so many districts which will be run by district management teams composed of the community physician, nursing and finance officers, administrators and two elected doctors — one a consultant, the other a GP' (*The Times*, 25 April 1974:1).

This complex structure has been criticised on several grounds but the Labour government, which was returned to power in 1974, regarded the organisation as insufficiently democratic. It is true that the Act specified certain bodies which must be consulted before appointments are made by the Secretary of State to the regional authorities. These include the relevant local authorities, trade unions and professional associations. At the district level 'management is in the hands of the professional staff, without any outside presence; but for each district there is a community health council which is supposed to represent the interests of the public' (*The Times*, 25 April 1974:1). Many commentators have regarded the latter as likely to be rather weak in the context of the organisation as a whole. Although it might have been more democratic to place the National Health Service under the local authorities, and this would probably have established more effective co-ordination between the health and welfare functions which are still separated, yet increased local authority representation may well enhance the democratic element at both regional and area level. 'But it would be futile to pretend that a large quota of local authority members can ever provide the same degree of democratic control as putting the whole service under local government.' Interestingly, the medical officer of health and his staff have been removed from local authority control under the new dispensation and incorporated in the National Health Service. Similarly, medical social workers who were hitherto in the control of the National Health Service have, at the insistence of the social work profession, been passed over to the control of the Social Services. The withdrawal of the last doctors from the orbit of local authority control marks the complete achievement of an objective which has for more than sixty years been pursued by the medical profession.

The formation of the Patients' Association and its increasing influence during the 1960s, from small beginnings, marks a noticeable increase in consumer interest in relation to medical matters and to the quality of service provided under the national health scheme. Governments may wish to strengthen the community health councils to increase the influence of the consumer interest. Clearly, if these councils are to be effective, then sufficiently spirited staff must be recruited to serve on them. It was with this in mind that the Labour government decided to withdraw their earlier suggestion by which it had been intended to fill these positions on the councils from among already retired but experienced National Health Service administrators. The other danger to be avoided is that of allowing councils to be drawn into the managerial establishment of the National Health Service. Another aspect of democracy, which the government may have in mind, is to make the service more responsive to those who work in it, especially those other than the medical profession who staff the service and who are not yet officially represented. Whether these steps will lead to better care of the patient can certainly not be taken for granted.

An important criticism which has been made of the reformed structure is that it has focussed too much on managerial efficiency, a term which has a profoundly adverse negative effect on doctors. On the one hand, the government clearly wishes to make sure that the £3,000 million a year spent on the health service is efficiently spent; on the other, the doctors fear that professional dominance will be weakened and that they will become subordinated to a management system over which they have little control. In *The Times'* opinion, the National Health Service does not have a history of strong administration and 'the real problem about managerial efficiency in the new service is that despite all the talk there is likely to be too little of it'.

'The theory of integration has been applied only in part. General practitioners will retain their treasured status as independent contractors under family practitioner committees which are in effect the old executive councils in modern dress' (*The Times*, 25 April 1974:1). In this sense it can be argued that the major effects of reform will be on the hospital service and the extent of the improvement in the relationship between the general practitioner and the hospital service remains problematic. The test of this will be the extent to which the district management teams will be able to achieve integration. There is not much sign at the moment that the average doctor is thinking in terms of integration. Family doctors are now able to elect their representatives into positions of managerial responsibility in the district teams and thus have more opportunity to influence day-to-day management than if they were merely in an advisory role. Such representatives will be paid £700 per annum which is intended to be some compensation for the time lost from general practice. 'The twin dangers of this exercise in syndicalism are that clinical practice will suffer without the elected representatives being able to devote enough time to management, and that they may be too timorous towards the prejudices of their electors – even when they do not actively share those prejudices' (*The Times*, 25 April 1974:1).

The lack of turmoil or controversy which accompanied the inception of the reformed National Health Service in April 1974 appeared to herald an era of renewed dominance on the part of the medical profession. The appearance belied a reality which was soon to indicate that the National Health Service was in a state of crisis. The crisis, as it unfolded, proved to contain an explicit challenge to the legitimacy of the existing role of the medical profession, both within the service, and in society generally. 1974 will be remembered as the year in which unionism and professionalism, the representative institutions of the working class and the successful middle class clashed within the arena of the National Health Service, or more specifically within the hospital service.

The summer of 1974 was a time when rapid inflation, then due mainly to the rise of world commodity prices (particularly oil), was having a drastic effect on the financing of the National Health Service and on the pay-levels of those employed within it. The return of the Labour government had not at once led to the disappearance of Phase III of the Conservative prices and incomes policy, but in anticipation of its end, the professions and unions engaged in the health service were not only making claims but pressing for their speedy satisfaction. Radiographers and technicians went on strike and doctors became concerned at the possibility of this action leading to the deaths of some patients. Eight big hospitals in the North-East were reported to have no X-ray services and the other forty-two in the region were restricted to emergency cover. Mr Essenhigh, a urologist at the Newcastle General, was reported as saying 'the radiographers have only a limited knowledge and probably do not understand the full consequences' (*The Times*, 14 August 1974:2). Nurses and midwives had put in a claim for thirty-eight per cent to the Halsbury Committee of Inquiry into nurses' pay, as well as demanding a cut in hours and the introduction of payment for overtime. Industrial action amongst hospital ancillary workers had become familiar during the previous year when there had been a strike lasting approximately six weeks. Increasingly the hospital was becoming the focus of union militancy, and the tradition among public service workers generally, and hospital workers in particular, namely, that the nature of their work precluded strike action, was further eroded. As a result of the six-week strike hospital waiting lists increased by 30,000 and admissions dropped by 91,000 in 1974. All those working within the National Health Service whether doctors, nurses or ancillary workers were agreed on one thing, that inflation was causing a deepening financial crisis from which the service could only escape by considerable additional funding from the government. Even the eleven Presidents of the Royal College, while explicitly stating they they dissociated themselves from the somewhat extreme view that the National Health Service was about to disintegrate, made a direct approach to Mrs Castle, the Minister of Health, and with a united voice pointed out the perilous state of the service. They affirmed that 'the Government has a duty to make it clear to the public what proportion of the national budget can be allocated to the service' (*Guardian*, 18 October 1974).

Disquiet among the general practitioners about the effects of Phase III of the prices and incomes policy was reflected in the fact that no less than 141 motions about remuneration were on the agenda at a conference of the British Medical Association's local medical committees which took place in June 1974. There was criticism of the delay in publishing the current report of the Review Body on Doctors' and Dentists' Remuneration. The expectation was that the recommendation would fall within the guidelines of Phase III and that general practitioners' incomes had fallen about eighteen per cent behind increases in salaries generally. At this stage there was a rejection of immediate action to call for doctors' resignations from the National Health Service but it was stated, after the ending of the statutory incomes policy in July, that doctors must decide how best to protect their standards of living. A new technique of industrial action was hinted at, but kept secret. It was stated that 'if reasoned argument failed then they [the doctors] would have to make the public realize the true cost, in present money values, of an effective level of medical care' (*The Times*, 13 June 1974:6).

Rumblings of discontent were heard from the general practitioners throughout the rest of the year, but the chief point of conflict came from an unexpected source, and focussed within the hospital service, on the fraught issue of private pay-beds. The Labour party had always contained a sizeable element of those who believed that Aneurin Bevan had never intended that private pay-beds should exist in the National Health Service but that he was forced to allow them as 'a part of the price that the various specialists within the medical profession exacted from him for their agreement to take part in Health Service'. The compromise was a wise one on Bevan's part because, as a result of it, he had 'the advantage of commanding the services of the most skilled and experienced members of a proudly independent, even prickly, profession'. However, 'this concession to the financial interests of one section of a profession has continued to rankle as a piece of private enterprise in the middle of an otherwise free, publicly-owned and administered and thus, in a sense, Socialist service' (*Observer* leader, 7 July 1974:8).

238

Reporting on the situation in July 1974 John Clare stated that until the action of Mrs Esther Brookstone, leader of the Charing Cross Hospital branch of the National Union of Public Employees, which withdrew services from thirty-one private patients, Labour Ministers did not believe that the government had any hope of phasing out pay-beds in the face of the implaccable opposition of the British Medical Association and the medical profession generally (*Observer,* 7 July 1974). The action, although quite clearly illegal, was seen by the consultants as successfully pre-empting the orderly negotiations in which they were already engaged on the phasing out of private patients. They believed that without this intervention they would have had every chance of retaining pay-beds, at least during the foreseeable future. As the *Sunday Times* put it,

> 'the underdog revolt against the privileged world of Floor 15 at Charing Cross Hospital was short, immediately effective and of immense significance for the future of British medicine . . . The hitherto unchallenged reign of the hospital consultants was shattered, only to be shakily restored by the intervention of a Secretary of State' (*Sunday Times,* 7 July 1974:4).

Leader writers in the major national newspapers unanimously condemned this illegal action and the *Observer's* response was typical when it stated that, while health service unions had every right to act as pressure groups on the issue, this was 'one more example of a trade union usurping the functions that belong to an elected Parliament and Government'. They concluded by saying that 'if we become a society in which every sectional interest tries to get its way by exploiting its nuisance value to the full, that will produce some grotesque results . . . such a society would be neither democratic nor socialist: it would be a form of brigandage' (*Observer,* 7 July 1974:8).

The action at Charing Cross Hospital was a result of a resolution which was passed *nem-con* at the National Union of Public Employees' Annual Conference in 1973 stating that private patients should be excluded from National Health Service hospitals. However, this local action took the union by surprise and caused some consternation, but eventually the union executive followed its rank and file. Part of the background to the situation was the rivalry between NUPE and the Confederation of Health Service Employees, the latter having waged a solitary campaign for nurses, derided for their pains by NUPE as 'amateur adventurers' seeking a bigger following among Britain's largely un-unionised 350,000 nurses. COHSE claimed the credit for the government pledge to grant the nurses an interim pay award if the Halsbury Enquiry was seriously delayed. COHSE had also run a campaign, in lower key, against private practice in the health service so NUPE was ready enough to try and exploit this issue. Mrs Castle, as Labour Minister, was in the unenviable position of believing that pay-beds should be phased out while having to condemn the illegality of direct action which soon spread to several other hospitals.

The doctors were not interested in the details of inter-union rivalry 'what was important to them was what they regarded as a cave-in to class warfare by the hospital authorities at Charing Cross and the weak reprimand to the union from Mrs Barbara Castle'. The grave difficulty for the doctors was that a joint working party had already been set up by the new Labour government under the chairmanship of Dr Owen, Under-Secretary of State for Health. The terms of reference linked hospital doctors' pay with the question of private practice. The doctors threatened militant action on the issue, and the threat was withdrawn only on the understanding that there would be no reduction in private beds at Charing Cross, or anywhere else, until the Owen working party had reported. Also that it would remain the policy of the government to permit pay-beds in health service hospitals and, moreover, no arbitrary reduction of pay-beds would be made. The British Medical Association and the government agreed to expedite the work of the Owen working party, both on the question of the consultant contract and on private practice. In the meeting of the British Medical Association with the government two representatives of the Hospital Consultants' and Specialists' Association, including their President, were present (*Sunday Times*, 7 July 1974).

By the end of September, before the Owen Committee had reported, Mrs Castle announced that the government intended to act on the matter within the present session of Parliament. The Owen Committee was said to be hopelessly split on the issues. A leader in *The Times* warned of the dangers of a clash between powerfully organised doctors and government, but thought that 'the profession would do itself incalculable harm in the eyes of the public if it endangered the whole basis of the NHS over a question in which self-interest is at least a substantial factor' (*The Times*, 4 November 1974).

The publication of the government's proposed new contract for National Health Service consultants was rejected by the profession on the grounds that it amounted to a full-time salaried service. The professional side of the Owen Committee was given a proposed new contract together with a time-table for phasing out most of the 5,000 National Health Service pay-beds within a year. The consultants thought the result would be a monopoly state hospital service within two or three years. Dr Derek Stevenson, secretary of the British Medical Association, said that 'since 1948 the profession has stood solidly behind the idea that doctors must not be compelled to take part in a whole-time service. What a doctor did in his spare time was his own concern' (*The Times*, 7 November 1974). The doctors objected particularly to the new concept of 'a full commitment allowance' which would intentionally create a disparity between rates of remuneration arising from National Health Service work as between part-time and full-time consultants. The new regulations proposed on pay-beds would also be likely to result in a rapid run-down from the existing levels of one or two per cent overall. Mrs Castle pointed out that forty-three per cent of consultants already work full-time for the National Health Service, and that if some consultants wish to work outside the National Health Service that is their privilege. There was no doubt, however, that the phasing out of pay-beds would restrict consultants' private practice.

Mrs Castle's statement about the phasing out of pay-beds was regarded by the profession as a pre-emption of the working party's finding on the issue. Dr Stevenson said 'the government has a lot to answer for by precipitating head-on confrontation while talks are still in progress' and he thought that the announcement had caused 'strongest resentment' among doctors (*The Times,* 4 November 1974). Mr Brownlow Martin, executive officer of the Hospital Consultants' and Specialists' Association which represents about 5,000 of the 12,000 consultants in Britain, said that 'feeling among his members was extremely high' and that while they were not likely to start any action at once they had contingency plans to do so. Either they might support British Medical Association action or take action of their own. Militancy among consultants was particularly strong in the North where most private patients were in health service hospitals because there were very few private nursing homes or hospitals. Thus, a consultant unable to use pay-beds in a National Health Service hospital could find it impossible to carry on private practice. It was for this reason that the consultants in the North decided not to wait for a decision from the British Medical Association in London, but to go it alone. A work-to-rule was started in the North-East region and it was thought that some four or five hundred of the 750 consultants in the area might be involved from 5 November 1974.

Feeling was now running high in the medical profession, and after personal criticism of Lord Halsbury, he resigned as chairman of the Review Body on Doctors' and Dentists' Remuneration which was considering an interim pay claim of eighteen per cent. The British Medical Association, while welcoming the resignation, said that most doctors, and certainly the BMA leadership, do not wish to lose the Review Body system (*The Times,* 13 November 1974:2). It was clear, however, that the Hospital Consultants' and Specialists' Association wanted to see the Review Body abolished. Mr John Riedel, secretary of the Association, said 'we want to discuss pay directly with the Department of Health' (*The Times,* 11 November 1974).

By the end of the year a warning was given by Mr Walpole Lewin, chairman of the Council of the British Medical Association that the dispute over the hospital consultants' contract may soon involve the whole medical profession. He said that 'we are fighting for the independence of the profession' (*The Times,* 31 December 1974). Just before Christmas the Owen working party talks finally broke down and shortly afterwards, in early January, most of the 12,000 hospital

241

consultants began to work to contract. The effect was not immediately apparent, but it was thought that as most consultants work fifty to sixty hours a week, well above the 31½ or 38½ hours for which they are contracted, patients were bound to be 'inconvenienced'. Dr McKim Thompson, secretary of the Junior Hospital Staff Group Council said that they would not fill in gaps that consultants had left. The British Medical Association's general medical services committee recorded its support for the consultants' stand and general practitioners working as part-time clinical assistants, of whom there are about 5,000, might well be involved (*The Times,* 31 December 1974). The work to contract was to last many weeks but action was limited to the consultants. The junior hospital doctors, up to and including senior registrars, were not directly involved. The threat of unified action by the whole profession seemed imminent in January 1975. When the Review Body rejected the doctors' interim pay demand of eighteen per cent, part of which was to be back-dated to April 1974, the possibility of surcharging National Health Service patients was discussed, but was judged to be illegal. It was thought, however, that a percentage of patients could be removed from doctors' lists as an act of protest. Dr Alexander, a member of the British Medical Association's general services committee, said that 'the Government has decreed that the BMA is a trade union. I feel that we can now use any method of industrial action we wish.' Dr Ball, another committee member said: 'I see any pay battle fought by the BMA as fundamentally on behalf of all the middle class of this country' (*Observer,* 5 January 1975:3). The Review Body found that family doctors had experienced a relative decline (*vis-à-vis* other professional groups) in their earnings of fifteen per cent since 1972, but it was felt that an interim award would break the 'Social Contract', which was Labour's replacement for the Conservative's prices and incomes policy. The doctors had already received an increase within Phase III and the fact that they had put in another claim, within a year, was one reason for the rejection of their claim.

In the event, the general practitioners were given assurances by Mrs Castle which led them to wait, if reluctantly, until April 1975 for their increases in remuneration. The implication was that these would be substantial. In their work to contract, the consultants found that for all practical purposes they were going it alone. Appeals for a direct meeting with the Prime Minister over the head of the Minister, Mrs Castle, were rebuffed and he gave her every support.

The question of pay-beds in National Health Service hospitals, plus the proposal to give consultants working full-time for the health service additional incentive remuneration, was felt by the consultants as a threat to make whole-time service so much more attractive that private practice would be seriously weakened. Dr Briggs, secretary of the militant Hospital Consultants' and Specialists' Association said 'private medicine is the yardstick by which we measure the health service'

(*Observer,* 5 January 1975:3). What is certainly germane is that part-time consultants, with their share in private practice, are a valuable measure against which the levels of remuneration of whole-time consultants may be assessed. It has been a useful lever in pay negotiations.

Another matter over which the consultants were greatly concerned was the system of merit awards. This system which goes back to the early days of the National Health Service was run by an advisory committee. At first Lord Moran, Sir Winston Churchill's doctor, was paid £3,000 a year to perform this function but subsequently the advisory committee have met in secret to disburse £10 million a year in merit payments. Part of Mrs Castle's plan was to correct the known imbalance between part-time consultants receiving these payments. About a third of all consultants receive a merit award ranging from the lowest level worth £1,506 *per annum* to £7,947 *per annum.* Under the existing system, part-timers were just as eligible as full-timers for this payment. Recently secrecy surrounding these awards has gradually been breached. Consultants at the Tavistock Clinic found that only one of them received a merit payment and it has become clear that some specialities such as psychiatry, geriatrics and anaesthetics have come off badly. The merit award system was designed to give the profession itself, rather than the National Health Service taken as an administrative organisation, the power to recognise the contribution of distinguished medical men within the whole professional field of medicine. It is possible to argue that the existing distribution of awards accurately reflects clinical distinction and that it is only to be expected that those practising in the teaching hospitals will be most favoured. In practice, however, the regional imbalance and the neglect of certain specialities has led the critics of the system to believe that it is less than impartial and secrecy exacerbates the feeling of the Medical Practitioners' Union that the 'merit award is a political weapon to keep people in line. Doctors won't speak out because they fear that they will be overlooked' (*Sunday Times,* 26 January 1975). The fact that Mrs Barbara Castle wished within the context of the proposed new contract to replace merit awards with payments which recognised special effort for the National Health Service, particularly where doctors worked under difficult conditions and with difficult patients, may seem to the outsider to be uncontentious but to the established organs of the profession it appears as yet another effort to undermine professional autonomy.

Another challenge to the established structure of the medical profession became apparent in 1972 two years before the clash between a Labour government and the consultants. As the *Spectator* put it

> 'the last entrenched stronghold of privilege, the very citadel of the Establishment, is under attack. This is the General Medical Council, the supreme disciplinary body of the profession.

Increasingly cries are heard, both young and old, claiming that it is old fashioned, arbitrary, undemocratic, expensive, and that something ought to be done about it' (Rowan Wilson, 24 June 1972:995).

The current reapparaisal of the role and structure of the General Medical Council has been, in part, an unintended consequence of inflation. Between 1858-1950 the General Medical Council was financed by an initial registration fee of £5 and no further payments were required from the registered doctor throughout his life. Subsequently the fee was raised several times but due to inflation the General Medical Council proposed in 1970 to introduce an annual retention fee of £2 which 'touched the doctors in a most delicate part of their anatomy' (Rowan Wilson, 24 June 1972:995). The medical protest which resulted raised the old question, which we have discussed earlier, of the elitist nature of the Council membership. The British Medical Association has always represented the conviction of the general practitioners about the lack of directly elected members from their own ranks. Equally, the junior hospital doctors made the same point but specifically argued for more representation for their own constituency. Changes were already being discussed in the General Medical Council's composition by a working party (under the chairmanship of Sir Brynmor Jones) the report of which suggested a widened membership, including five lay members, but 'the militants — who significantly carried with them the majority of delegates at this summer's [1972] annual representative meeting of the BMA — are not satisfied by these concessions'. Essentially they 'want to do more than first change the balance of power in the GMC' (Klein 1972:400). What was wanted, in their view, was a more radical reform of the General Medical Council's functions, particularly in the disciplinary machinery.

Public attention has always been focussed on the disciplinary function of the General Medical Council which gives the misleading impression through press reporting of cases that it is concerned almost exclusively with adultery and abortion. Klein and Shinebourne's analysis of disciplinary proceedings shows that this is something of a myth and that 'the picture is far more complex than this stereotype suggests'. The traditional phrase 'infamous conduct' has been replaced by the Medical Act, 1969, and it is now the statutory duty of the General Medical Council to deal with 'serious professional misconduct'. The process by which cases are filtered through to the General Medical Council is rather elaborate and very likely uncertain. The Council cannot act as a police force and seek out cases, nor was it intended to do so. It has no inspectorate as does the Pharmaceutical Society; it must rely on such outside sources as the police, who may report convictions of doctors in the Courts or upon reports from professional colleagues, executive councils, government departments, patients or their aggrieved friends or relatives. The penal cases committee, by virtue of its screening role, is perhaps more crucial than the disciplinary committee, which because of its public sittings, is more widely known. The majority of complaints are dismissed before they reach the disciplinary committee because they are judged not to raise any question of professional misconduct. There appears to have been a gradual change in the uses made of the disciplinary committee by the profession. Originally, after the 1858 Act, its principal purpose was to deal with quacks and to maintain the 'respectability' and standing of the profession in the era of stuffy Victorian sexual morality. Hence the reputation for being solely concerned with doctors' sexual misdemeanors. In the latter part of the nineteenth century the disciplinary machinery was used to regulate self-advertisement and competition within the profession but apart from the problems of the abortion business, this appears to be no longer such an important category in an era when quacks 'can no longer compete on price' and when the National Health Service has taken 'the pressure off doctors to compete for customers' (Klein 1972:401). There has been a growth in recent years in the proportion of cases connected with drug offences which have replaced drink as the single largest category coming before the General Medical Council. Most cases arise from prior convictions in a court of law and it is now the case that those arising from complaints by patients or other members of the profession are in a minority. 'The overall impression left by examining a long run of cases is that the disciplinary committee is very largely dealing with social casualties, the down-and-out fringe of the medical profession.' The myths about the General Medical Council cannot thus be substantiated, but a further criticism that it is a private court acting 'not only as prosecutor, judge and jury but also as Director of Public Prosecutions' remains (1972:401). Another weakness, it has been argued, arises from the General Medical Council's particular statutory function; dealing with the deviant fringe of the profession is quite a different thing from a continuing inspection or surveillance of the post qualification competence throughout a doctor's medical career. The British Medical Association itself has discussed the question and it has been mooted that the existing work of the General Medical Council should be divided between two public bodies dealing respectively with complaints on the one hand, and continuing competence to practice, on the other.

The Merrison Report (Merrison 1975) disposed of the idea of two public bodies and recommended that the General Medical Council remain independent of the government and of the National Health Service. Perhaps surprisingly, in a committee which was composed of doctors and laymen in equal proportions, it sustained the principle of the General Medical Council as a predominantly professional body with only ten lay members. It did, however, propose that the balance of representation within the profession itself should be altered ensuring a larger voice for young doctors, including young hospital doctors and for general practitioners. It favoured the use of the system of the single transferable vote and insisted upon a more democratically constituted Council in which elected members would exceed all other members by ten. On the question of the finance of the General Medical Council, it was proposed that it should continue to be financed by the medical profession with an unhypothecated government contribution. Contrary to the protests of the medical profession which led originally to the appointment of the committee, the annual retention fee, which the General Medical Council had earlier tried to enforce, was recommended together with the sanction that a doctor's registration should be withdrawn for failure to pay.

The report offered a thorough analysis of issues relating to registration and education, the problem of standards among overseas doctors as well as a discussion of the principles of professional conduct and the control of the sick doctor. From our point of view the most interesting aspect of the report is its assertion of professionalism as the fundamental principle upon which the control of the medical profession should continue to be organised. We have noted that during the 1970s there has been a challenge emanting from several quarters to the legitimacy of the entrenched organisations and institutions of professional autonomy in medicine. The Merrison Report presents a reasoned case for maintaining the independence of the General Medical Council as the regulating body of the medical profession in Britain, and as a result, makes it more difficult for those who would seek a permanent weakening of the strong position established by the medical profession during the past century. It is still possible that the medical profession, which itself called in question the traditional role of the General Medical Council, may well find its 'exclusive professional control' will be moderated by increasing lay representation and thus a diminution of professional autonomy. It remains to be seen whether the government will act simply to implement the recommendations of the report, or whether it will significantly alter them in subsequent legislation. While professionalism itself no longer has the unquestioned legitimacy which it hitherto enjoyed, the Merrison Report provides a rationale for a well organised profession which continues to have a very powerful base for maintaining a high degree of control over the health field, although much depends on the extent to which it can find the resources of leadership and solidarity to withstand contemporary pressures upon its established position.

PART III

11. CONCLUDING SUMMARY AND SOME IMAGES OF THE FUTURE

Concluding Summary

Collective social mobility has been neglected as an object of enquiry by sociologists in Western countries despite the fact that the study of individual social mobility has been a major research interest of the discipline during the past twenty-five years. The reasons for this lie in the fundamentally liberal values which have inspired the researchers and in the related methodological individualism which focussed attention upon the mobility of individuals. Social mobility in Western countries has come to mean no more than individual mobility: where reference is made to collective mobility, it is generally regarded as an integral feature of traditionalism of which the process of sanskritisation within the Indian caste system is used as a prime example. A reader of the literature might conclude that collective mobility in the West is such an unusual phenomenon, inimical as it is to liberal individualism, that there is no requirement to study it if, indeed, there is anything to study.

Taking a wider perspective we suggested that studies of social class which have dealt with either the Marxian thesis of proletarianisation or the counter-thesis of *embourgeoisement* may both be seen as hypotheses about downward and upward social mobility respectively. Contrary to Lopreato, we offer evidence which supports the view that social mobility need not always be a dissociative variable, eroding social class structure, but may also be an associative one. When related to class consciousness social mobility can be important in its collective aspects in the process of class formation. Analysing the studies of Lockwood and Goldthorpe, we noted in particular the tendency in sociology to conceive of classes in terms of ideal types — the working class following collective modes of action and the middle class essentially individual modes inimical to collective action. We asserted that while this model may well have been appropriate for Lockwood's study of clerical workers, it hardly characterises adequately the core of the middle class. In our view, there is a considerable weight of evidence to support the contention that the rise of the middle class in English society has been very much dependent on collective action and collective social mobility. Our case study of the medical profession as an archetypal case is presented as a demonstration of this point of view.

The study of the professions, we noted, has been important in sociological writing but has been largely divorced from an analysis of class structure. Increasingly this separation has been marked by the emergence of a special sub-discipline, the sociology of professionalisation. Originally, in the work of Durkheim, the professions were identified as a means of redressing the balance against individualism. Professional ethics were regarded as a means of asserting moral standards in an industrial world about which it was believed that the de-regulation of society through the impact of individualism was leading to moral decline. This theme had a continuing impact, particularly between the wars, but since the Second World War sociologists have preferred to concentrate on the narrower question of professionalisation, and this has resulted, as Johnson points out, in the rather sterile approach of the 'trait theorists'. At the same time, the level of analysis most often selected has been micro-sociological. It has been concerned with role relationships, socialisation and related matters rather than with the broader macro-sociological issues relating the professions to social structure, particularly class structure. Ben-David appears at first sight to address himself to this question but, in fact, as we have argued, his perspective and method of approach lead him away from a conception of professionalism as a form of collective social mobility into a comparative analysis of the rates of individual social mobility. In short, he conceives of the professions, as did Sorokin, merely as vehicles utilised by people for their individual mobility.

More recently, there has been a return to a focus on the problem of professionalism at the macro level by such writers as Prandy, Turner and Johnson. Johnson's study, in particular, offers a critique of the post-war developments in this area of sociology but fails to deal with the question of professionalism and class structure which we have conceptualised in this book, beginning with the concept of collective social mobility. This may seem surprising in view of the centrality of power to his analysis. Freidson, too, stresses the importance of power and particularly, what he calls professional dominance. Johnson defines professionalism as control over clients. Freidson speaks of it in terms of control over organisations and institutions but we have suggested that the defining characteristic is the control which professional associations themselves develop over professional colleagues who are formally equal. This is the basis for professional control over education, markets for service and organisations over which a profession may achieve dominance.

If the study of professionalism has been to a large extent separated from the theories of social class, so it is equally true that writers who have contributed to the development of class theory have failed adequately to explore and explain the relationship of professionalism to social class. Marx briefly addressed the problem in *Das Kapital* but the text breaks off at the very point where he is about to reveal his view of the matter (Marx 1962:863). Generally, however, varieties of Marxian conflict theory have tended to regard the study of the working class as the vanguard of future historical development and the capitalist class as the chief barrier to such a development. For this reason the middle class is conceived of as both transitory and dependent, and the professions

248

have been thought of as peripheral to the class struggle. Weber, writing in the German context, was more fully aware of the professional 'secure in a bureaucratic position' than of the concept of the 'free professional', which has been more important in Anglo-Saxon countries. Giddens presents perhaps the most sophisticated version of class theory to date. He rightly points out that the key problem in developing Weber's class theory is that of articulating the relationship between 'market capacity' and 'class as a structured form'. Giddens uses the concept of 'closure' as a means of identifying the process of class formation which he describes by use of the term 'structuration'.

It is a weakness of Giddens' position that he fails to develop his theory adequately, especially the concept of closure. His discussion of social mobility remains conventional because it is entirely concerned with individual mobility and does not touch upon the important question of collective social mobility, which we regard as integral to the study of closure as a social process. The question of the relationship of professionalism to class theory is mentioned by Giddens only to be dismissed as presenting no problem for class theory. In our view, closer attention to professionalism would have offered Giddens the opportunity to understand and develop his central concept of closure, which would in turn have led to a greater adequacy of theorisation about social class. Giddens, like Johnson wishes us to understand the importance of power in his analysis. We suggest that power is fundamental to the problem of uncertainty in industrial societies and to the development of social structure, including class structuration. In the classical social science of economics, Rothschild has argued, the question of power was pushed from the centre of analysis. The market mechanism could offer us a self-equilibrating system of production and distribution which would be fair to all. Unlike a situation of oligopoly and monopoly, where human agents may collectively rig the market in their favour, the perfect market would require no collective political action and hence prevent maldistribution through the unbalancing effects of power conflicts. Power must be brought forward as a central rather than a peripheral concept.

Durkheim objected to the individualism inherent in liberal economic theory because, in his view, it is society which is the repository of moral value and which, by the exercise of constraint over the individual, shapes and sets bounds to man's insatiable desires. Only under conditions of social constraint can a moral framework be provided which will uphold established values in a stable social order. Without the exercise of the generalised power of society, which functions to contain the urgent quest of individuals for self-satisfaction, society would collapse into an anarchy of competing interests. The erosion of normative constraint would produce a situation of *anomie*, or normlessness, and high rates of social pathology. Durkheim would have preferred a political system based upon occupational associations rather than upon the individualism of the franchise and the secret ballot. Such a corporate form of representation, he believed, would help to avert the danger of extreme individualism arising from the application of liberal democratic theory. Durkheim had only a marginal interest in class theory as such. He stressed the impact of individualism on society taken *as a whole* and was little concerned with class conflict, which he believed could be overcome by the individual's attachment to corporate occupational associations serving to transcend class divisions. The thrust of Durkheim's sociology led him to be concerned with power as a generalised control emanating from the collective reality of society itself and independent of the wills of individuals or the purposes of particular organised vested interests.

Marx and Weber did not regard power in this generalised sense as problematic because they did not share Durkheim's view of the causes of social disorganisation. They regarded capitalism as a structured social form and derived alternative theories of power and control from their different conceptions of the relationship between the state and the economy. Marx typically regarded the state as subordinate to the interests of private property owners. Weber stressed the independent and autonomous position of the state *vis-a-vis* private property, defining the state in terms of its monopoly of power within a given territorial area. Both focussed on the horizontal class divisions, which unlike Durkheim, they regarded as fundamental to capitalism. Subsequent theorists have combined elements of both positions in different ways. For example Dahrendorf utilised the Weberian analysis of bureaucracy as a basis for attempting a reconstruction of Marx's theory of class as applied to advanced industrial societies. Goldthorpe and Lockwood developed the Weberian class analysis for the purpose of examining problems of class consciousness and class structure in the mid-twentieth century. In our view, neither the neo-Marxist nor the neo-Weberian positions take sufficient account of the importance of the free occupational association in the development of class structure in capitalist societies, particularly in the cases of the USA and Britain. The study of unionism has usually been identified with the development of the working class, but little attempt has been made to locate it along-side other forms of free occupational association, such as professionalism. These types of association are themselves an expression of the existence of 'free association' as an institutionalised feature of Western capitalism, a feature which has been both preserved and extended in Western democracies. It was, for example, strengthened after the allied victory in Western Germany in 1945. The varieties of industrialism include cases of social democracy, fascism and state socialism where in the latter two cases the principle of free association is either denied or fundamentally curtailed.

Collective action is an important element in class structuration and, as Lukes has suggested, must be taken into account in any analysis of power. He marks out the limitations of the one-dimensional approach which focusses on decision-making alone, and the two-dimensional approach which includes the study of non decision-making. These approaches, in his view are tied to a behavioural perspective which is subject to all the problems which arise from methodological individualism. A three-dimensional approach, which includes as the third element collective forces and social forces, Lukes believes is essential to the sociological conceptualisation and study of power. These would include the Durkheimian case of generalised constraint, where social forces may be utilised for particular political objectives, and also the cases of action by a collectivity, such as the ones in which we are interested, namely professionalism and unionism. Lukes is well aware of the difficulties which arise from attributing power to collectivities, especially in an intellectual ethos in which the terrain of debate has been dominated by behaviourism and methodological individualism. He suggests that it is essential to provide an adequate conceptualisation of the degree of structural determination on the one hand, and openness for political action, on the other. The exercise of power can only take place where individuals or collectivities are faced with a genuine choice. It is not possible to speak of the exercise of power in a situation which is completely determined. Such a view is fully compatible with the definition of power as the exercise of degrees of control exerted by collectivities, such as occupational associations, which is integral to the study of collective social mobility undertaken by the present authors.

In capitalist societies there are no legal sanctions against social mobility as such. Collective action, directed towards collective social mobility, is typically based upon occupation which in turn is rooted in market relationships. Occupational association is fundamental to an understanding of class structuration in so far as it is concerned with a choice of strategies to close off occupational opportunities against outsiders. Such strategies are not necessarily connected with aspirations towards upward social mobility, as is professionalism, but may be concerned with the defence of a particular occupational position, as in the case of craft unionism. Indeed, there is evidence to suggest that unionism can serve to inhibit upward collective social mobility, although some of the 'individual-mobility aspirations' may be present in individual unionists and their wives. Unionism and professionalism may be seen as alternative occupational strategies which are concerned with the collective manipulation and control of particular types of market capacity. Collective social mobility requires, in Goldthorpe and Lockwood's terms, not merely similar levels of income but assimilation in the normative sphere and in relational patterns. Where this occurs, there is the emergence of a shared style of life. Goldthorpe and Lockwood's conception of the middle class as essentially characterised by individualism is incorrect, if by this they mean that there is little

251

readiness to adopt collective strategies for the control of the market, as opposed to working class solidarity expressed in the collective activity of unionism. Professionalism is one typical collective strategy of the middle class, or of those with aspirations to join the middle class. It involves control of an occupation by colleagues who, in a formal sense, are equal and who set up a system of self-government for which they seek the legal recognition of the state. Such a conception of professionalism has been particularly important in the British and North American context. By contrast, there is the notion of the professional 'secure in a bureaucratic position', to which Weber drew attention in the case of Germany before the First World War. It is essential to distinguish between these two institutionalised conceptions of professionalism in industrial society.

The relationship between professionalism and class formation, we believe, is an important problem for class theory. While agreeing with Giddens' general theoretical position, we note that he fails to understand the key role of professionalism as an area of study which has the potential of assisting sociologists in the development of class theory. He rightly draws attention to the difficulty of making the transition from market capacity to class as a structured form as the central problem in contemporary class theory. He proposes the notion of closure as the connecting concept but fails to offer a satisfactory account of the *processes* by which closure is achieved. In our view, a realisation of the *general* theoretical importance of occupational association in the process of closure is fundamental to the understanding of class formation and maintenance. Like other sociological writers he discusses individual social mobility but does not identify collective social mobility, which is one of the processes by which closure is achieved.

Parkin pinpoints some of the important elements in the process of closure and reminds us that Weber recognised that collectivities are concerned to keep opportunities and rewards within the grasp of a limited circle of eligibles. He suggests that we should distinguish between the processes of exclusion and solidarism which are clearly general categories embracing what we have termed professionalism and unionism. We are dubious about his particular terminology because of the sociological convention which tends to connect solidarism exclusively with communal action and which often is identified only with the working class. In an associational society both professionalism and unionism may tap resources of communal solidarity under appropriate conditions. In the formation of the English class structure occupational associations, which have become identified with strategies of professionalism or unionism or indeed associations of businessmen, have themselves played a fundamental role in class formation. In the early nineteenth century these forms of association were not so markedly differentiated by their typical strategies as they have subsequently become.

The concept of *structuration*, we suggest, ought not to be defined simply in terms of *class structuration* because the study of social structure requires that we introduce other elements such as those of sexual divisions and religion. There is a tendency in sociological studies to assert a claim at the outset to be studying social structure. One notices however, that the focus of analysis is quickly reduced to that of 'class structure'. This derives from the domination of the debate by the notion that economic activity is both a separable and fundamental element in social life. Our view is that other structural elements cannot be reduced without residue to economic considerations, and must therefore be given due theoretical consideration in sociological analysis. We have used the term *social structuration* to embrace this wider conception of the process by which social structure is formed and have applied this perspective to the history of the medical profession in England.

In 1800 the practice of medicine in England was still divided into three occupations of physicians, surgeons and apothecaries. The system of orders was breaking down as part of the general decay of guild control which, in 1815, saw a last flourish in the Apothecaries' Act. From the 1790s onwards there was a movement among the emerging general practitioners of medicine to increase their share of the market for medical care and to improve their status in society by a process of upward assimilation into the ranks of the gentleman physician. During this period the general practitioners espoused and developed the ideology of professionalism. They created a successful movement which achieved unification of the orders of medicine within a single profession in 1858. This was the first and major step in a process of successful upward collective social mobility.

The objective of the newly founded General Medical Council, after 1858, was the cultural incorporation into the unified profession of the large body of general practitioners, a process which was, in fact, already underway. They were determined to produce a homogeneous profession in terms of social background and recruitment, purging the remnants of commercialism inherent in the trade-derived apothecary, and replacing it with the ethic of the cultured gentleman. The conflict between the consultant and the general practitioner was increased by unification because all practitioners were now in a formal sense equal as registered practitioners. The hospital, which was becoming increasingly important, proved to be the basis for the establishment of elite consultant control, especially through the control of education, and it was during this period that the referral system was hammered out. Under the new educational arrangements apprenticeship was phased out thus cementing the educational dominance of the hospital school. Apart from the growth of the voluntary hospital movement,

253

new special hospitals began to proliferate and a public hospital system began to emerge from the Poor Law infirmaries. A counter move by general practitioners was expressed in the foundation of the cottage hospital movement. Under the Poor Law system general practitioners, who were Poor Law medical officers, were dissatisfied with their situation. Equally, the growth of Friendly Society and Provident Club medicine threatened the autonomy of the general practitioner. The British Medical Association was chief among medical associations which strove to protect the general practitioner and enhance his status and position in society. It condemned the evils of contract practice, Poor Law and local authority employment, and led the negotiations on behalf of general practitioners which resulted in the establishment of a state-financed national health insurance scheme. This had the effect of redressing the balance towards greater professional participation and control through greater representation and effective power within the state machinery.

The nineteenth century saw the culmination of a process, which was already strongly apparent in the eighteenth century, which excluded women from the emerging medical profession. Women were confined either to domestic and factory employment or to the leisured life of a lady, serving as a symbol of the pecuniary success of their menfolk. Involvement in associations outside the family, particularly occupational associations, was a rarity. Even in midwifery which had always been a female mystery the woman was increasingly excluded by the man-midwife. Midwifery became of vital importance to the young surgeon or apothecary — the general practitioner — seeking to establish himself in practice. The unified medical profession of 1858 was a male monopoly which strongly resisted the efforts of the feminist movement to open it to women practitioners. Midwifery was nearly extinguished in England as an occupation for women and modern nursing was created as a 'handmaiden' occupation strictly subordinated to the authority of the male-dominated medical profession. General practitioners, in particular, stood out against the registration of midwives and also against the introduction of district nurses whom they regarded as a source of competition for medical business. Even today equality between the sexes within the medical profession is still a somewhat distant prospect and the relationship between nurses and doctors remains as an institutionalised example of the conception of the appropriate relationship between the sexes as it existed in the mid-nineteenth century.

The fact that the doctors were well organised prior to the major entry of the state into the field of personal health care, was a crucial factor in the success of the negotiations with Lloyd George over the principles and administration of the National Health Insurance Act of 1911. Private practice was preserved except for those least able to pay. The poorer general practitioner had his income secured, and remuneration was paid at a higher rate than previously. Participation by doctors in the committee structure administering the service guaranteed considerable influence and, in some aspects, undoubted control. Between the wars there was a feeling that the profession was well-established and well-respected in the community. It was staunchly middle class and largely recruited from the homogeneous product of the public school. The Second World War saw the introduction of the Emergency Medical Service which laid the foundations for the inclusion of the hospital system within the newly-created National Health Service in 1948. The doctors' fears of a socialist government led them to press strongly, particularly through the Royal Colleges, for an administrative structure which would preserve their interests, particularly in relation to private practice. The National Health Service has largely been dominated by the doctors, and it was only in 1974 that a new administrative structure founded on 'managerial' principles was introduced.

Even this structure did not touch the established rights of the profession with regard to private practice including the admission of private patients to National Health Service hospitals, but shortly afterwards, in a time of acute inflation the lower paid hospital workers clashed with organised doctors. Here was an instance of a direct conflict between professionalism and unionism. The National Health Service inherited the incipient conflicts between general practitioners and hospital doctors, and junior hospital doctors and consultants. These conflicts originated far back in the formation of the modern medical profession and in the origins of the hospital service. They have more to do with the inherited organisation of the profession than with the National Health Service *per se*. The industrial action by consultants in the National Health Service against the proposed new contract put forward by Barbara Castle, and the appointment of the Merrison Committee which reported in 1975 were indicative that the powerful institutional controls exercised by the complex of organisations and associations representing the medical profession have been under considerable pressure. This has opened up at least the possibility of change through party political action in the position and power of the profession both within the National Health Service and in society. It should not be thought that radical changes can be introduced easily without conflict and without the agreement of the established interests within the medical profession. On the other hand there has been a shift in the balance of power between the medical profession and the state which may well result in doctors, like teachers and other groups in the public sector, relying increasingly in future upon union action rather than professionalism, however unpalatable this may be to those of the old guard in medicine who are ideologically antipathetic to unionism.

Some Images of the Future

In this book we have examined in some historical depth the way in which a particular occupation, the medical profession, has achieved unity and an established place in the middle class through a process of collective social mobility. We have placed our case study in the context of a theoretical and conceptual scheme which enables us to understand this process as part of a wider movement of class structuration and indeed of social structuration. It now remains for us to look to the future and envisage some of the possible as well as the likely outcomes of the present situation. We do not wish to claim predictive powers although we judge some developments to be more likely than others, but we wish rather to discuss briefly some of the alternative futures which have been recommended or predicted.

Ivan Illich, well known for his advocacy of the deschooling move-ment (Illich 1970) exhorts us to engage in de-professionalisation. His claim is that from just before the First World War doctors have had in their hands more and more specifically effective treatments for disease. 'Since then', he says,

> 'medicine has gone on to define what constitutes disease and its treatment. The Westernised public learned to demand effective medical practice as defined by the progress of medical science. For the first time in history, doctors could measure their efficiency against scales which they themselves had devised . . . Paradoxically, the simpler the tools became, the more the medical profession insisted on a monopoly of their application, the longer became the training demanded before a medicine man was initiated into the legitimate use of the simplest tool and the more everyone felt dependent on the doctor' (Illich 1973:633).

Illich suggests that from the 1950s onwards iatrogenic (doctor-induced) disease became an important factor and techniques of extending life at high cost became increasingly possible. He believes that the process of monopolisation of medical practice by professionals increasingly excluded the *care* of relatives and non-professional helpers creating a greater dependency on professional services. 'Simultaneously, more conditions were defined as needing treatment by creating new specialisations or para-professions to keep the tools under the control of the guild' (1973:633-4). Illich argues that this process is by no means confined to medicine but to many other institutions of industrial society. While at first science and technology are applied to the solution of a clearly stated problem and the new efficiency can be clearly measured, this achievement is then used 'as a rationale for the exploi-tation of society by one of its self-certifying professional elites'. Illich makes the point that this can be a self-defeating process because often the poor application of recently acquired knowledge generates further problems which then require the application of further technological solutions to rectify the mistakes.

A new alternative is suggested by Illich who argues that science should be used 'to simplify tools and to enable the layman to shape his immediate environment to his taste. The time has come', he says, 'to take the syringe out of the hand of the doctor, as the pen was taken out of the hand of the scribe during the reformation in Europe' (1973:634). The simplification of medical diagnosis can even now, according to Illich, enable the medical treatment of most curable sickness to be put into the hands of the layman. He believes that 'people find it so difficult to accept this statement because the complexity of medical ritual has hidden from them the simplicity of its basic procedures' (1973:634). He wishes to see an expansion of lay therapy and the concomitant reduction of professional medicine but he observes that the main obstacle to this is the exaggerated value placed on standard products, uniformity, and certified quality in industrial society, as well as the vested interest of the health professions in their monopoly.

The prospect of de-professionalisation to this extent and on this scale seems to us to be an unlikely future for the medical profession in particular and for most other professions, although Illich's argument is interesting because it reflects an increasing tendency to challenge the legitimacy of the ideology of professionalism, which has been noticeable during the last few years. The likelihood is, however, that this challenge will increasingly result in demands for lay participation and control in the institutions and organisations of medical care. If something like Illich's hopes for the future were to be realised, they would be bound to have a radical effect on the class position of the professions, including medicine.

At a recent conference of the British Sociological Association,[1] Terence Johnson presented a paper in which he developed the argument of his earlier book (we discuss this work in Chapters 2 and 3) and addressed himself to the problem of the professions in the class structure (Johnson 1975). He himself recognised the criticism which we have made of his book when he said 'it is now clear that the weakness of this analysis lay in the failure to anchor the conditions for such ideological and political forms [e.g. professionalism] in an adequate theory of class relations' (1975:10). He proposed a theory of the relationship between the professions and the class structure utilising the Marxian perspective developed by Carchedi (Carchedi 1975). Unlike the approach adopted in this book, which Johnson would probably recognise as owing much to the Weberian tradition, Johnson argues that Giddens is wrong to suggest that the emergence of the 'new' middle class cannot be adequately coped with by the development of Marxian theory. He believes that a theory of the type proposed by Giddens is likely to reach misleading conclusions and 'that this general failure is directly related to the inadequacies of those Weberian solutions now dominant in sociology' (1975:1). We too have had occasion to be critical of Giddens' failure to explore the relationship between professionalism and class, but have attempted to develop the theory rather than turn to an alternative Marxian theorisation, as Johnson has done. Johnson does however examine two views of the future of the professions which are currently being advanced. For this purpose he examines the work of Oppenheimer and Freidson neither of which claim that 'the views of the professions they present describe an existing situation; rather they set out to extrapolate from existing *trends* affecting professional employment, a view of the professionals' future' (1975:2). Oppenheimer believes that the professional and white-collar worker is increasingly subject to pressures of proletarianisation which involves the extensive division of labour and the fragmentation of tasks so that the typical worker performs only one or few tasks in a total process. There is at the same time an increasing subordination of the worker to some higher authority — public or private — which determines the conditions of work. The work is devalued and the worker becomes more and more dependent on his wage. In order to withstand the probable deterioration of living and working conditions, the worker engages in collective bargaining rather than in individual face to face bargaining. Oppenheimer's thesis is that professional work is increasingly incorporated and subordinated within bureaucratic structures with fixed rules and jurisdictions controlled by others in a hierarchical command structure. Rather than autonomous professional control of certification, examinations are employed as means of testing competence for advancement within a bureaucracy. Oppenheimer envisages that a severe disjunction will occur arising from the conflict between expectations generated during the long professional training and the fragmented and stunted scope of the tasks which will be performed in practice. He envisages that for this reason professionals will become ready to identify with political movements which are anti-establishment particularly where they are concerned to resist state oppression.

As we have noted in Chapter 3, Freidson takes a different view: he argues that authority is based on institutionalised expertise in post industrial society. He asserts that knowledge-based labour is likely to be resistant to the process of rationalisation inherent in the traditional Weberian forms of bureaucratic organisation governed by the rules of legal rationality. In the case of the provision of health care, the division of labour is ordered and co-ordinated not by management or bureau-cratic principles but by the dominant profession of medicine. Johnson asks the question 'why should this radical transformation of the authority structure occur?' He tells us that 'Freidson is forced back to the conventional "post-industrial" thesis of the growing significance of knowledge in the production process'. The argument may be finally summed up by saying that 'knowledge then has its own inherent logic determining the emergence of specialised functions which are themselves resistant to other forms of authority' (1975:4).

The views of Oppenheimer and Freidson present 'two views of present trends and future states which have completely antithetical implications for any evaluation of the professionals' place in the class structure'. Either professions face a future of subordination to bureaucratic authority, becoming increasingly subject to proletarianisation and, in consequence, espousing unionism and becoming 'potentially capable of revolutionary political activity', or professionals will achieve domination of the bureaucratic structure 'thus creating the conditions for the emergence of knowledge-based occupational groups as the dominant class — some form of technocracy' (1975:4). Johnson regards it as evident that these contradictory views of the future both share important assumptions in common and both appear to have some empirical justification. Indeed the division between Oppenheimer and Freidson amounts to only one thing — namely, that Freidson believes that knowledge-based occupations are by their nature resistant to the rationalising and routinising effects of bureaucratic authority while Oppenheimer believes that such authority can and will undermine the existing knowledge-base of such occupations. Johnson argues that these conflicting conclusions arise from a neglect of what he believes to be a

> 'central dualism or contradiction in the organization of knowledge as work and that its expression in "professional" work activities is an instance of the basic dualism characterizing the capitalist mode of production. The neglect of these dual processes which express themselves in relations of production derives from a Weberian analysis in which the relations of production are conflated with the social division of labour and authority identified with the conditions of imperative co-ordination alone' (1975:5).

This statement is, we think, somewhat unfair to the multi-dimensionality of Weber's thought because while it is true that Oppenheimer develops the logical consequences of Weber's concept of legal rational authority, Freidson's conception of professional dominance is also derived from the Weberian tradition and is akin to the notion of closure. The fact that Johnson identifies both Oppenheimer and Freidson as part of the Weberian tradition and tells us that they drew his attention 'unwittingly' to 'the contradiction characterizing the organization of professional knowledge', itself suggests that the problem may be at least posed within a Weberian frame of reference (1975:5).

Following the work of Jamous and Peloille (Jamous, Peloille 1970:111-53) and utilising what they call the 'indetermination/technicality ratio' as a means of characterising the nature of the duality in any occupation process, Johnson proceeds to apply the concepts to the professions. Technicality comprises those aspects of professional knowledge which may be identified, in terms of the primacy of cognitive rationality, and which Johnson asserts is the basis of the idea in the 'conventional sociology of the professions' that the professional expert is 'autonomous'. Quite contrary to this idea is the view of Jamous and Peloille who 'stress the fact that technicality is the condition for external intervention'. The very rationality of technical knowledge, its systematic nature, allows it to be communicated as a set of rules, procedures, and solutions which may be passed from one generation to the next (Johnson 1975:5). The rationality of knowledge, which offers a basis for codification, legitimation and certification, also make it vulnerable, as Oppenheimer claims, to bureaucratic rationality. Rather than preventing the intervention of non-expert outsiders, the increasing rationality of knowledge is held inevitably to lead to opportunities for intervention by lay outsiders in the affairs of the professional.

Indetermination is one of two elements which make up the duality of the indetermination/technicality ratio. The concept of indetermination refers to 'those aspects of the professional organization of knowledge which function as barriers to intervention'. In other words, technical knowledge is complemented by other forms of knowledge relevant to the organisation of a profession. 'The bases of [professional] mystique, the sources of its legitimations, which . . . underpin its monopolistic position and successful resistance to external authority' (1975:5). The duality of indetermination and technicality are both essential, in the view of Jamous and Peloille to the 'problems of the role and functions of the professions in modern societies' (Jamous, Peloille 1970:118). Thus, any study which neglects one term of this duality is bound to be distorted so that Oppenheimer and Freidson, who respectively stress technicality or indetermination, risk the failure of their analyses to cope with the problem. For example, as Johnson points out, 'Freidson stresses indetermination and yet seeks the conditions for its existence in technicality: the duality collapses and the possibility of distinguishing between professions and the variations, in the forms of institutionalized control they are subject to, evaporate' (1975:6).

Johnson identifies a failure of explanatory power in the work of Jamous and Peloille which is, he believes, 'their inability to theoretize the conditions for *indetermination*'. They focus on the historical variability of indetermination but Johnson wishes to be more precise for he asserts that the conditions for indeterminacy are however, the very conditions which will enable us to identify the class characteristics

260

of the professions as an element of the 'new' middle class. For Johnson, it is not simply that Oppenheimer and Freidson are wrong but that each stresses only one aspect of a duality which underlies the professional organisation of knowledge. He says,

'what is noticeable about both positions is their *insufficiency*. Even if Oppenheimer's argument for proletarianization was an adequate description of certain contemporary socio-economic trends it still remains on the level of description, without ever explaining the process, in which case such extrapolated trends *may* or *may not* be significant' (1975:6).

Johnson suggests that an adequate theorisation of the problem can only be offered in terms of the relations of production and for this purpose he utilises the work of Carchedi. This Marxist analysis focussed on the capitalist mode of production, which is conceived of as a dualistic structure involving 'the labour process', on the one hand, (creating real use value) and, on the other hand, the surplus in the production process which is peculiar to capitalism. The characterisation of capitalism in terms only of ownership and non-ownership of the means of production is regarded by Carchedi as a vulgar Marxist usage which must be supplemented by additional dichotomies such as producer and non-producer and labourer and non-labourer. These round out the understanding of the relationship between the class of those who produce surplus value and those who appropriate it. Capitalism is seen in terms of stages of development in which the first stage is simply the formal subordination to capital. In the second stage this is followed by a continuous technical revolution in which the division of labour, involving the application of science and technology, creates a complex labour process. Manual labour power is frequently extended or replaced by activities carried out by agents who are not necessarily themselves engaged in manual work, but are agents of what is called the *collective labourer*. In this way, the Marxian theory of Carchedi incorporates routine white-collar workers as part of the proletariat through involvement in the socio-technical system called the collective labourer. There is at the same time a parallel process by which the individual capitalist is replaced in the second stage by the collective capitalist. The emergence of the collective capitalist involves the sub-division, on a rational basis, of the operations of capital into numerous specialist tasks and the outcome is the collective appropriation of surplus value by capital. This process is referred to as the *global functions of capital*. The separation of legal and economic ownership, which critics of Marxism have used as evidence for the replacement of capitalism by a post-capitalist form of industrialism is taken, in this version of Marxist theory, to be simply an extension of capitalism into a third stage called monopoly capitalism. Under

261

monopoly capitalism the global functions of capital are carried out through a complex organisation structure by agents who are not themselves the owners of the means of production. The global functions of capital involve the growth of bureaucratic organisation, not merely for the purpose of co-ordinating the social division of labour for production, but for control and surveillance in respect of the production of surplus value. In brief, the application of the dual ideas of the collective labourer and the global functions of capital allows an analysis of the new middle class in which certain professional occupations are seen as agents of both the collective labourer and of global capital. They are, then, part of a class which carries out the global functions of capital without owning the means of production and are therefore distinct in relation to a capitalist class. At the same time, and in various ratios they are also carrying out the functions of the collective labourer — they are both labourer — non-labourer, exploited and exploiters (1975:9). In the case of the medical profession, for example, Johnson argues that the institutions sustaining 'autonomy' are directly related to the monopolisation of 'official' definitions of illness and health.

> 'The doctor's certificate defines and legitimises the withdrawal of labour. Credentialism, involving monopolistic practices and occupational closure, fulfils ideological functions in relation to capital and reflects the extent to which medicine in its role of surveillance and the reproduction of labour power is able to draw upon powerful ideological symbols in the creation of indetermi-nation' (1975:10).

Among professional workers one may usually find that they carry out functions of supervision and control but in differing ratios. Thus among accountants one may find class divisions within a heterogeneous occupation in which 'a small high-status elite may be largely the agents of global capital; themselves creating the conditions for the routinised work activities of colleague-subordinates'. Johnson concludes that professionalism

> 'involving the colleague control of work activities, can arise only *where the ideological and political processes sustaining indetermination coincide with the requirements of capital*; that is where core work activities fulfil the global function of capital with respect to control and surveillance including the specific function of the reproduction of labour power' (1975:10).

The following criticisms may be made of Johnson's position. First, when the argument is reduced to its elements, indetermination appears to be linked solely with the global functions of capital. Essentially the class position of professionals depends upon their participation as agents of authority. Professions which are fragmented by the application

262

of increasing rationality have a small group of those exercising authority in one (presumably upper-middle-class position) while the remainder, divested of their authority, become simply technicians — that is part of the collective labourer. This view is extraordinarily reminiscent of the Weberian analysis of legal-rational bureaucracy in which the professional, secure in a bureaucratic position wields authority as an agent of a bureaucracy. It follows that there is a close approximation to Dahrendorf's conception of class divisions based on authority. Furthermore, as Gouldner put it in a verbal comment on the paper, such an analysis would be equally appropriate to the Soviet as to the Western capitalist case. In other words the analysis paradoxically tends to support the post-capitalist thesis which asserts that there has been a convergence between the structures of 'capitalist' and 'socialist' which can both be characterised as industrial societies.

This is the chief weakness of Johnson's theory and the source of his difficulty stems from his treatment of the concept of indeterminacy. He rightly identifies this as the core problem for any understanding of the relationship between professionalism and social class. Yet there is a surprising identity of view on the role of the professional as an agent of control and surveillance in Marxist and Weberian writings. This conception is prominent also in the work of functionalist writers such as Parsons, and the major dispute between the functionalist and Marxist writers is not over the fact of the social control function of professionals but over whether this function is viewed as politically benign or malevolent in state socialist and capitalist societies.

We believe that Johnson correctly identifies a duality in capitalist society which he reaches via the opposed theses of Oppenheimer and Freidson, and which has been specifically identified by Jamous and Peloille in terms of the concepts of indetermination and technicality. The specific weakness of Johnson's argument lies in the fact that he reduces the concept of 'indeterminacy' to participation in authority — surveillance and control — that is part of the global function of capital. In every industrial society, as Gouldner has pointed out, the function of social control is exercised to a greater or lesser extent by professionals. This is as true of the doctor, lawyer or accountant in the Soviet Union, or in modern China as it is in Western Europe or the United States. The concept of technicality applies in industrial societies, whether capitalist or socialist and so does indeterminacy in so far as it derives from participation in authority. Johnson's analysis, though couched in the framework of contemporary Marxism, actually fails to identify any elements of indeterminacy which are specific to the capitalist social democracies as such and which would distinguish them from state socialist societies.

Our theory, we believe, does enable an identification of the distinguishing features which relate 'indeterminacy' to class structuration under capitalism. At the general level, as Giddens points out, capitalism may be characterised by the separation of the state and the economy, although the relationship between them is subject to continuing change in each of the capitalist societies. We wish to draw attention to a specific duality of the social democratic capitalist societies which distinguish them from fascism and state socialism, namely the principles of imperative co-ordination on the one hand and free association on the other. A good deal of attention has been paid to the principle of imperative co-ordination which, following Weber may be said to be one of the principal features of capitalist society, indeed of industrial society. It is integral to Weber's concept of rational-legal authority. Perhaps too little theoretical attention has been paid to an alternative principle of organisation, namely 'free association'. The free association is characterised by the existence of free, independent persons who come together to form an association in which they are formal equals. This type of association remains characteristic of capitalist society except in its fascist forms. The political party, the business association, the private company, the professional association and the trade union are all typical free or voluntary associations. The principle of free association contrasts with that of imperatively co-ordinated association,[2] and the two together make up a duality which is characteristic of capitalism, under social democracy. It is this form of association which distinguishes them from the imperative co-ordination typical of the state socialist and fascist societies. Professionalism, where it has been used successfully in obtaining a high degree of institutionalised autonomy, derives much of what Johnson refers to as indeterminacy from this fact. We can observe then two modes by which professionals can be related to social structure. One where the professional – the person with special expertise – is incorporated within the structure of an imperatively co-ordinated association. This is what Weber referred to as 'the professional secure in a bureaucratic position'. The other we may call 'free professionalism', where the exericse of power is generated by colleague control on the basis of independent professional association. Professionalism, in this second sense, was originally a product of a society in which the state performed minimum functions of regulation and control, not only over economic activity but over the free association of citizens for a wide variety of purposes. Where the state is or becomes dominant through its control of economic activity and the subordination or destruction of free associations, then professionals are likely to find themselves seeking such security as they can obtain in a bureaucratic position within imperatively coordinated associations.

An important duality of capitalism then is manifested in alternative principles of imperatively co-ordinated association and free association. The elimination of one of the terms of this duality would signal the end of capitalism. This was presumably what Marx hoped for when he suggested that the state after the revolution would eventually wither away. Weber clearly believed that imperative co-ordination of a legal-rational type was an essential feature of capitalism and indeed of industrial society. His rejection of the Marxian analysis rested heavily on his belief that the benefits of industrial society could not be obtained if imperative co-ordination were done away with. A society without imperative co-ordination would not be a capitalist society because the essential terms of the duality of capitalism are free association *and* imperative co-ordination. State socialism and fascism extinguish the duality by retaining imperative co-ordination but rejecting free association. Every capitalist society stands as an example of the attempts of men to accommodate the contradiction between these two principles and much of the political debate and social practice centres on questions arising from this duality.

In order to understand the phenomenon of collective social mobility, we must relate it to this wider question of the duality of capitalism. The case study we have examined in the second part of our book, that of the medical profession, demonstrates a case of collective social mobility via the strategy of professionalism and explores the growth and extent of its dominance of the institutions and organisations of medical care, as well as its changing relationship with the state. Elsewhere, we have examined the case of the failure of the strategy of professionalism among teachers, especially in relation to the state (Parry 1974:160-85). It should not however, be thought that we would wish to exclude the possibility of forms of collective social mobility within imperatively co-ordinated structures. We believe that it would be possible to chart the collective mobility of particular groups within the imperatively co-ordinated state systems of Eastern Europe and the Soviet Union and within the capitalist societies. Such an additional enterprise has not been possible within the confines of this book which has set out with the objective of establishing that collective social mobility is an important but neglected subject of study and reinte-grating it with a theory of social class. The case study of collective social mobility which we have presented focussed on the ideology of professionalism, but in this regard we have also had to leave aside systematic consideration of the mobility of organisations. This would be worth following up elsewhere. For example, Halsey has demonstrated the attraction of the high status universities of Oxford and Cambridge in setting aspirations for the British higher education system. A process of mobility of individual university teachers is matched by the aspirations and movement of universities and colleges within a hierarchical pecking order. The process of 'academic drift' by which colleges tend to shed 'lower level' work and take on that of a higher level has been noted by a number of writers, but especially by Burgess and Pratt who explored the assimilation of the colleges of

265

advanced technology into the British university system (Burgess, Pratt 1970). They offer some evidence for the view that a similar process is already at work in the case of the polytechnics (Pratt, Burgess 1974).

On a related theme Burrage has suggested that the professional ideal is manifested as a British cultural preference in the establishment of public corporations, such as the BBC or the nationalised industries. This preference has been shared by both the Conservative and Labour parties. Tawney, whose work was particularly influential in Britain in the middle decades of the twentieth century, believed that

> 'public ownership . . . is a means to a new moral order, but there are, within existing capitalist societies, several occupations which already embody elements of this new order, namely judges, academics, doctors, soldiers and other professions. The attitude of these professionals to their work, their clients and their colleagues is, for Tawney, the model of what relationships within industry ought to be, and he argues that state ownership is the means by which such relationships may be established in industry' (Burrage 1973:254).

There has been a conception, within English socialism, of the essential 'kinship between professions and crafts'. Burrage suggests that the disagreement within the Labour party between those who have seen crafts or professions as alternative models of what work relationships ought to be, is in the end, 'a disagreement about the existing system of social stratification, or the choice of agents for the reform of capitalist society' (1973:255). It is worth keeping in mind this British cultural preference when examining the contribution of Wedgewood Benn to British social and industrial reform. It is clear that the ideal of the 'free association' based on normative principles is a fundamental institution in British society. The study of collective social mobility must then be broader than we have been able to undertake. A range of cases require to be studied. The relationship between technological change and collective social mobility would need a more extensive treatment than we have been able to offer. Technical change or the impact of rapid inflation may both produce rapid collective mobility. It would be especially worth while to examine any cases of downward collective mobility, including the dissolution of particular groups, if and when they occur. For our part we have tried in writing this book to correct an imbalance which we discerned in the study of social mobility and which has caused an over emphasis in the measurement of individual social mobility at the expense of collective social mobility. We trust that we have demonstrated that the study of collective social mobility in advanced industrial societies is a phenomenon worth studying not only in its own right but by reason of the benefits which can be derived for the development of sociology and social policy. We hope that for those who have read the book but who are not specialists in the relevant conventionally defined subject areas, the material presented and the perspective through which it has been presented has enabled an understanding to be attained of some important issues of contemporary society and of the social forces which are operating to shape them.[3]

Notes

1. At which we also presented a paper utilising some of the material from this book on collective social mobility.
2. Imperative co-ordination refers to relationships of superordination and subordination within a hierarchy of command.
3. Thanks are due to Gordon Causer for his helpful comments on our paper to the British Sociological Association Annual Conference, March 1975. Several of these are incorporated in this concluding section.

BIBLIOGRAPHY

Abel-Smith, B. *A History of the Nursing Profession*. London: Heinemann 1960.
The Hospitals 1800 – 1948. London: Heinemann 1964.
Allen, B.M. *Sir Robert Morant. A Great Public Servant*. London: Macmillan 1934.
Ashe, I. *Medical Education & Medical Interests*. Dublin: Fannin 1868.
Bachrach, P., and Baratz, M.S. 'The Two Faces of Power' in *American Political Science Review* (1962), 52: pp. 947-52.
Power and Poverty. Theory and Practice. New York: Oxford University Press 1970.
Bain, G.S. *The Growth of White-Collar Unionism*. Oxford: Clarendon Press 1970.
Banks, J.A., and O. 'A Case Study of a Social Movement' in G.K. Zollschan & W. Hirsch (eds) *Explorations in Social Change*. pp. 547–69. London: Routledge and Kegan Paul 1964.
Barber, B. *Some Problems in the Sociology of Professions*. pp. 669–88. Daedalus 92(4) 1963.
Becker, H.S. Greer, B., Hughes, E.C., and Strauss, A. *Boys in White: A Study of Student Culture in Medical School*. Chicago: University of Chicago Press 1961.
Ben-David, J. 'Professions in the Class System of Present-day Societies' in *Current Sociology*, (1963–4) 12 (3): pp. 246–98.
Bennion, F.A.R. *Professional Ethics*. London: Charles Knight 1969.
Brand, J. *Doctors and the State*. Baltimore, Maryland: John Hopkins, 1965.
Briggs, A. 'The Language of "Class" in Early Nineteenth-Century England' in A. Briggs and J. Saville (eds) *Essays in Labour History*. pp. 43-73. London: Macmillan 1967.
Browne, J. *The Accoucheur: a letter to the Rev. Mr Tattershall of Liverpool on the Evils of Man-Midwifery*. London 1859.
Burgess, T., and Pratt, J. *Policy & Practice: The Colleges of Advanced Technology*. London: Allen Lane 1970.
Burnham, J. *The Managerial Revolution*. London: Harmondsworth 1945.
Burrage, M. 'Nationalization and the Professional Ideal' in *Sociology* (1973) 7 (2), May: pp. 253–72.
Carchedi, G. 'On the Economic Identification of the New Middle Class' in *Economy & Society* (1975) 4 (1): pp. 1–86.
Carlin, J.E. *Lawyers' Ethics, A Survey of the New York City Bar*. New York: Russell Sage Foundation 1966.
Carlyle, T. 'Chartism' in *Essays – English and other Critical Essays*, Vol. 2. London: Dent 1967.
Carr-Saunders, A.M., and Wilson, P.A. *The Professions*. Oxford:

Oxford University Press 1933.

Cassels, A. *Fascist Italy*. London: Routledge and Kegan Paul 1969.

Champney, T. *Medical & Chirurgical Reform proposed from a review of the healing art throughout Europe, particularly Great Britain*. London: J. Johnson 1797,

Christie O.F. *The Transition from Aristocracy 1832 – 1867*. London: Seeley 1927.

Clark, A. *The Working Life of Women in the 17th Century*. London: Routledge and Sons 1919.

Coxon, A.P.M. 'Patterns of Occupational Recruitment: the Anglican Ministry' in *Sociology* (1967), 1 (1), January: pp. 73-9.

Dahrendorf, R. *Class & Class Conflict in Industrial Society*. London: Routledge and Kegan Paul 1959.

Dale, W. *The State of the Medical Profession in Great Britain and Ireland*. Dublin: J. Atkinson 1875.

Dock, L.L., and Stewart, M.I. *A Short History of Nursing*. London: G.P. Putnam. 4th Edition (1938). (First published in 1920)

Donnison, J. *The Professional Development of the Midwife in England from 1850 – 1902*. University of London Ph.D. 1974

Dumont, L. *Homo Hierarchicus* London: Paladin 1972.

Durkheim, E. *Professional Ethics & Civic Morals*. London: Routledge and Kegan Paul 1957.
The Division of Labour in Society. New York: Free Press 1964.

Eckstein, H. *The English Health Service. Its Origins, Structure, and Achievements*. Cambridge (Massachusetts): Harvard University Press 1959.
Pressure Group Politics. The Case of the British Medical Association. London: Allen and Unwin 1960.

Ede, J.F. *History of Wednesbury*. University of London M.A. Thesis 1962.

Etzioni, A., and E. (eds) *Social Change*. pp. 481–97 New York: Basic Books 1964.

Ferris, P. *The Doctors*. London: Victor Gollancz 1965.

Fogarty, M.P., Rapoport, R., and Rapoport, R.N. *Sex, Career and Family*, London: Allen & Unwin 1971.

Foot, M. *Aneurin Bevan. A Biography* Vol. 2: 1945-1960. London: Davis-Poynter 1973.

Forsyth, G. 'Solving the General Practice Crisis' in *New Society* 181, 17 March 1966: pp. 10–13.

Franklin, F.E. *Medical Education & the Rise of the General Practitioner. 1760–1860*. University of Birmingham Ph.D. 1950.

Freidson, E. *Professional Dominance: The Social Structure of Medical Care*. Chicago/New York: Atherton Press 1970.
'Professionalization & the Organization of Middle-Class Labour in Post-Industrial Society' in P. Halmos (ed) *Professionalization and Social Change. The Sociological Review Monograph* 20 December 1973, Keele: University of Keele pp. 47–59.

269

Galbraith, J.K. *The New Industrial State.* New York: New American Library 1968.

Geiger, T. *Aufgaben und Stellung der Intelligenz in der Gesellschaft* (Functions and position of the Intelligentsia within Society). Stuttgart: Ferdinand Enke 1949.

Gerth, H.H., and Wright Mills, C. *From Max Weber: Essays in Sociology.* London: Routledge and Kegan Paul 1948.

Giddens, A. *Politics and Sociology in the Thought of Max Weber* London: Macmillan 1972.
The Class Structure of the Advanced Societies. London: Hutchinson 1973.

Gilbert, B.B. *British Social Policy 1914-1939.* London: Batsford 1970.

Glass, D. (ed) *Social Mobility in Britain.* London: Routledge and Kegan Paul 1954.

Goldthorpe, J., Lockwood, D., Bechhofer, F., and Platt, J. *The Affluent Worker: Industrial Attitudes and Behaviour,* 1968a.
The Affluent Worker: Political Attitudes and Behaviour, 1968b.
The Affluent Worker in the Class Structure. Cambridge: Cambridge University Press 1969.

Gosden, P.H.J.H. *Friendly Societies in England 1815-1875.* London: Kelley 1961.

Gouldner, A.W. *Patterns of Industrial Bureaucracy.* New York: The Free Press 1964.

Gramsci, A., *Selections from the Prison Notebooks of Antonio Gramsci.* Edited & translated by Q. Hoare & G. Nowell-Smith. London: Lawrence and Wishart 1971.

Gray, R.Q. 'The Labour Aristocracy in the Victorian Class Structure' in F. Parkin (ed) *The Social Analysis of Class Structure.* London: Tavistock 1974.

Gretton, H.R. *The English Middle Class.* London: Bell 1919.

Halèvy, E. *A History of the English People in 1815.* London: T Fischer Unwin 1924.
A History of the English People 1830-1841. London: T Fischer Unwin 1927.

Halmos, P. *The Personal Service Society.* An Inaugural Lecture delivered at University College, Cardiff. Wales: University of Wales Press 1966.
The Personal Service Society. London: Constable 1970.

Harrison, E. *Address to the Lincolnshire Benevolent Medical Society* London: R. Bickerstaff 1810.

Haug, M.R., and Sussman, M.B. 'Professionalization & Unionism: A Jurisdictional Dispute?' in E. Freidson (ed) *The Professions & their Prospects.* Beverly Hills: Sage Publications 1973.

Hill, A.B., and Roy, J. 'The Doctor's Day & Pay: Some Sampling Inquiries Into the Pre-war Status' in *Journal of the Royal Statistical Society* (1951), CXIV (23): pp. 1—34.

Hill, M. *The Religious Order: A Study of Virtuoso Religion and its Legitimation in the 19th Century Church of England.* London: Heinemann 1973.

A Sociology of Religion. London: Heinemann 1973.

Hodgkinson, R.G. *Origins of the National Health Service: Medical Services of the New Poor Law, 1834-1871.* London: Wellcome Institute of History 1967.

Holloway, S.W.F. 'Medical Education in England, 1830-1858: A Sociological Analysis' in *History* (1964), 49: pp. 299-324.

'The Apothecaries Act, 1815: A Reinterpretation' in *Medical History*: 10 July 1966 part I: pp 107-29 and 11 July 1966 part II: pp. 221-36.

Honingsbaum, F. 'Struggle for the Ministry of Health, 1914-1919' in *Social Administration Occasional Papers.* London: Bell 1971.

Hope, K. 'The Analysis of Social Mobility: Methods and Approaches' in *Oxford Studies in Social Mobility.* Oxford: Clarendon Press 1972.

Hughes, E.C. *The Sociological Eye: Selected Papers* Chicago/New York: Atherton 1971.

'Professions' in Daedalus 92(4) (1963), Fall: pp. 655-668.

'The Social Significance of Professionalization' in H.M. Vollmer and D.L. Mills *Professionalization* pp 64-70 Englewood Cliffs N.J.: Prentice Hall 1966.

Illich, I. *Deschooling Society.* New York: Harper Row 1970.

'The Professions as a form of Imperialism' in New Society, 25 (571), pp 633-5 13 September

Jamous H., and Peloille, B. 'Professions or Self-Perpetuating Systems: Changes in the French University – Hospital System' in J.A. Jackson (ed) *Professions and Professionalization* pp 111-152. Cambridge: Cambridge University Press 1970.

Johnson, T. *Professions and Power.* London: Macmillan 1972.

'Imperialism & the Professions' in P Halmos (ed) *Sociological Review Monograph 20,* December 1973, Keele: University of Keele, pp 281-309 *The Professions in the Class Structure.* A paper presented at the British Sociological Association Annual Conference, University of Kent 1975.

Klein, R. 'An Anatomy of the N.H.S.' in *New Society,* 24 (560), 28 June pp 739-41.

Klein R., and Shinebourne, A. 'Doctors' Discipline' in *New Society,* 22 (528) 16 November 1972: pp. 399-401.

Klingender, F.D. *The Condition of Clerical Labour in Britain.* University of London Ph.D. thesis 1935.

Laffan, T. *The Medical Profession.* Dublin: Fannin 1888.

Lees, D.S. *The Economic Consequences of the Professions.* London: Institute of Economic Affairs 1966.

Lewis, R., and Maude, A. *The English Middle Classes.* London: Phoenix House 1949.

Professional People. London: Phoenix House 1952

Lindsey, A. *Socialized Medicine in England & Wales. The National Health Service, 1948-1961.* The University of North Carolina Press: Chapel Hill 1962

Lipset, S.M. and Bendix, R. *Social Mobility in Industrial Society.* Berkeley, California: University of California Press 1959.

Little, E.M. *History of the British Medical Association 1832-1932* London: British Medical Association 1932.

Lockwood, D. *The Blackcoated Worker.* London: Allen & Unwin 1958. 'Social Integration and System Integration' in G.K. Zollschan and W. Hirsch (eds) *Explorations in Social Change* pp. 244-57. London: Routledge and Kegan Paul 1964.

Lopreato, J., and Hazelrigg, L.E. *Class, Conflict and Mobility. Theories & Studies of Class Structure.* San Francisco: Chandler Publishing Company 1972.

Luckmann, T. *The Invisible Religion.* New York: Macmillan 1967.

Lukes, S. *Emile Durkheim. His Life & Work – A Historical & Critical Study.* London: Allen Lane 1973.
Power. A Radical View. London: Macmillan 1974.

Lynn, K.S. Introduction to the issue, 'Professions' in Daedalus 92 (4) (1963), Fall: pp 649-54

Lyttelton, A. *Roots of the Right. Italian Fascisms: From Pareto to Gentile.* London: Jonathan Cape 1973.

Macrae, D.G. *Weber.* London: Fontana 1974.

Manchester Medico - Ethical Association 'Tariff of Medical Fees' in *Medical Tracts 1830-79* 3rd Edition 1879. (First published in 1865, subsequently revised.)

Mannheim, K. *Ideology & Utopia.* London: Routledge and Kegan Paul 1936.

Manton, J. *Elizabeth Garrett Anderson.* New York: Dutton 1965.

Marshall, D. *The English Poor in the 18th Century* London: Routledge and Kegan Paul 1969.

Marshall, T.H. 'The Recent History of Professionalism in Relation to Social Structure and Social Policy'. *Canadian Journal of Economics and Political Science,* 5 August: pp. 325-340.

Marx, K. *Poverty of Philosophy.* Moscow: Progress Publications 1955. *Das Capital* Vol. III. Moscow: Foreign Language Publishing House 1962.

Marx, K., and Engels, F. 'Manifesto of the Communist Party' in *Selected Works.* London: Lawrence and Wishart 1968.

Merton, R.K. *Social Theory & Social Structure.* New York: The Free Press 1957.

Middleton, C. 'Sexual Inequality & Stratification Theory' in F. Parkin (ed) *The Social Analysis of Class Structure.* London: Tavistock 1974.

Mill, J.S. 'On Miss Martineau's Summary of Political Economy' in Monthly Repository (ed W.J.Fox) *New Series* (1834) Vol 8: pp318-22.

Millerson, G. *The Qualifying Associations. A Study in Professionalization.* London: Routledge and Kegan Paul 1964.

Mitchell, J. *Woman's Estate.* London: Pelican 1971.

Moore, N. *History of St Bartholomew's Hospital.* Vol. II London: Pearson 1918.

Newman, B. *Social Stratification.* Unpublished Manuscript 1974.

Newman, C. *The Evolution of Medical Education in the 19th Century.* Oxford: Oxford University Press 1957.

Nichols, J.G. (ed) *The Autobiography of Anne, Lady Halkett.* London: Camden Society 1875.

Oppenheimer, M. 'The Proletarianization of the Professional' in P. Halmos (ed) 'Professionalization and Social Change' *The Sociological Review Monograph* 20, December 1973. Keele: University of Keele, pp. 213-27.

Parkin, F. 'Strategies of Social Closure in Class Formation' in F. Parkin (ed) *The Social Analysis of Class Structure.* London: Tavistock 1974.

Parry, N.C.A. 'How to Win Friends and Influence the Boss' in *Clare Market Review* (Magazine of the London School of Economics Students Union), Spring Edition 1963: pp 15-19.
Power, Class and Occupational Strategy. A paper presented at the British Sociological Association Annual Conference, University of Surrey 1973.

Parry, N.C.A., and Johnson, D. *Sexual Divisions in Lifestyle and Leisure.* A paper presented at the British Sociological Association Annual Conference, University of Aberdeen 1974.

Parry, N.C.A., and Parry J. 'The Teachers and Professionalism; the Failure of an Occupational Strategy' in M. Flude & J. Ahier *Educability, Schools & Ideology* pp. 160-185. London: Croom Helm 1974.

Parsons, T. *The Social System.* London: Routledge and Kegan Paul 1951.
'The Professions and Social Structure' in *Essays in Sociological Theory.* Glencoe, Illinois: The Free Press 1954.
'The American Family: Its Relation to Personality & Social Structure' in T. Parsons, and R.F. Bales *Family: Socialization and Interaction Process.* Glencoe, Illinois: The Free Press 1955.
'Some Considerations on the Theory of Social Change' in *Rural Sociology,* (1961) XXVI(3): pp 219-39.

Phelps Brown, E.H. *The Growth of British Industrial Relations.* London: Macmillan 1959.

Poulantzas, N.'The Problem of the Capitalist State' in *New Left Review,* 58 November-December 1969: pp 67-78.

Power, E. 'Women Practitioners of Medicine in the Middle Ages' in Proceedings of the Royal Society of Medicine 1921.

Prandy, K. *Professional Employees: A Study of Scientists and Engineers.* London: Faber 1965.

273

Pratt, J. and Burgess, T. *Polytechnics: A Report.* London: Pitman Publishing 1974.

Reader, W.J. *Professional Men. The Rise of the Professional Classes in Nineteenth-Century England.* London: Weidenfeld and Nicholson 1966.

Reeney, M.F. *The Medical Profession.* Dublin: Browne and Noland 1905.

Ridge, J.M. (ed) Mobility in Britain Reconsidered. *Oxford Studies in Social Mobility* Vol. II Oxford: Clarendon Press 1974.

Rivington, W. *The Medical Profession.* Dublin: Fannin 1879.

Rothschild, K.W. (ed) *Power and Economics.* London: Penguin 1971.

Rowan Wilson, J. 'Outdated Citadel' in *The Spectator* 24 June 1972. 'Hidden GPs' in *The Spectator* 27 January 1973.

Ryan, M. 'Health Centre Policy in England and Wales' in *British Journal of Sociology* 19 (1) March 1968: pp 34-46.

Schumpeter, J.A. *Imperialism and Social Classes.* Oxford: Basil Blackwell 1951.

Sorokin, P. *Social Mobility.* New York: Harper Bros. 1927.

Sprigge, S.S. *Medicine and the Public.* London: Heinemann 1899.

Srinivas, M.N. 'A Note on Sanskritization & Westernisation' in R. Bendix & S.M. Lipset *Class, Status & Power* pp 552-560. London: Routledge and Kegan Paul 1967.

Stevens, R. *Medical Practice in Modern England. The Impact of Specialization & State Medicine.* New Haven: Yale University Press 1966.

Tawney, R.H. *The Acquisitive Society.* London: Allen & Unwin 1972.

Titmuss, R.M. (ed) *Essays on the Welfare State.* London: Allen & Unwin 19

Turner, C., and Hodge, M.N. 'Occupations and Professions' in J.A. Jackson (ed) *Professions & Professionalization* pp 19-50. Cambridge: Cambridge University Press 1970.

Turner, E.S. *Call the Doctor.* London: Michael Joseph 1958.

Veblen, T. *Engineers and the Price System.* New York: B.W. Huebsch 1921.

Waddington, I. 'The Role of the Hospital' in *Sociology,* 7 (2), May 1973: pp 211-25

Wade, J. *History of the Middle & Working Classes* 1842. (First published in 1833).

Webb, B. *The State & the Doctor.* London: Longmans, Green & Co. 1910.
'Special Supplement on Professional Associations' (Part II) in *The New Statesman,* IX (211), 21 April 1917: pp. 1-24.
Our Partnership. (edited by Barbara Drake, Margaret Cole). London: Longmans, Green & Co. 1948.

Weber, M. *Economy & Society* (eds G. Roth and C. Wittich). New York: Bedminster Press 1968.

Weightman, G. 'Centres of Health' in *New Society,* 31 (650), 20 March 1975: pp. 727-8.

Woodward, J.H. *To do the sick no harm: a Study of the British Voluntary Hospital System to 1875.* London: Routledge and Kegan Paul 1974.

Wright Mills, C. *White Collar. The American Middle Classes.* New York: Galaxy 1956.

The Power Elite. New York: Galaxy 1959.

Young M., and Willmott, P. *The Symmetrical Family.* London: Routledge and Kegan Paul 1973.

Government Publications

1871 Royal Commission on the Operation of the Sanitary Laws, *Reports 1869-1871,* C 281.HMSO

1928 Royal Commission on National Health Insurance, *Report,* Cmd 2596 HMSO

1960 Royal Commission on Doctors' and Dentists' Remuneration 1957-1960, *Report,* Cmnd 939. HMSO (Pilkington)

1968 Royal Commission on Medical Education 1965-1968, *Report,* Cmnd 3569. HMSO (Todd)

1968 Royal Commission on Trade Unions & Employers' Associations, *Reports 1965-1968,* Cmnd 3623. HMSO (Donovan)

1955 Ministry of Health, Annual Report of the Ministry of Health. Including an address by the Minister to the Annual Meeting of the Executive Councils' Association, 21st October. Cmd 9857, HMSO

1961 Ministry of Health, Annual Reports of the Ministry of Health. Report of the Joint Working Party on the Medical Staffing Structure in the Hospital Service. HMSO (Platt)

1944 Ministry of Health, Department of Health for Scotland, A National Health Service, Cmd. 6502, HMSO (The 1944 White Paper)

1946 Ministry of Health, Department of Health for Scotland, Report of the Inter-departmental Committee on Remuneration of General Practitioners, Cmd 6810, HMSO (Spens)

1948 Ministry of Health, Department of Health for Scotland, Report of the Inter-departmental Committee on the Remuneration of Consultants & Specialists, Cmd 7420. HMSO (Spens)

1957 Ministry of Health, Department of Health for Scotland, Report of the Committee to Consider the Future Numbers of Medical Practitioners and the Appropriate Intake of Medical Students. Cmnd 32-444. HMSO (Willink)

1973 Department of Health and Social Security, Scottish & Welsh

Offices Private Practice in National Health Service Hospitals, Cmnd Cmnd 5270. HMSO

1974 On the State of the Public Health. Annual Report of the Chief Medical Officer of the Department of Health and Social Security for the year 1973 London: HMSO (Dr Yellowlees)

1868 Poor Law Board, Twentieth Annual Report 1867-68, HMSO

1879 Local Government Board, Eighth Annual Report, 1878-1879, C 2372. HMSO

1905 Report from the Select Committee on Registration in Respect of Recruitment & Training of Nurses. Parliamentary papers (263)

1912 Report of Sir William Plender to the Exchequer on the result of his investigation into existing Conditions in respect of medical attendance and remuneration in certain towns. Parliamentary papers 1912-1913, Vol 78, Cmd 6305. HMSO

1920 Consultative Council on Medical & Allied Services, Interim Report on the Future Provision of Medical & Allied Services Cmd 693. HMSO (Dawson)

1922 PRO Cab. 23/29, Cabinet 20 of 1922, Meeting 22nd March. Quoted by B.B. Gilbert British Social Policy p. 272.

1942 Sir William Beveridge Social Insurance & Allied Services, Cmd 6404, HMSO

1942 Draft Interim Report of the Medical Planning Commission. See *British Medical Journal,* Vol 1: pp 743-53

1956 Central Health Services Council, Committee of Enquiry into the Cost of the National Health Service, Report, Cmd 9663. HMSO (Guillebaud)

1963 Committee on Higher Education, Higher Education, Report of the Committee Appointed by the Prime Minister under the Chairmanship of Lord Robbins 1961-1963, Cmnd 2154 HMSO

1970 Monopolies Commission, *Report.* Professional Services: a Report on the General Effect on the Public Interest of Certain Restrictive Practices in relation to Supply of Services, Cmnd 4463 HMSO

1975 Report of the Committee of Inquiry into the Regulation of the Medical Profession, Cmnd 6018. HMSO (Merrison)

Newspaper Articles

The Times 3 July 1893, 25 April 1974, 13 June 1974, 14 August 1974, 4 November 1974, 7 November 1974 11 November 1974, 13 November 1974, 31 December 1974 16 January 1975

Sunday Times 7 July 1974, 12 January 1975, 26 January 1975
The *Guardian* 18 October 1974
The *Observer* 7 July 1974, 5 January 1975

Medical Journals

British Medical Journal – 28 January 1853, 2 August 1858,
10 April 1875, 13 October 1894, 22 July 1905, 3 July 1909,
23 February 1935, 4 September 1937, 5 March 1949
The *Lancet* – 16 January 1830, 9 January 1858, 3 August 1861,
2 June 1866, 6 April 1946, 31 January 1948, 25 March 1950,
23 November 1957
The *Nursing Record* – 2 March 1893

INDEX

Abel-Smith, B. 138, 142, 143, 144, 145, 146, 182, 188, 227
achievement, 4, 16, 30-31
altruism, 30-31
anomie, 63, 249
Apothecaries, 104-16, *passim*. 120, 122, 131, 137, 142, 165
Apothecaries Act, (1815) 111-16
apprenticeship, 113, 116, 133
Armed Forces, the 147
artisans *see* craftsmen
ascription, 30-31
Ashe, I. 131-2
Associated Apothecaries, 111
Association for the Improvement of the London Workhouse Infirmaries, 141
associational society, 63
authority, 47-8, 53, 68-70, 258-9
autocracies, 6

Bachrah, P. 71
Bain, G.S. 70
Banks, J.A. and O. 93-4
Baratz M.S. 71
Barber, B. 26-7
Barrie, James 173
Becker H.S. 21
Ben-David, J. 29-37, 248
Bendix, R. 10, 39
Bevan, Aneurin, 202-11, 215
Beveridge report (1942), 213
Blackwell Elizabeth, 173-4
Brain Sir Russell 222
Brand, J. 157, 160
Briggs, A. 89-90
British Hospitals Association, 200
British United Provident Association, 230
Butler, Josephine, 172-3
Butler, R.A.B. 22
Bradlaugh, Charles 178
British Medical Association, 43, 254; consultants, 185, 224, 241-3; free health care 143, 160; general practitioners, 185, 202, 214, 216-8, 224; influence, 147, 254; junior hospital doctors 231; medical registration, 123, 125; midwifery, 178-80; National Health Insurance Act, 187-94; National Health Service, 202-11; Poor Law Hospitals, 146-7; reform movement, 126-30; role in pay negotiations 190-99, 223 *see also* remuneration
British Nurses' Association, 181-4
bureaucracies, 22, 46-7, 252; expertise of 83; legal rational

67-70 *passim,* 99, professional work in 258-65 *passim*
Burgess, T. 265-6
Burnham, J. 31-2
Burrage, M. 266

capitalism, 44, 60, 162-4; labour market, 12-13, 54-9; Marxist view of, 250; social class, 70, 85-93, 261-5; Weber's view of 248-53; working class consciousness, 17
Carchedi, G. 257-8, 261
careers, 81, 137-42
Carlin, J.E. 48
Carlyle, T. 90
Carr-Saunders, A.M. 22, 23, 28, 29, 31-2
'cash nexus', 90
Castle, Barbara 239-43
Champney, T. 107-8
chemists, 109, 115
Chessa, F. 7
churches, the 99-103
Clark, A. 162-4, 166-7
class consciousness, false, 11, 13, 18, 38, 69-70, 90
class theory, 33-5, 84-99, 248-53
clerks, 12, 13-14
clients' needs, 44
closure, 85-7, 131, 249, 251-3
collective bargaining, 82, 194 *see also* remuneration
collective social mobility, 8, 10, 18, 52, 247, 251, 265; and the market, 56-7, 77, 85-6; conditions for, 78-88; downward, 86, 266; upward, 86, 251
Collings, Dr. 217
community health councils, 235, 236
Confederation of Health Service Employees, 239
conflict, 38-9, 66, 69
consultants, 134, 185, 253; and general practitioners, 135, 199, 210, 214, 218-19, 223-4; merit awards 243; National Health Service, 206, 209-11, 218, 232-4; power, 137-9; remuneration, 137, 210-11, 219, 221-2
consumption patterns, 57-8
contract practice, 151-4
Cowper, W.F. 124-5
Coxon, A. 102
craftsmen, 79, 80, 88, 89, 91

Dahl, R.A. 71
Dahrendorf, R. 39, 53, 55, 64, 68-70, 250, 263

al, 37, 50, 77, 83-4
Illich, I. 256-7
immigrant doctors, 227-8
imperative co-ordination, 264-5
Incorporated Medical Practitioner's
     Association, 185
indetermination, 260-63
India, 3, 9, 72
individual social mobility, 10, 85,
     248, 252
individualism, 18, 30, 163; ideology
     of, 14, 16, 60-61, 247-8; liberal,
     11, 249-50
industrial action, 241-2, 255
instrumental collectivism, 14, 15
insurance, private, 148-54
interest groups, 68-9
Italy, 11, 22

Jamous, H. 259-63
Japan, 67
Jensen, A. 10
Jex Blake, Sophia 172, 175
Johnson, D. 162
Johnson, T. 20, 21, 24-6, 27, 40-42,
     45, 46, 51-2, 248, 249, 257-63
Junior hospital doctors, 146, 230,
     231-2, 242, 255
Junior Hospital Doctor's Association

Klein, R. 213, 244
Klingender, F.D. 12, 18
knowledge, 27, 29, 51, 256-7

lifestyle, 15
Labour Party, 200, 266
Lewis, R. 22, 34, 90
liberal economic theory, 62, 249-50
liberalism, 96-7
Lipset, S.M. 10, 39
Little, E.M. 127, 129, 130, 151
Lloyd George, David 187-8, 190
local authorities, 202, 213, 236
Local Government Board, 155-7, 172,
     193
Local Government (Board) Act
     (1871), 155
local health executive councils, 207-8
Lockwood, D. 12-18, 64, 68, 79, 80,
     81-2, 85, 92, 247, 250
London School of Medicine for
     Women, 172
Lopreato, J. 11, 247
Luckmann, T. 99-100
Lukes, S. 71, 73-4, 251
Lynn, K.S. 22-3
Lytton, B. 91

MacRae, D.G. 23
Mannheim, K. 33
Manton, J. 164
manual labour, 89
market, the 53-9, 70; capacity, 56-7;

control over, 64, 74, 77-9;
     ideology, 95; Marxist view of,
     52-9, 64-85; relations, 12, 61,
     251; status 77, 253; Weber's
     concept of, 53-4, 64, 85
Marsh, 20
Marshall, T.H. 33
Marxist perspectives 1; bureaucracy,
     65; class, 11, 17, 52-9, 64-7,
     247-9; power, 63-75 *passim;* social
     change 38-9; social structure 92;
     the market, 52-9, 64, 85; middle
     classes 37-40; the state, 65;
     women, 94-5
Maude, A. 22, 34, 90
medical aid associations, 152-3
medical officers of health, local 147,
     158-9
medical practice, 151-4; lay partici-
     pation in, 256-7; unqualified,
     109-10, 180
Medical Practitioners' Union, 243
medical profession, 50, 117, 126;
     and other occupations, 43-4;
     control of, 229; entry, 131-4,
     224-9; middle class nature, 198
     see also professions
Medical Reform Committee, 129
medical registration, 117-30
Medical Registration Act (1858),
     129-31
Medical Services Review Committee,
     234
medical social workers, 235-6
Merrison report (1975), 245-6
Merton, R.K. 16, 23
Metropolitan Asylums Board, 141
middle classes: and the working
     classes, 15, 80, 88, 91; and
     theories of social class 34-5, 53;
     assimilation of people into 15;
     clerks' identification with 12, 13;
     conception of society, 16; Marxist
     view of 37-40 *see also* professions
Middleton, C. 94-6
midwifery, 144-5, 167-72; legislation
     on, 177-81
Midwives Institute, 176-7, 178-9
Miliband, R. 73
Millerson, G. 24, 82-3
Ministry of Health, 156-7, 202-11
     passim
Mitchell, J. 94, 97, 99
monopoly, professional 59, 83
moral orders, 62-3, 249
Morant, Robert, 188-92
Mosca, G. 55
Murphy, P.K. 217

National Association of General
     Practitioners in Medicine, Surgery
     and Midwifery, 128
National Health Insurance Act (1911)

sanitary legislation, 154-5
Schumpeter, J. 36, 56
Scotland, 105-14 *passim*
secularisation, 99-100
sexual divisions, 92-9; and
    class, 97-8; and medicine,
    162-85
Shinebourne, A. 244
Simon, John 124, 154-6
skills, 54
Smith, Adam 27
social change, 28, 38-9
social class: and status 39-44, 46,
    58-9; and structure, 91-3, 97-8,
    250-53; as an economic interest
    group, 36; awareness, 58; conflict,
    38-9 66; consciousness, 58;
    defined, 52; formation of, 79;
    Marxist view of, 52-9, 64-74
    248-9; professionalism, 20-59,
    84-6, 257-65; sexual divisions,
    97-8; theories of 33-5, 84-99,
    248-53; transitional 53; Weber's
    view of, 64-74 *passim*
social distance, 40-41
social mobility, 5-10; chances, 56-7
    75; class structure, 3-19 *see also*
    collective social mobility
social structuration, 55-60, 85-6, 91,
    98-9, 251-3
social structure, 33, 60-74; and class,
    91-3, 98, 250-53; and social
    mobility 76-103; and the profes-
    sions 248, 252-3
Socialist Medical Association, 200
society, 65
Society of Apothecaries, 107, 108,
    112, 119, 165, 169, 174; and
    education, 132-3, 136
Society of Medical Officers of Health
    147, 158-9
solidarism, 87, 252-3
Sorokin, P. 5-10, 56, 248
Spens report (1946), 205, 210,
    219, 221, 223
Stansfeld, Mr. 172
state, the: and doctors, 154-9, 212;
    and personal health services,
    159-60, and society, 65-6; and
    economy, 13, 66-7, 264; as
    mediator, 44; Marxist view of
    64-5
status, 38-9, 49, 58, 64; and social
    class, 39-44, 46, 58-9; and the
    market, 77; defined, 76; of
    doctors, 126, 133, 195, 212, 225,
    253; transmission of, 7
Stevens, R. 208, 220, 232
Stevenson, Derek, 240-41
stratification, 55, 68
structural functionalism, 93-4
'style of life', 58-9, 64, 76, 77, 225
surgeons, 104-17, *passim*, 131

Tanner, Dr. 178
Tawney, R.H. 22, 266
Taylor, Lord 217
technicality, 260-63
technology, 256-7
trade unions, 1, 5, 16, 70, 76, 259;
    and professional associations,
    39-40, 79-82, 250, 255; and
    reduction of conflict, 32-3
Turner, C. 40

U.S.A. 9-10, 25, 29, 67
U.S.S.R. 67
uncertainty, 60-74, *passim,* 249
unionism *see* trade unions
universities, the 105, 121, 136
unskilled workers, 12

values, 28, 88
Veblen, T. 23

Waddington, I. 106
Wade, J. 90
Wakley, Thomas 117-18, 120, 121,
    122, 126, 127, 128, 141
Warburton, Mr. 117-18, 122
Webb, B. 156, 159-60, 187, 193
Weber, Max 1, 13, 23, 34, 75, 101;
    concept of the market, 52-9, 64,
    67, 85, 249; distinction between
    class and status 46; his class
    theory 249; his view of bureau-
    cracy, 65, 67-70 *passim,* 250, 252,
    258-65; his view of power, 63-74
    passim; 'style of life' 58-9, 64
Webster, George 127
White, Jessie M. 173
white collar workers, 35
Whitley Council machinery, 219, 221
Willink report (1957), 2-3, 226, 228,
    229
Willmott, P. 96
Wilson, P.A. 22, 28, 29, 31-2
women, 93-4, 162-85, 254
Woodward, J. 136
working class, 15-18, 88; and revo-
    lution 66; and middle class 15,
    80-81, 88, 91; conception of
    society, 16; proletarianisation of
    12-13, 17, 258-61
Worshipful Company of Apothecaries
    104-16
Wright Mills, C. 23, 34

Yellowlees, Dr. 228
Young, Dr. 228